Ocular Telehealth

Ocular Telehealth

A Practical Guide

EDITED BY

APRIL MAA, MD
Associate Professor,
Department of Ophthalmology
Emory University School of Medicine,
Atlanta, GA, United States
Tele-Specialty Care Director,
Regional Telehealth Services,
Clinical Resource Hub,
Veterans' Integrated Service Network (VISN) 7,
Atlanta, GA, United States

ELSEVIER

Elsevier
1600 John F. Kennedy Blvd.
Ste 1800
Philadelphia, PA 19103-2899

OCULAR TELEHEALTH, FIRST EDITION

ISBN: 978-0-323-83204-5

Notice

Library of Congress Control Number: 2021946069

Publisher: Sarah Barth
Acquisitions Editor: Kayla Wolfe
Editorial Project Manager: Sam Young
Production Project Manager: Poulouse Joseph
Cover Designer: Miles Hitchen

Printed in the United States of America

Last digit is the print number: 9 8 7 6 5 4 3 2 1

Working together
to grow libraries in
developing countries

www.elsevier.com • www.bookaid.org

Dedication

I have always had aspirations to publish a book, and therefore I am very excited about this textbook as it combines both my passion for telehealth and my love for literature. The work of telehealth truly takes a village, so first, this book is dedicated to my awesome telehealth team (TECS National Team, Regional Telehealth Services, VA Office of Connected Care, VA Office of Rural Health, and HEROIC COIN, among others). The telehealth team members who deserve special recognition are our amazing ophthalmology technicians who are excellent at their craft and whose daily hard work is extremely critical to our success. These dedicated and talented technicians are our "eyes and ears" and without them, none of our telehealth care is possible. Second, I wish to recognize my fellow VA optometry and ophthalmology in-person and telehealth colleagues who are true innovative leaders, paving the way for the future of eye care. I have learned so much from them, and I am blessed to work with all these wonderful individuals. Together, we are preventing blindness by providing care from 'anywhere to anywhere'. Third, I dedicate this book to my Veteran patients; it is a true honor to "serve those who have served." Last, I wish to acknowledge my mentors who have helped me grow in more ways than I ever thought possible. MGL, my "work mom", RN and IKW, my supervisors, and last but not least, my husband, David Brandon, MD. He has celebrated my successes, encouraged me after my failures, tackled problems with me by providing so many useful suggestions, and has been an absolutely amazing pillar of support. He also knows more about eyes after 17 years of marriage than most non-eye physicians! This book is really my dream come true, and no words can express my gratitude to all who contributed and inspired me throughout this journey.

Contents

Contributors

Akshar Abbott, MD
Staff Physician, Minneapolis VA Healthcare System, Department of Veterans Affairs, Minneapolis, MN, United States

R.V. Paul Chan, MD, MSc, MBA
The John H. Panton Professor of Ophthalmology, Chair, Department of Ophthalmology, University of Illinois College of Medicine, Chicago, IL, United States

Alejandra Torres Diaz, BS
Research Specialist, Department of Ophthalmology and Visual Sciences, University of Wisconsin School of Medicine and Public Health, Madison, WI, United States

Elaine Downie, MD
University of Wisconsin-Madison, Department of Ophthalmology and Visual Sciences, Madison, WI, United States

Annette L. Giangiacomo, MD
Associate Professor, Eye Institute, Medical College of Wisconsin, Milwaukee, WI, United States

Bharat Gurnani, MD
Aravind Eye Hospital and Post Graduate Institute of Ophthalmology, Pondicherry, India

Thao M. Harris, OD, FAAO
Staff Optometrist, Atlanta VA Healthcare System, Department of Veterans Affairs, Atlanta, GA, United States

Matthew S. Hunt, BS
Department of Ophthalmology, University of Washington, Seattle, WA, United States

Washington University School of Medicine, Saint Louis, MO, United States

Carolyn Ihrig, OD, FAAO
Staff Optometrist, Buffalo VA Western New York Health Care System, Department of Veterans Affairs, Buffalo, NY, United States

Li Jianjun, MD, PhD
Beijing Institute of Ophthalmology, Beijing Tongren Hospital, Capital Medical University, Beijing, China

Anney Joseph, OD, FAAO
Staff Optometrist, Technology-based Eye Care Services (TECS) Subsection, Regional Telehealth Services, Clinical Resource Hub, Veterans' Integrated Service Network (VISN) 7, Atlanta, GA, United States

Melissa W. Ko, MD
Associate Professor, Departments of Neurology, Neurosurgery, and Ophthalmology, Indiana University School of Medicine, Indianapolis, IN, United States

Kevin E. Lai, MD
Assistant Professor, Department of Ophthalmology, Indiana University School of Medicine, Indianapolis, IN, United States

Aaron Y. Lee, MD, MSCI
Associate Professor, Department of Ophthalmology, University of Washington, Seattle, WA, United States

Daniel Lee, BA
Medical Doctoral Candidate, Morehouse School of Medicine, Atlanta, GA, United States

Yao Liu, MD, MS
Assistant Professor, Department of Ophthalmology and Visual Sciences, University of Wisconsin School of Medicine and Public Health, Madison, WI, United States

Loren J. Lock, MS
Researcher, Department of Ophthalmology and Visual Sciences, University of Wisconsin School of Medicine and Public Health, Madison, WI, United States

Xiaoqin Alexa Lu, MD
Assistant Professor of Ophthalmology, Emory University School of Medicine, Atlanta, GA, United States
Staff Physician, Technology-based Eye Care Services (TECS) Subsection, Regional Telehealth Services, Clinical Resource Hub, Veterans' Integrated Service Network (VISN) 7, Atlanta, GA, United States

April Maa, MD
Associate Professor, Department of Ophthalmology, Emory University School of Medicine, Atlanta, GA, United States
Adjunct Associate Professor for Research, W.K. Kellogg Eye Center, University of Michigan, Ann Arbor, MI, United States
TeleEye Co-Lead, Office of Connected Care, Department of Veterans Affairs, Washington, DC, United States
Tele-Specialty Care Director, Regional Telehealth Services, Clinical Resource Hub, Veterans' Integrated Service Network (VISN) 7, Atlanta, GA, United States

Robert Morris, OD, FAAO
Chief, Tele-Eye Section, Optometry Service, Salisbury VA Health Care System, Department of Veterans Affairs, Salisbury, NC, United States
Assistant Professor of Clinical Practice, College of Optometry, The Ohio State University, Columbus, OH, United States

Charles F. Palmer, MD
Staff Physician, Technology-based Eye Care Services (TECS) Subsection, Regional Telehealth Services, Clinical Resource Hub, Veterans' Integrated Service Network (VISN) 7, Atlanta, GA, United States

Gerald Selvin, OD, FAAO
Retired TeleEye Lead, Department of Veterans Affairs, Washington, DC, United States
Adjunct Faculty, Massachusetts College of Pharmacy Health Sciences University School of Optometry, Boston, MA, United States

Ankoor Shah, MD, PhD
Assistant Professor, Massachusetts Eye and Ear, Department of Ophthalmology, Harvard University School of Medicine, Boston, MA, United States

Ravilla D. Thulasiraj, MBA
Executive Director, Lions Aravind Institute of Community Ophthalmology, Madurai, Tamil Nadu, India

Suzanne van Landingham, MD
Assistant Professor, University of Wisconsin-Madison, Department of Ophthalmology and Visual Sciences, Madison, WI, United States

Rengaraj Venkatesh, MD
Aravind Eye Hospital and Post Graduate Institute of Ophthalmology, Pondicherry, India

Stephanie J. Weiss, DO
Clinical Assistant Professor (Adjunct) in the Lewis Katz School of Medicine at Temple University, Department of Ophthalmology, Philadelphia, PA, United States
Adjunct Assistant Professor of Ophthalmology in the Associated Faculty of the Perelman School of Medicine at the University of Pennsylvania, Philadelphia, PA, United States
Wilmington and Philadelphia VA Medical Centers, Department of Veterans Affairs, Site Director for TECS, Wilmington, DE, United States

Preface

APRIL MAA
Associate Professor, Department of Ophthalmology, Comprehensive Division, Emory University
School of Medicine, Atlanta, GA, United States
Tele-Specialty Care Director, Veterans Integrated Service Network (VISN) 7 Regional Telehealth
Services, Veterans Health Administration, Washington, DC, United States

As I write the preface to this book, *Ocular Telehealth*, the world is drastically different from what it was 1-2 years ago. Society is in the midst of the coronavirus pandemic, which has fundamentally altered the landscape of life. As the world works toward social and economic recovery, my thoughts turn toward the Zulu philosophy of Ubuntu, the belief that we, in our humanity, are all fundamentally intertwined. In a similar vein, Helen Keller once said:

> "The welfare of each is bound up in the welfare of all"

I believe this statement is very apropos in our current time because in order to promote the overall well-being of our society, we need to improve the well-being of each individual.

Promoting a high quality of life is one way of achieving well-being, and this is one of the reasons it is so rewarding to be an eye health provider. Protecting and restoring sight has a tangible, immense positive impact on a patient. Several studies show that patients care more about preserving their vision than keeping a physical limb, and going blind is, for some, a fate worse than death.[1] Visual impairment leads to increased falls, social withdrawal, increased depression, and increased morbidity and mortality.[2,3] In the current pandemic environment, however, patients may be foregoing important preventative or chronic ophthalmic care that may have devastating future consequences. Furthermore, as eye providers, we may not have the capacity to meet the future demands of an aging, sicker population if we do not fundamentally change the way we approach patient care. My esteemed co-authors and I passionately believe that telehealth is the future of eye care delivery, and we hope this book will show you the why and how of ocular telehealth.

It might surprise you to know that telemedicine, while an incredibly hot topic in the 21st century, actually has long-standing roots, with the first glimmers potentially arising in 1876, when Alexander Graham Bell invented the telephone.[4] From there, capabilities expanded, for example, in the 1940s when a radiology image was transmitted between two sites in Pennsylvania via telephone lines.[4] Telemedicine really "took off" when NASA, desiring to deliver health care to astronauts in space, began integrating methods of telemedicine technology into their spaceships and into spacesuits to monitor the health of astronauts.[5] Other landmark moments in telehealth occurred in 1964, where the Nebraska Psychiatric Hospital provided telemedicine consults to the Norfolk State Hospital, 112 miles away, or the 1972 Space Technology Applied to Rural Papago Advanced Health Care (STARPAHC) to deliver health care to remote, underserved regions such as those inhabited by the Papago Indians.[5]

As telecommunications, internet, and smart phone technology advances, the possibilities for telemedicine are endless, and patient demand for this type of healthcare experience grows. The COVID-19 pandemic has only added fuel to the fire; now telehealth is an indispensable, critical tool that allows providers to care for our patients while maintaining their safety and our own.

An old Chinese proverb comes to mind during these challenging times:

> A wise man adapts himself to circumstances, as water shapes itself to the vessel that contains it.

I encourage you, the reader of this textbook, to think of telehealth as a versatile, flexible tool in your armamentarium to reach your patients and provide them with what they need, no matter where they are located.

Whether you are curious, just starting the practice of ocular telehealth, or you run a large eye telehealth program and are looking for additional information, this book will meet your needs. My co-authors and I designed this textbook to be practical in nature, starting with common definitions, then providing specific use cases, and finally discussing "how to": implementation, monitoring quality, billing/coding for financial sustainability, and future directions.

> A small group of thoughtful people could change the world. Indeed, it's the only thing that ever has.
> - Margaret Mead

The new healthcare world post pandemic needs us to revolutionize the way medical care is provided to our growing global population. Ocular telehealth is a tool we believe eye providers should adopt because it will promote health equity, reduce health disparities, and improve access for all. Ultimately, innovators such as you, the reader, will transform your practice and advance the quality of life for your patients, one telehealth visit at a time.

REFERENCES

1. Luckie R, Leese G, McAlpine R, et al. Fear of visual loss in patients with diabetes: results of the prevalence of diabetic eye disease in Tayside, Scotland (P-DETS) study. *Diabet Med.* 2007;24(10):1086–1092.
2. Eichenbaum JW, Burton WB, Eichenbaum GM, Mulvihill M. The prevalence of eye disease in nursing home and non-nursing home geriatric populations. *Arch Gerontol Geriatr.* 1999;28(3):191–204.
3. Eichenbaum JW. Geriatric vision loss due to cataracts, macular degeneration, and glaucoma. *Mt Sinai J Med.* 2012;79(2):276–294.
4. la Folla T. *History of Telemedicine Infographic*; 2021. https://blog.evisit.com/virtual-care-blog/history-telemedicine-infographic. Accessed 1/18/2021.
5. Allen R. *A Brief History of Telemedicine*; 2006. https://www.electronicdesign.com/technologies/components/article/21770508/a-brief-history-of-telemedicine. Accessed 18 January 2021.

Acknowledgments

We acknowledge Paul Lee, MD, JD; Linda Harrison, PhD with OMIC; and Ronald Pelton, MD, PhD, for their expert review of Chapters 14 and 15. We also thank Stephen Herman, COT, for his photographic expertise, and Jennifer Damonte, MS, who took photographs, coordinated efforts for permissions with figures, and also provided a review of Chapter 13.

CHAPTER 1

Background, Definitions, and An Introduction to Ocular Telehealth

ROBERT MORRIS, OD, FAAO

INTRODUCTION TO GENERAL TELEHEALTH

A consistent challenge in healthcare is the disparity in demand for services, and access to healthcare providers. Certainly, this is true for developing countries but even developed countries struggle with this disparity in both rural and urban areas. Telehealth provides a promising opportunity to increase access to care, connecting remote patients to healthcare providers. There are many definitions for "telemedicine" and "telehealth" with significant cross-over between the two terms. The American Telemedicine Association (ATA) practice recommendations for diabetic retinopathy referenced the World Health Organization (WHO) definitions which state that: *Telehealth* programs are "designed to integrate telecommunications systems into the practice of protecting and promoting health," whereas "*Telemedicine* programs are designed to integrate telecommunications into diagnostic and therapeutic intervention."[1] In this book, "telehealth" will be used to represent both terms and serve to encompass all aspects of remote healthcare, healthcare-related education, diagnostic, and therapeutic management.

Some of the earliest telehealth endeavors include testing the ability to send electrocardiogram readings over telephone lines in 1906 and using microwave video links for medical consultations and continuing education in 1959 at the University of Nebraska.[2] For the most part, early telehealth programs were unsustainable due to four main reasons: high technology cost, poor image quality, poor adoption of services, and inability to integrate with mainstream healthcare.[3]

However, due to extremely specific clinical needs, some unique programs saw notable telehealth growth in the mid-1970s to late 1980s. These programs shared the significant challenge of providing medical care to remote and inaccessible individuals. These special areas included the United States National Aeronautics and Space Agency (NASA), Antarctic explorations, offshore oil rigs, and the military.[3] These programs had special needs that justified the substantial cost of establishing and maintaining a telehealth program as the alternatives were to provide no medical care or costly evacuation.

Since that time, telehealth has evolved due to numerous factors including significant technological advances and increased patient comfort with technology. Telehealth is becoming a common method of delivering healthcare, with most hospitals and clinics offering virtual means for patients to connect with the healthcare team. Before social distancing mandates were put in place as a response to the 2019 SARS-CoV-2 (COVID-19) pandemic, 74% of patients were unaware of a telemedicine option in their physicians' practices.[4] The COVID-19 pandemic transformed the healthcare environment, with some leading telehealth platforms reporting telehealth patient visits increasing by 257%–700%.[4] The United States based National Committee for Quality Assurance (NCQA) Taskforce for Telehealth Policy was charged to evaluate the rapid transition to telehealth during COVID-19. Their statements provide a great perspective of the state of telehealth in the fall of 2020. "Telehealth is healthcare's natural evolution

Ocular Telehealth. https://doi.org/10.1016/B978-0-323-83204-5.00001-9

into the digital age, not another type of care. Telehealth can be a critical tool in advancing a well-coordinated, patient-centered, value-optimized healthcare system."[5]

Saleem et al. provided valuable perspective on ocular telehealth during the COVID-19 pandemic: Previously, ocular telehealth was typically reserved for rural or underserved areas. During this pandemic, everyone became remote and underserved, making telehealth mainstream.[4]

INTRODUCTION TO OCULAR TELEHEALTH

Ocular telehealth is becoming a more common method of delivering eye care when access to a provider is limited, to screen for ocular findings in at-risk individuals, or to monitor patients with known eye conditions. Historically, the evolution of ocular telehealth trailed other medical specialties largely due to limited ability to capture high-quality images and information technology challenges with speed and security of data transmission and storage. One of the earliest ocular telehealth programs evaluated the ability to monitor retinal vessels during a 1987 Space Shuttle Columbia mission. The Johnson Space Center in Houston, Texas developed a portable video funduscope that transmitted real-time images to provide ophthalmic advice remotely.[6] Since the 1980s, however, advancements in digital imaging with near loss less data transfer have allowed high-quality information to be sent via high-speed data transfer to a remote provider.[7] In addition, the growing availability of high-speed internet connectivity allows providers to connect to patients in places previously never thought possible. This near-everywhere connectivity combined with secure data transmission and storage is creating new opportunities for ocular telehealth. The development of high-quality ocular telehealth programs is a result of integrating technological advancements with innovative ways of delivering eye care.

The benefits of ocular telehealth are numerous. First, reducing travel burden, including time, distance, and cost savings for patients to receive care is significant as the information travels instead of the patient.[6] Second, there is an imbalance between supply and demand for eye care which results in significant challenges to accessing eye care. Location is a key reason; traditionally this was viewed as an issue for rural patients, but those in an urban setting also face limited access to eye care. For example, India, with a population of well over a billion people, only has one ophthalmologist for every 107,000 individuals[8] and has a shortage of over 60,000 Optometrists to meet the national need for eye providers according to a 2016 study from the India Vision Institute.[9] An ocular telehealth program can reach more patients than would be possible using a traditional clinic-visit model and is a cost-effective method to monitor at-risk individuals. A telehealth visit can also reduce risk for vulnerable individuals including immunocompromised patients and those with mental health conditions who may be hesitant or uncomfortable in a traditional clinic setting. Furthermore, telehealth may be the only realistic option to care for individuals in remote or high-risk areas.[6] Third, ocular telehealth is a potential solution to address many important patient eye care needs ranging from screening to monitoring chronic, potentially blinding conditions. Worldwide there are many cases of preventable blindness from conditions that can be evaluated by ocular telehealth. Cataract, glaucoma, age-related macular degeneration, diabetic retinopathy, and retinopathy of prematurity are the most common causes of blindness in many countries and can be screened and monitored through ocular telehealth.[10] Similarly, curable conditions like uncorrected refractive error and cataracts were estimated to be 75% of all visual impairments around the world in 2010 and can be assessed through ocular telehealth.[10]

The most widely recognized ocular telehealth programs screen for diabetic retinopathy. These programs help improve the frequency of retinal evaluation by making retinal screening more readily accessible to patients. Retinal screening may be available in a variety of locations, among the most common include primary care clinics, endocrinology clinics, or community health centers. Future predictions estimate that by 2030 more than a half-billion individuals will have diabetes worldwide, which would require 2000 exams per minute just to provide an annual diabetic eye examination for everyone in need.[11] The benefit of consistent diabetic retinal screening is well established. A study from northern Europe reported that for patients with diabetes not screened in a timely manner, there was an increased rate of developing referable retinopathy, and specifically, those with a 3 year or more delay in screening had a 4 times higher risk of developing proliferative retinopathy.[12] Diabetic retinal screening via ocular telehealth provides another opportunity to meet the eye care needs of these individuals. Chapters 2 and 6 delve into diabetic teleretinal screening in greater depth.

THE "REAL WORLD" USE OF OCULAR TELEHEALTH

There are many challenges to developing and implementing any new healthcare strategy or method of delivering care. Telehealth is not immune to these challenges and ocular telehealth faces numerous aspects unique to a program that is dependent on incorporating new technology and working with remote sites. Some key aspects to evaluate when implementing a new program include feasibility, clinical outcomes, financial resources, human resources, ease of access, equity, cultural barriers, quality assurance, and patient satisfaction.[10] One of the most challenging elements is related to individual, both patient and provider, acceptance for a new program. Provider buy-in to a new method of delivering care is often wide ranging. Early adopters buy-in quickly and typically lead the change for their peers. The early adopters may be more comfortable in the new program for many reasons including meeting a clinical need they have directly encountered or their relative high comfort level with emerging technology. Other providers may be hesitant to try new methods and lag behind the early adopters as moving to an ocular telehealth visit disrupts the usual practice models to which they are accustomed. A survey of eye physician attitudes towards ocular telehealth provides perspective: The majority (82%) reported they would be willing or extremely willing to participate in ocular telehealth in a consultation role for reading and interpreting photographs. A remarkably high number (91%) responded that ocular telehealth was underutilized in ophthalmology with 60% believing it would have a positive effect on their practice yet 59% had low confidence in using remote screening for making a decision on appropriate eye care.[13,14]

In addition to possible provider barriers in ocular telehealth, one must remember that patients have varying desires to virtually connect with their eye provider. There are many factors that may make ocular telehealth appealing to a patient with convenience consistently ranked near the top of the list. Convenience could take numerous forms including reducing the time and distance required to attend an in-person eye appointment. The physical burden to travel to an in-person clinic appointment is a difficult task for some with limited mobility, chronic medical conditions, vision loss or blindness, or mental health conditions that impact their ability to feel safe in certain environments. Furthermore, a telehealth visit could be an appreciated alternative when time away from work or other responsibilities, including care for family or friends, limits their ability to access traditional in-person care. Telehealth may directly save a patient money, for example, a person who is homebound with medical transport requirements for in-person clinic appointments may benefit from the convenience of an at-home telehealth visit and the associated cost savings.

Another important factor to consider is a patient's comfort level with technology and access to technology. Many patients may describe themselves as technologically challenged, with the thought of connecting virtually to their provider unrealistic. Discomfort with technology is more likely to occur with advanced age, and with older patients having a higher need for regular eye care, ocular telehealth may not be the best option for some.

Furthermore, the gap in available technology and connectivity for some individuals has been referred to as the digital divide. This commonly describes the limitations for some patients to connect to a provider through a telehealth visit. The divide can include limited access to devices including computer, laptop, smartphone, or tablet or it can reference limited access to internet connectivity based on Wi-Fi or cellular availability. Some telehealth programs overcome this by taking the necessary equipment and technology closer to the patient in a satellite clinic, mobile telehealth unit, or in their home. Chapter 12 discusses implementation strategies in detail.

Another factor that needs to be fully evaluated is medical malpractice liability in telehealth. This is reported as a significant reason for provider hesitation.[14,15] However, there are protective elements to reviewing and interpreting digital images in ocular telehealth as they provide objective documentation regarding the quality and representative nature of the patient.[14,15] Moreover, legal considerations include the patient-provider relationship and how a telehealth visit compares to an in-person visit. The criteria to identify a patient-provider relationship is typically dependent on state statutes. Provider state licensure permits a provider to deliver care for a patient that resides in the state where the provider is licensed but not across state lines. Statutes related to care across state lines are slowly evolving to catch up to current telehealth practices. Chapter 15 discusses these topics in greater depth.

In addition, variability and challenges with reimbursement for care provided virtually is another significant factor limiting the expansion of ocular telehealth. For many years, telehealth was not reimbursed at a consistent level with in-person care, and the United States Medicare system only reimbursed telehealth services in rural areas and did not cover asynchronous care except in Hawaii and Alaska.[15] To reduce this challenge during the COVID-19 pandemic, Medicare relaxed many of the reimbursement restrictions on telehealth. Chapter 14 details billing and coding for telehealth visits.

Finally, aside from the factors listed above, there are additional technical aspects that are important to identify and navigate to safely establish and manage an ocular telehealth program. There are standards related to image capture, data transfer, and storage such as Digital Imaging and Communications in Medicine (DICOM) compliance standards and Health Insurance Portability and Accountability Act (HIPAA) regulations. Labiris et al. identified key items that limit the expansion of ocular telehealth: lack of teleconsultation infrastructure, cost of necessary equipment, the capability of the equipment to capture high-quality data, staff training, deficiency in guidelines, and protocols, and safety and security of personal health information.[6] The choice of equipment is also important, as the goal of the program will influence what equipment is necessary. Chapter 13 delves into technology considerations for ocular telehealth programs.

The future of ocular telehealth is almost limitless. The explosive rate of technological innovations will provide new opportunities for patients to connect to a remote eye provider. Smart device advancements may allow patients to acquire diagnostic level information from home and submit it to an eye provider from their personal devices. The expansion of internet connectivity with rapid and secure data transmission is creating new opportunities to provide eye care to patients around the globe.

DEFINITIONS

Throughout this book, the following standard terms will be utilized to describe aspects of an ocular telehealth program. The terms telemedicine and telehealth are used interchangeably in this textbook.

1. *Telehealth:*
   a. WHO definition: designed to integrate telecommunications systems into the practice of protecting and promoting health.[1]
2. *Telemedicine:*
   a. WHO definition: designed to integrate telecommunications into diagnostic and therapeutic intervention.[1]
3. *Ocular telehealth:*
   a. Telehealth focused on screening, consultation, monitoring, and education of ocular conditions.
4. *Telehealth visit:*
   a. Used to identify a synchronous or asynchronous interaction between the patient and provider.
5. *Asynchronous telehealth:* (also known as Store-and-Forward Telehealth or SFT)
   a. Refers to a telehealth modality where health information for a patient is acquired and

transmitted to a secure location, to be reviewed by a distant provider at a different time (ranging from minutes to days).
   b. Example
      i. At a primary care visit, a patient with diabetes is identified as due for diabetic retinal evaluation. At that visit, a telehealth facilitator captures and transmits undilated retinal images to a secure storage location. A remote provider accesses and reviews the clinical information and images and provides a recommendation for follow-up eye care.
6. *Synchronous telehealth:* (also known as live or interactive telehealth)
   a. Refers to either a clinic-based, or home-based, telehealth visit where the patient and provider are meeting in real-time via video conferencing, live chat, or telephone.
   b. Examples
      i. A low vision eye provider connects with a patient over video telehealth. The patient is in a remote clinic setting (clinic-based telehealth) where a telehealth facilitator assists the distant eye provider with low vision device evaluation and instruction.
      ii. An eye provider connects with a patient over video telehealth and the patient is logged in at home (home-based telehealth) to discuss lab results and to determine a plan of care.
7. *Hybrid telehealth:*
   a. Refers to a telehealth visit that incorporates both asynchronous and synchronous modalities.
   b. Example
      i. Ocular telehealth visit where clinical information and images are captured & stored (asynchronous portion) followed by a synchronous video telehealth visit (synchronous portion) to discuss the findings, plan, and provide health education directly with the patient.
8. *Clinic-based telehealth:* (also known as in-the-clinic telehealth)
   a. Patient participating in an asynchronous or synchronous telehealth visit in a clinic-based setting (as opposed to home-based telehealth), often with a clinical staff member (i.e., nurse, technician, or telehealth facilitator) supporting the telehealth visit.
9. *Home-based monitoring telehealth:* (also known as in-home monitoring)
   a. Refers to a patient participating in telehealth from home or a nonclinical setting where the

patient collects and/or submits physiologic information to a provider to monitor, typically as part of ongoing management of a known condition.

10. *In-person care:* (also known as a traditional patient-provider visit)
    a. This is the traditional clinical or healthcare visit where the patient and provider are in the same physical location at the same time for the purpose of a clinical visit. In-person care is not telehealth.
11. *Patient site:* (also known as spoke site or originating site)
    a. The physical location of the patient when connecting with the distant telehealth provider or where clinical information is obtained, could be at home or in a clinic.
12. *Provider:*
    a. In this book, the term provider will be used to identify the clinician or healthcare professional, often a physician or other licensed practitioner who is providing clinical care as part of the telehealth visit.
13. *Provider site:* (also known as hub site or distant site)
    a. The physical location of the provider at the time of the telehealth visit.
14. *Referring provider:*
    a. The referring provider sends the patient to another healthcare professional for care including a second opinion. Common referring providers to an ocular telehealth program include Primary Care provider, Eye provider, Neurology provider, Rheumatology provider, or Endocrinology provider.
    b. Examples
        i. A Primary Care Provider may refer a patient with diabetes for an ocular telehealth visit to assess diabetic retinopathy.
        ii. An eye provider may refer a patient to a subspecialist for telehealth consultation for their opinion on the patient's glaucoma status.
15. *Teleconsultation:*
    a. Refers to a synchronous or asynchronous telehealth visit using information and communication technology to overcome geographical and functional distance to obtain a clinical opinion from another provider, often a specialist. A teleconsulting provider does not assume care or liability for the patient.[16]
16. *Telehealth encounter:*
    a. Represents a discrete episode of care event regardless of the modality of care.
17. *Telehealth technician or facilitator:*
    a. Refers to the clinical support staff at the patient site who assists with the telehealth visit. This role may include connecting the patient and provider for a synchronous telehealth visit or capturing and transmitting clinical data as part of an asynchronous telehealth visit.
    b. Common telehealth facilitators include technicians, imagers, nurses, and other medical professionals.
18. *Telehealth modality:*
    a. Refers to the format and structure of telehealth visits. The most common telehealth modalities include asynchronous, synchronous, or home-based.
19. *Telehealth platform:*
    a. Refers to the application or software that connects a patient and provider during a telehealth visit. Common applications for synchronous telehealth include: Zoom, FaceTime, Facebook Messenger video chat, Google Hangouts video, Go-To-Meeting, Skype, and others.[17]
20. *Telehealth provider:*
    a. Refers to the clinical provider that delivers the care or clinical recommendation for the patient as part of the telehealth visit.

REFERENCES

1. Li HK, Horton M, Burseel SV, et al. Telehealth practice recommendations for diabetic retinopathy, 2nd edition. *Telemed J E Health.* 2011;17(10):814–837.
2. Murdoch I. Telemedicine. *Br J Ophthalmol.* 1999;83:1254–1256.
3. Darkins AW, Cary MA. *Telemedicine and Telehealth.* New York: Springer; 2000.
4. Saleem SM, Pasquale LR, Sidoti PA, Tsai JC. Virtual ophthalmology: telemedicine in a COVID-19 era. *Am J Ophthalmol.* 2020;216:237–242.
5. National Committee for Quality Assurance (NCQA). *Taskforce for Telehealth Policy Final report.* National Committee for Quality Assurance website; 2020. Accessed 15.02.21 https://www.ncqa.org/wp-content/uploads/2020/09/20200914_Taskforce_on_Telehealth_Policy_Final_Report.pdf.
6. Labiris G, Panagiotopoulou EK, Kozobolis V. A systematic review of teleophthalmological studies in Europe. *Int J Ophthalmol.* 2018;11(2):314–325.
7. Newton MJ. The promise of telemedicine. *Surv Ophthalmol.* 2014;59:559–567.
8. Paul PG, Raman R, Rani PK, Deshmukh H, Sharma T. Patient satisfaction levels during teleophthalmology consultation in rural South India. *Telemed J E Health.* 2006;12(5):571–578.
9. Optometry in India. India Vision Institute. Accessed 16.11.21 https://www.indiavisioninstitute.org/resources-files/1730Optometry%20in%20India%20report_February%202016.pdf.

10. Mohammadpour M, Heidari Z, Mirghorbani M, Hashemi H. Smartphones, tele-ophthalmology, and VISION 2020. *Int J Ophthalmol.* 2017;10(12):1909–1918.

11. Silva PS, Aiello LP. Telemedicine and eye examinations for diabetic retinopathy a time to maximize real-world outcomes. *JAMA Ophthalmol.* 2015;133(5):525–526.

12. Sim DA, Mitry D, Alexander P, et al. The evolution of teleophthalmology programs in the United Kingdom: beyond diabetic retinopathy screening. *J Diabetes Sci Technol.* 2016;10(2):308–317.

13. Woodward MA, Ple-plakon P, Blachley T, et al. Eye care providers' attitudes towards tele-ophthalmology. *Telemed J E Health.* 2015;21(4):271–273.

14. Shaw J. Teleophthalmology: ready for prime time? *Eyenet.* 2016;6:41–45.

15. Rathi S, Tsue E, Mehta N, Zahid S, Schuman JS. The current state of teleophthalmology in the United States. *Ophthalmology.* 2017;124:1729–1734.

16. Deldar K, Bahaadinbeigy TSM. Teleconsultation and clinical decision making: a systematic review. *Acta Inform Med.* 2016;24(4):286–292.

17. TeleOphthalmology. *How to Get Started.* American Academy of Ophthalmology website; March 23, 2020. Accessed 10.04.21 https://www.aao.org/practice-management/article/teleophthalmology-how-to-get-started.

CHAPTER 2

Comprehensive Eye Telehealth

GERALD SELVIN, OD, FAAO • ANNEY JOSEPH, OD, FAAO

SECTION I: DIABETIC TELERETINAL SCREENING: THE FOUNDATIONAL OCULAR TELEHEALTH PROGRAM—GERALD SELVIN OD, FAAO

Introduction

Comprehensive ocular telehealth encompasses eye telemedicine programs that are (1) geared toward population health management (primarily focused on screening for a common eye condition(s)), or (2) provide a general ocular health assessment (for example, correction of refractive error and a full ocular exam). The authors will begin this chapter with an in-depth discussion about how comprehensive ocular telehealth programs are used in population health management. This particular section will provide a detailed discussion about diabetic retinopathy (DR) screening since this is the first and most robust eye telehealth program in the world. Other expanded eye telehealth programs covered in this textbook, such as tele-glaucoma, are built upon the same principles and infrastructure of DR screening. Thus, this chapter will begin by outlining the most successful use case of telehealth population health management—the screening for DR. Using DR as a case study, this section will highlight important principles that are conserved across all eye telehealth.

Diabetic Retinopathy (DR)—The Goal of Population Screening With An Ocular Telehealth Method

As chronic disease increases in the global population and as innovative technology increasingly enables analysis of individual risk for vision loss without the requirement of increasing resources (space, equipment, and to degree, personnel), it is reasonable to consider broad population screening utilizing telehealth. In diabetes mellitus, using eye telehealth for mass population screening for DR has demonstrated efficacy and ability to bring the highest risk patients more promptly to subspecialists for in-person examinations, thereby enabling these specialists to treat potentially vision-threatening conditions earlier and often more successfully. However, when beginning to develop any eye telehealth program, some basic and critical questions must be answered.

First, the goal of the telehealth program should be clearly articulated and address a significant need. The goal of DR screening is to detect asymptomatic patients at risk of vision loss from diabetic retinopathy. Clinically, it is an extremely relevant problem to address since diabetes mellitus (DM) creates an increased risk of vision loss and in fact, DR is the leading cause of vision loss in the US working-age population as well as elderly retired.[1] Population studies from prior decades have established that reasonably better glycemic control along with frequent eye screening can potentially stave off the worst effects of DR.[2,3] However, there is definitely a need to find alternative ways to screen patients for vision-threatening DR because less than 50% of diabetics receive their recommended eye screening if patients are managed solely by traditional in-person care.[4]

In order to effectively accomplish the goal of DR screening with telehealth methods, certain criteria must be met, including a program that is accurate, safe, and convenient. The most important tenet of any eye telehealth program is the assurance of patient safety. What is the risk that screening can cause "misses" resulting in increased patient and societal burdening of disease? The best way to assure patient safety is through rigorous scientific validation. Fortunately, validation has shown that DR screening is indeed safe and the "misses" that may occur are comparable with in-person care.[5] Most importantly, there is strong evidence for the actual equivalence between DR screening via telehealth to in-person care with respect to the assessment of vision threats from DR.[2,3,5,6]

Second, DR screening programs should be convenient and reduce barriers to access, such as lessening travel distance and wait times that are associated with traditional in-person care. One of the easiest ways to accomplish this task is to house the DR screening in the primary care clinics so that patients can have a "one-stop shop" and receive eye screening at the same time as a primary care visit. Accordingly, following these two principles above, many DR programs such as the Joslin Vision Network (JVN), the Department of Veterans Affairs Diabetic Teleretinal Imaging Program (VA TRI), EyePACS, INOVEON, Wisconsin Reading Center, and others have established asynchronous telehealth methods at the primary medical care home to screen patients with diabetes for DR and subsequently refer some for in-person care at the appropriate time frame depending on the findings from the eye telehealth screening.[7–11]

Another important consideration for any eye telehealth program and DR screening is the ease of actual implementation. One of the reasons that DR screening has flourished over the past 20 + years is the beauty of technology. Digital fundus photography is a simple and relatively inexpensive technology. The only requirement is enough resolution and DICOM (digital imaging and communication in medicine) ability to

transmit images from the local device to a secure server for review by remote readers.

As technology advanced in the past 20 years, most modalities produced images with DICOM capability enabling remote review. Moreover, DR screening programs have been ubiquitously successful because they are focused on attracting the largest number of patients with the disease. These programs reach out only to those with defined risk in a specific population and these programs do everything possible to avoid redundancy. For example, avoidance of patients with recent in-person eye care is strongly adhered to.

More importantly, as mentioned in Chapter 1 and more in-depth in Chapter 12, DR screening telehealth program processes are patient-centric and appealing to people with limited time. With any eye telehealth program including DR screening, the question of patient acceptance must be considered. One would think this is a so-called "no brainer". Patients have strongly embraced telehealth. This is particularly relevant in the age of COVID-19. However, long before the COVID-19 pandemic, patient acceptance of DR screening via telehealth has been high.[12]

Another key component contributing to the wide success of DR screening is the emphasis on education—both on the provider and patient side. Many programs educate technicians to serve as the liaison between the patients and providers at the patient site and readers at the provider site. These technicians can range from Eye Technicians (Ophthalmology or Optometry), Licensed Practical Nurses, Registered Nurses, to name a few. A subsequent important outcome of patient education can be improved diabetes self-care with better glycemic outcomes. The reduced cost and burden on the healthcare system from better outcomes with less complicated or no diabetic eye disease substantiate the need for care coordination in all patient care environments.[13]

Additional aspect to consider with DR screening is technology, a topic discussed in depth in Chapter 13. As stated above, DICOM enhanced the ability to do DR screening via asynchronous telehealth because images can easily be transferred to a secure server for a remote reader to read at a different time point than when the patient presents. The typical technology used in DR screening programs is nonmydriatic fundus imaging. This technology will have a percentage of studies that are ungradable, but that fraction should dramatically drop utilizing wide-field fundus imaging. Soliman et al. reduced the ungradable rate to 0.5% in a study of 200 subjects in 2012 imaged with wide-field nonmydriatic imaging.[14] The negative aspect of wide-field is cost vs standard fundus photography. Wide-field imaging, while less costly vs 10 years ago still would typically cost about 2–3 times what a standard nonmydriatic fundus camera would. Essentially, in a world of always limited resources, for every 2–3 screening locations using standard fundus photography, the same resources would allow only 1 wide-field unit. For instance, in the VA TRI program, there are roughly 1000 imaging locations in use, the vast majority being standard nonmydriatic fundus cameras. Replacing 1000 cameras with wide field would cost $60 million plus. Logically wide-field imaging should yield more gradable studies in the assessment of diabetic retinopathy.[14] However, in comparison to in-person exams, eye telehealth screening, regardless of technology and start-up costs, is always more cost-effective to maintain in an ongoing fashion. A full-time reader without ancillary staff can manage multiple imaging locations and provide care to a larger number of patients than the number an in-person provider would be able to see in one clinic session.

VA TRI: A Case Study of a Comprehensive Eye Telehealth Program

To understand how successful large and small telehealth programs may be deployed, let's do an analysis of the VA Teleretinal Imaging (TRI). The VA TRI program was modeled after the Joslin Vision Network (JVN) experience, including image composition, patient education, and care coordination. When the VA deployed its program, referral criteria received strong emphasis. Not only did the referral criteria need to be clinically relevant, they had to be patient-centric. Safe referral intervals validated by sound science without regard to monetary gain by any stakeholder were practiced.

The Department of Veterans Affairs has had for decades, a robust multi-disciplinary nationwide electronic medical record (EMR), and a telehealth emphasis on providing the right care in the right place at the right time. The referral criterion choice for VA TRI had been the International Classification of Diabetic Retinopathy and Maculopathy, which marries clinical pertinence with clinical classification using the Early Treatment Diabetic Retinopathy Study (ETDRS).[15]

In order to deploy the VA TRI program, multiple stakeholders must "buy-in". Failure to involve the entire team managing patients with diabetes (e.g., primary care providers, eye providers, administrative personnel) will at the very least slow the process to the extent that fewer patients can access the program. At worst, the program will be stuck at the "starting gate". Every healthcare system or clinic has management. Administrative leaders must support the telehealth program or it is likely doomed to sub-par performance. With regard to the VA TRI program, obtaining "buy-in" required repetitive education starting with the pitch to upper-level management such as the Chief of Staff. Once management support was obtained, the next group to educate and obtain concurrence from was the Eye Care Team, including Ophthalmologists, Optometrists, Technicians, and Eye Care Administrative Leaders. Despite the education of providers on the advantages of a program utilizing sound science, individual biases also needed to be overcome. Frequent education utilizing clinical demonstration of the DR screening process was conducted. This way, the clear advantages, including the impact on patients and providers, can be experienced first-hand by the key clinical stakeholders. Since the eye care providers were ultimately responsible for the management of all patients going through VA TRI and were active partners in the process, it significantly increased the likelihood of program success. Increased referrals initially to eye clinics represent patients either lost to follow-up or are underserved. Sometimes this increase in workload is a deterrence to Eye Clinics. Well-established referral criteria should be established with the assurance that it does not deviate from published and accepted clinical standards.

Concurrence and active participation of the Primary Care Team-whether in one consolidated multidisciplinary environment or a private setting was also crucial to the VA TRI program's success. Since the goal is for better outcomes for a Primary Care Team's patients, the acceptability to Primary Care Providers must be ascertained, particularly when education and literature are reviewed. In addition, the VA ocular telehealth team was willing to repeat the provider education as often as needed (since there were also frequently rotating residents) until it became ingrained into the daily operation of the clinic. Experience has shown that failure to prioritize this education can lead to front-line providers not utilizing the program and fewer at-risk patients being screened for vision-threatening disease.

Since any eye telehealth requires information technology (IT) coordination, any organization considering the deployment of an eye telehealth program requires partnership with the IT team from the beginning. Most who have successfully or unsuccessfully organized an eye telehealth program understand how critical it is to partner with IT from the conceptualization of the program. This includes the Biomedical Engineers who will be working with IT to provide seamless image transmission for "plug and play" provider application. The VA TRI program incorporated Biomed, IT, and clinical applications coordinators to ensure a seamless transition of information from the remote site to the reader, and an ability to easily convey results of screening within the EMR framework.

Before the national rollout of VA TRI, it was understood that IT and Biomedical Engineering must be at the center of the plans from the beginning. When IT understood what the needs of the program were, imaging modalities including coordination of images from devices to local hospital EMR systems to national systems could be accomplished *with collaboration.* Having been in the room from the beginning of the national roll-out, this writer (Dr. Selvin) is convinced that the success of the Diabetic Teleretinal Imaging Program was due to the extraordinary collaboration between multiple disciplines but most importantly IT/Biomedical Engineering partners!

Even though literature has validated the accuracy and safety of DR screening programs, another way the VA assures that the TRI program is indeed safe for patients and clinically relevant, is to use peer review instruments. The frequency of these reviews typically is biannual and included with the re-credentialing process occurring biennially. On a programmatic level, there should be an assurance of standardization and adherence to stated standards which can be applied to each location deployed. Quality Management staff review the VA TRI program periodically using established metrics for standardization. The VA ensured that Quality Management was highly prioritized.[16] More details about how to establish a quality monitoring program are discussed in Chapter 16.

Additional Diseases Suitable for Telehealth Population-Based Screening

Population screening for DR was able to be accomplished due to many fortunate factors that are inherent in diabetic retinopathy. Early imaging devices had much lower resolution (2.1 megapixels), yet the typical ungradable rate was still below 20%. The unique ability to enhance retinal photos through image manipulation (e.g., red filter, increasing contrast) such that hemorrhages and microaneurysms (MAs) can be more easily detected, gave diabetic risk assessment a major advantage. However, it became quickly clear that non-diabetic eye disease could also be incidentally detected from the same set of fundus photos. For example, the ability to recognize diabetic disease may be dependent on whether or not there are ocular media obscurations. A patient with media opacity should be referred for an in-person exam and may have an improvement in life quality with cataract surgery.

Since the fundus photos also incorporate images of the macula and optic nerve, the DR screening program can also detect other high prevalence conditions such as Age-Related Macular Degeneration (AMD) and Glaucoma. The burden of AMD is high and growing.[17] With the increased efficacy of treatments for all forms of AMD, early detection and placement of patients to eye clinics should result in better outcomes. The discussion on how to employ eye telehealth in the screening of those most at risk for AMD is ongoing. Risk factors include age, race, smoking history, family history, body mass index (BMI), and comorbid disease. If these risk factors of patients in a given practice or healthcare system are extractable by electronic means, then those at the highest risk can be identified and screened first. Can plain fundus images give enough information? What are the measures that should be obtained to result in the best referrals for in-person care? A collaborative approach among providers should answer those questions. However, starting with what's available in a program's infrastructure can enable a healthcare system to identify more patients with higher risk of AMD.

Glaucoma occurs at an increased frequency as the population ages. Those at highest risk for glaucoma (by age, race, and family history among others) can be screened via eye telehealth with a referral for in-person care at an interval based on risk factors observed in the eye telehealth encounter.

The above examples of other high prevalence/high morbidity conditions being screened by eye telehealth illustrates a potential comprehensive eye care delivery model for the future. Providers, particularly specialists and subspecialists are often co-located in urban areas frequently clustered in large academic medical centers. Rural-based patients may not easily have access to all of these subspecialty providers in the traditional clinic-visit model, but may have improved access via ocular telehealth. Only with the full collaboration and cooperation among many stakeholders can this important improvement in access for all patients, regardless of their location, be accomplished. As our healthcare systems and individual practices continue to understand the burden of disease and the poor distribution of providers between urban and rural areas a lifeline can be provided to those most in need. The COVID-19 pandemic has taught providers across all disciplines the value of virtual care. This virtual care is likely to continue to grow and society will probably not revert back to the same level of in-person care post-pandemic.

The Impact of Machine Learning on Population Health Management

Chapter 18 discusses machine learning and artificial intelligence (AI) in greater detail. AI is a frontier that is just in the early stages of use in population health management. As AI ability becomes more robust, more and more care may become virtual, with "instantaneous" preliminary reports, more efficient reading workflow, and tailored therapies.[18]

Summary of Population Health Management Using Ocular Telehealth

A huge part of comprehensive eye telehealth focuses on screening for common disease conditions in order to identify patients at the highest risk and triage those to receive necessary in-person care while providing an important and necessary lifeline for the underserved populations to achieve better access to risk management. The goal of these screening telehealth programs is to minimize the possibility of vision loss. While the eye care field is still early in the broad application of ocular telehealth, the development of stronger eye telehealth messaging for eye providers is important and needs to be a priority to not only care for the increasing number of patients (baby boomer generation continues to age with the oldest reaching age 75 in 2021), but also as an efficient, safe, and patient-centric way to support the management of vision-threatening disease.

SECTION II: COMPREHENSIVE EYE TELEHEALTH FOR COMPLETE OCULAR HEALTH ASSESSMENT—ANNEY JOSEPH, OD, FAAO

Introduction

As mentioned above, the second goal of comprehensive eye telehealth, aside from population screening, is to provide an ocular health assessment. The components of a traditional, in-person comprehensive eye exam are typically standard across platforms and continents. The components of general ocular telehealth programs aim to provide a complete ocular health assessment, therefore, are directed toward methods of gathering similar information as in-person care.

Components of a Complete Ocular Health Assessment via Telemedicine

An eye exam typically begins with reviewing a patient's chief complaint and past medical, ocular, and social history. In a traditional in-person exam, a patient fills out a hard copy of a review of systems in the waiting room with an ophthalmic technician and/or eye care professional reviewing the document with the patient in the exam room. Newer intake methods allow a patient to answer these questions prior to coming in for an eye appointment via a secure portal. Alternatively, patients may fill out these forms on a tablet while waiting for their exam to begin in a traditional waiting room.

Gathering history in a comprehensive ocular telehealth program can be accomplished in a similar manner.

After the history, visual acuity testing and refraction are performed. Visual acuity assesses how well a patient can see the details of a letter or symbol at a specified distance. In an in-person exam visual acuity is measured with a Snellen Acuity chart placed at 6 m (20 ft) away or with a modified corrected distance eye chart. With the advent of virtual visits, depending on whether the telehealth encounter is clinic-based or home-based, the measurement of visual acuity may vary. For at-home telehealth encounters (e.g., via a Zoom or FaceTime video call) visual acuity charts are readily available to print from a variety of websites. Directions state to place the chart on a wall, with no windows nearby, at 10 ft (3 m) away; cover each eye and read the lowest line without squinting. There are also online vision screening checks, for example on the Zeiss website, to test visual acuity, contrast, and color vision. Once linked, the patient moves the required distance from their home computer screen and then identifies the sequence of Landolt C targets until no longer possible, at which point their acuity is recorded.[18] A small study out of India, with a sample size of 96 subjects, compared traditional, face-to-face visual acuity measurement with a virtually controlled, digital method called "computerized logMAR" (COMPlog; http://www.complog-acuity.com). The COMPlog system also utilizes Landolt C optotypes. The study concluded that visual acuity measurement via telehealth-at-home model can be as reliable as a conventional, face-to-face method.[19] Chapter 13 on Technology provides more details about technology to test visual acuity.

In both in-person and telehealth eye care, autorefraction is an invaluable tool as an objective starting point for manifest refraction. Traditional autorefractors measure lower order aberrations (sphere, cylinder, and axis) whereas the newer wavefront autorefractors measure higher-order aberrations (spherical, coma, and trefoil). Literature is conflicting on which type is more accurate. A study that compared the Canon RK-F2 (traditional) to the Carl Zeiss Vision i.Profiler (wavefront) showed that the traditional autorefractor was more accurate in determining cylinder power and that the wavefront autorefractor tended to over-minus, inducing "instrument myopia."[20] Other studies (see Chapter 13) show greater accuracy with wavefront autorefractors. Either type of autorefractor is useable in a comprehensive ocular telehealth program or other attributes such as portability may play a factor in which device is chosen. After auto-refraction, conventional manifest refraction begins with entering either the auto-refraction or a previous spectacle prescription in the phoropter or trial frames. A certified technician or eye care professional refines the manifest refraction by changing lenses with subjective responses from the patient. If the manifest refraction is being performed by an ophthalmic technician, then the measurements must be sent to a licensed eye care professional for clinical evaluation. There is now technology that enables manifest refraction to occur remotely from the patient. For example, newer technology utilizes binocular wavefront aberrometer with a phoropter to perform dynamic refraction. The Eye Refract system by Luneau Technology (Eye Refract™, Visionix-Luneau Technologies, Chartres, France) is one such system. Unlike a traditional autorefractor, Luneau's system tests and makes adjustments binocularly. It utilizes artificial intelligence-powered binocular and dynamic refraction using two Hartmann-Shack aberrometers running simultaneously. According to their literature, reducing the time spent in refraction is a proper method to increase clinical efficacy. This system showed similar results to conventional subjective refraction in terms of spherical and cylindrical components, visual acuity, and visual satisfaction.[21]

One study out of the Netherlands that studied web-based refraction, called Easee BV, showed mild agreement with conventional subjective refraction in healthy, mildly myopic eyes.[22] Topcon has also developed a web-based application (RDx) that can now remotely control their automated phoropter, CV 5000, and allow for remote refractions in a synchronous, clinic-based telehealth method.[23] Whatever the mode of manifest refraction, if the comprehensive ocular telehealth program is going to perform refraction on the patient, the patient is usually participating in a clinic-based telehealth encounter as there is no well-validated and acceptable program for patients to "self-manifest refract" from home. A company, Visibly (formerly Opternative), had attempted to design a vision test and refraction at home but was removed from the market and is not available at this time.

The next part of a comprehensive eye exam involves the ocular health assessment. During an in-person visit, an eye care professional checks pupillary response and uses diagnostic eye drops and biomicroscopy to accomplish this assessment. An anesthetic eye drop is used to obtain intraocular pressure (IOP) via Goldmann applanation tonometry or any number of handheld devices. Traditionally, a slit lamp biomicroscope is used to view anterior and posterior ocular structures. The eye provider then performs a dilated exam using biomicroscopy and/or indirect ophthalmoscopy. In a comprehensive eye telehealth exam, this ocular assessment can be accomplished in a variety of different ways.

One way is to utilize certified ophthalmic technicians as telehealth facilitators in clinic-based telehealth to check pupils and IOP in the same fashion as above. In addition, this technician can capture anterior segment photos or video and send it to the reviewing provider. Posterior pole and peripheral retina assessment in an ocular telehealth exam can be accomplished by having the telehealth facilitator or technician take fundus photos for the eye care professional to review. The number and quality of fundus photos are dependent upon the technology available, the goal of the program, the protocol used, and the practice setting. Ancillary testing, such as optical coherence tomography (OCT) and visual field testing, can also be utilized in ocular telehealth programs and sent for review by eye care professionals. Advancements in technology that can be utilized for telehealth, such as virtual reality visual field testing, are discussed at length in Chapter 13.

Communication with patients is key whether it be a traditional in-person exam or via telehealth. Patients' questions and concerns must be addressed regardless of the way the exam is conducted. In a telehealth eye exam, the eye care professional may be able to communicate with their patients in real-time via high-definition video conferencing (synchronous) or they may call the patient on the phone after reviewing exam results (hybrid model—asynchronous review of information followed by a synchronous telehealth visit). During this time, the eye care professional can also enter orders for spectacle prescription, any ocular medical prescriptions, return to the clinic and/or follow-up orders. According to the American Academy of Ophthalmology's "Telemedicine for Ophthalmology Information Statement," timely reporting must be HIPAA-compliant, provide verifiable transmission and receipt, and allow for secure and persistent storage of the data report.[24] Typically, a comprehensive ocular telehealth program that allows for the prescription of spectacles or medications is a telemedicine model, where the licensed eye provider assumes ownership of the patient's care.

Representative Cases for a Comprehensive Ocular Telehealth Assessment

Comprehensive ocular telehealth uses a wide variety of telehealth modalities, asynchronous, synchronous, or a hybrid model. One example of an asynchronous, (store-and-forward), telehealth eye care platform is the Department of Veterans Affairs (VA) Technology-based Eye Care Services (TECS). The TECS program is a telehealth eye care delivery model based at the VA primary care clinics, designed to screen patients for cataract, macular degeneration, glaucoma, and diabetic retinopathy, while also providing eyeglass prescriptions to correct refractive error. The platform is a clinic-based telehealth visit staffed by certified ophthalmic technicians who perform all aspects of the telehealth exam including history, vision, refraction, IOP, and fundus photos. Refraction is obtained using a combination of an autorefractor and then manifest refraction via trial lenses/frames or a standard phoropter. An example of a TECS clinic site set up can be seen in Figure 2.1A and B. All information is transmitted to a licensed eye care provider remotely through the VA's EMR, Computerized Patient Record System (CPRS) and the eye provider prescribes eyeglasses (if appropriate) and medications if necessary. Results are communicated to the patient via letter or a subsequent follow-up telephone or video call. The TECS program appears to improve access for Veterans for basic eye care services, allowing for earlier disease diagnosis and treatment.[25]

While TECS is predominantly asynchronous telehealth, there are several comprehensive ocular telehealth programs that primarily use synchronous methods within a clinic-based telehealth encounter. Two well-known entities will be outlined here, in no particular order. Digital Optometrics utilizes live, remote, high-definition video conference between a licensed eye provider and patient. Assessment of general medical and visual health history, including current medications, occurs via tablet or a kiosk. According to their website, a qualified ophthalmic technician checks refraction using a phoropter and performs noncontact

tonometry. The external and anterior segment portion of the eye exam is accomplished via anterior segment video, and the posterior segment exam is accomplished through nonmydriatic retinal imaging. Other components, such as checking peripheral vision, are done via confrontation visual fields performed by the technician, or by a computerized visual field analyzer.[26]

Another company currently in operation at the time of writing is 20/20 Now. 20/20 Now is a hybrid comprehensive eye telehealth model, incorporating both asynchronous and synchronous elements. Patients complete a questionnaire electronically to capture their medical history and establish their initial file in the 20/20 Now electronic medical record. An on-site optical assistant with minimal training performs auto-refraction and auto-lensometry, if the patient currently wears glasses. A certified ophthalmic technician then remotely performs subjective refraction in real-time via high-definition video conferencing (synchronous element). This company utilizes proprietary exam software and scientific algorithms to help guide the subjective refraction to arrive at the spectacle prescription. The optical assistant then performs the eye health assessment including ocular alignment and motility via cover test, pupil function, color vision, digital slit lamp images with video, noncontact tonometry, and nonmydriatic fundus photography (45–60 degree images of the posterior pole and 30-degree images centered on the optic nerve). The assistant will also check visual field via automated

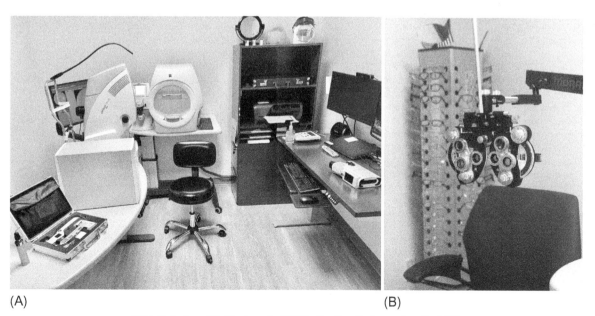

(A)   (B)

FIG. 2.1 A and B: Photos of a TECS site. Credit: Aaron Jerrells, LPN.

perimeter; according to one of 20/20 Now's representatives, they prefer using technology that can integrate well with easy to update software such as Olleyes and Oculus Easyfield. This information is transferred to the medical record (asynchronous element). While the patient waits, a remote licensed eye provider reviews all the information gathered, finalizes the spectacle prescription and provides medical counseling for the patient via real-time high-definition video conferencing. The finalized spectacle prescription is then signed by the eye provider and printed out for the patient.[27]

CONCLUSION

All comprehensive eye telehealth modalities aim to remove barriers to accessibility while bridging the gap in service delivery by reaching remote and underserved areas, including reducing conventional travel time and expense for patients. Whether the comprehensive eye telehealth program is targeted for population health management through focused screening or aiming to provide a general ocular health assessment, these programs are safe, high-quality, and have high patient satisfaction and acceptance in numerous teleeye care studies. As mentioned previously, early detection, accurate evaluation, and timely, evidence-based treatment and follow-up care are critical in reducing risk of vision loss in the general population either through focused screening or comprehensive eye telehealth exams.[28–32, 33, 34]

REFERENCES

1. Nguyen M, Waller M, Pandya A, Portnoy J. A review of patient and provider satisfaction with telemedicine. *Curr Allergy Asthma Rep.* 2020;20(11):72. https://doi.org/10.1007/s11882-020-00969-7. PMID:32959158. PMCID: PMC7505720.
2. Diabetes. https://www.who.int/news-room/fact-sheets/detail/blindness-and-visual-impairment.
3. Cavallerano AA, Cavallerano J, Katalinic P, et al. Use of validated Joslin Vision network digital-video nonmydriatic retinal imaging to assess diabetic retinopathy in a diabetes outpatient intensive treatment program. *Retina.* 2003;23:215–223.
4. Bursell S-E, Cavallerano JD, Cavallerano AA, et al. Stereo Nonmydriatic digital-video color retinal imaging compared with early treatment diabetic retinopathy study seven standard field 35-mm stereo color photos for determining level of diabetic retinopathy. *Ophthalmology.* 2001;108:572–585.
5. Bursell S-E, Clermont A, Cavallerano J, Cavallerano AA, Aiello LP, Aiello LM. Validation of stereo-non-mydriatic video retinal imaging for diabetic retinopathy assessment in a telemedicine environment. *IOVS.* 2000;41:S166.
6. Conlin PR, Asefzadeh B, Pasquale LR, Selvin G, Lampkin R, Cavallerano AA. Accuracy of a technology-assisted eye exam in evaluation of referable diabetic retinopathy and concomitant ocular diseases. *Br J Ophthalmol.* 2015;99(12):1622–1627.
7. https://www.joslin.org/patient-care/eye-care/joslin-vision-network.
8. https://www.va.gov/communitycare/docs/news/VA_telehealth_services.pdf.
9. https://www.eyepacs.com.
10. https://www.inoveon.com/index-4.html.
11. https://www.ophth.wisc.edu/research/fprc/.
12. Soliman AZ, Silva PS, Aiello LP, Sun JK. Ultra-wide field retinal imaging in detection, classification, and management of diabetic retinopathy. *Semin Ophthalmol.* 2012;27(5–6):221–227.
13. Rawlins WS, Toscano-Garand MA, Graham G. Diabetes management with a care coordinator improves glucose control in African Americans and Hispanics. *J Educ Health Promot.* 2017;6:22.
14. Wu L, Fernandez-Loaiza P, Sauma J, Hernandez-Bogantes E, Masis M. Classification of diabetic retinopathy and diabetic macular edema. *World J Diabetes.* 2013;4(6):290–294.
15. Darkins A, Foster L, AndersOn C, Goldschmidt L, Selvin G. The design, implementation, and operational management of a comprehensive quality management program to support national telehealth networks. *Telemed J E Health.* 2013;19(7):557–564.
16. Wong WL, Su X, Li X, et al. Global prevalence of age-related macular degeneration and disease burden projection for 2020 and 2040: a systematic review and meta-analysis. *Lancet Glob Health.* 2014;2(2):e106–116.
17. Hansen MB, Abràmoff MD, Folk JC, Mathenge W, Bastawrous A, Peto T. Analysis for Detection of Diabetic Retinopathy from the Nakuru Study, Kenya. *PLoS One.* 2015;10(10):1–5.
18. https://www.zeiss.com/vision-care/us/better-vision/vision-screening.html.
19. Srinivasan K, Ramesh SV, Babu N, et al. Efficacy of a remote based computerised visual acuity measurement. *Br J Ophthalmol.* 2012;96:987–990.
20. Lebow KA, Campbell CE. A comparison of a traditional and wavefront autorefraction. *Optom Vis Sci.* 2014;91(10):1191–1198.
21. Carracedo B, Carpena-Torres C, Serramito M, et al. Comparison between aberrometry-based binocular refraction and subjective refraction. *Trans Vis Sci Tech.* 2018;7(4):11.
22. Wisse RPL, Muijzer MB, Cassano F, et al. Validation of an independent web-based tool for measuring visual acuity and refractive error (the manifest versus online refractive evaluation trial): prospective open-label noninferiority clinical trial. *J Med Internet Res.* 2019;21(11):e14808.
23. https://topconhealthcare.com/wp-content/uploads/2021/03/Refraction-Solutions-Brochure-MCA4313.pdf.
24. Silva PS, Cavallerano JD, Aiello LM, et al. Telemedicine and diabetic retinopathy: moving beyond retinal screening. *Arch Ophthalmol.* 2011;129(2):236–242.

25. Maa AY, Wojciechowski B, Hunt KJ, et al. Early Experience with Technology-Based Eye Care Services (TECS): A Novel Ophthalmologic Telemedicine Initiative. *Ophthalmology.* 2017;124(4):539–546.

26. https://digitaloptometrics.com/what-a-patient-can-expect-at-a-visit-conducted-with-tele-optometry-technology/.

27. https://for2020now.com.

28. Mechanic OJ, Persaud Y, Kimball AB. Telehealth systems [Updated 2020 Sep 18]. In: *StatPearls [Internet].* Treasure Island (FL): StatPearls Publishing; 2020. Available from: https://www.ncbi.nlm.nih.gov/books/NBK459384/.

29. https://www.aao.org/clinical-statement/telemedicine-ophthalmology-information-statement.

30. https://www.ncbi.nlm.nih.gov/pmc/articles/PMC7187969/.

31. Sreelatha OK, Ramesh SV. Teleophthalmology: improving patient outcomes? *Clin Ophthalmol.* 2016;10:285–295.

32. Sommer AC, Blumenthal EZ. Telemedicine in ophthalmology in view of the emerging COVID-19 outbreak. *Graefes Arch Clin Exp Ophthalmol.* 2020;258:2341–2352.

33. Caffery LJ, Taylor M, Gole G, et al. Models of care in tele-ophthalmology: a scoping review. *J Telemed Telecare.* 2019;25(2):106–122.

34. Patel J, Morettin C, McLeod H, et al. Patient experience of tele-optometry in the comprehensive eye examination: a pilot study. *Invest Ophthalmol Vis Sci.* 2020;61(7):1596.

CHAPTER 3

Oculoplastic and Orbital Surgery Telehealth

ELAINE DOWNIE, MD • SUZANNE VAN LANDINGHAM, MD

INTRODUCTION

Oculoplastic surgery is a subspecialty within ophthalmology that focuses on reconstructive and cosmetic procedures involving the ocular adnexa and face. Due to the focus on external disease, in oculoplastics, there is a limited need for slit lamp examination, visualization of the ocular fundus, or ophthalmic imaging. Oculoplastic assessment is also highly visual, similar to dermatology and plastic surgery, which makes it uniquely amenable to the incorporation of telemedicine.

HISTORY OF OCULOPLASTIC TELEHEALTH

Review of the literature suggests that the use of telemedicine in oculoplastics has been minimal until recently. There are a small number of studies published prior to the coronavirus pandemic examining the feasibility of telehealth for oculoplastics and its use in a select set of circumstances. However, none of these earlier studies address its use in routine clinical practice.

One early study by Rayner et al.[1] looked at the practicality of using telemedicine for ocular adnexal evaluation. A small number of patients in the United Kingdom were initially evaluated remotely by an ophthalmologist through a synchronous home-based video visit, and then subsequently assessed in-person. The clinical outcomes from both types of visits were documented independently and then reviewed for correlation. The authors found that while some conditions, such as ptosis, could be accurately evaluated using telehealth methods, other complaints, such as nonspecific orbital pain or socket issues after enucleation were more challenging to evaluate remotely.

In 2009, Verma et al.[2] in India demonstrated that telehealth may have a useful role in expanding access to care for patients with orbital and adnexal disease in rural areas. In this study, optometrists using a mobile ophthalmic exam vehicle, obtained slit lamp and external photographs of patients which were then transferred using satellite technology, (due to poor internet connectivity in the villages), to a tertiary eye hospital. Images and other available clinical data were reviewed by specialists who then had synchronous video visits with both the patient and the optometrist. Any patients with potential sight or life-threatening problems were then transferred to the tertiary hospital for further management. Approximately one-third of patients who were evaluated during the course of the study required referral to the eye hospital. These results showed promise for use of telemedicine to expand access to oculoplastic specialists for patients in remote locations.

Ocular Telehealth. https://doi.org/10.1016/B978-0-323-83204-5.00003-2

Telemedicine has also been employed by the United States (U.S.) Army to facilitate access to ophthalmic care. A review was performed of the army's ocular teleconsultation services from 2004 to 2009.[3] Consults were performed via email between health care providers at remote locations, mostly in Iraq and Afghanistan, and domestic military ophthalmologists. Teleconsultation was used to assist in the evaluation of a variety of types of ocular problems, including evaluation for orbital and adnexal concerns, which made up 23.9% of consult requests. Within oculoplastics, the most common concerns requiring consultation were eyelid disease and possible orbital mass or fractures. Consults mostly consisted of requests for management recommendations or diagnostic support, however, consultants also facilitated evacuation in the cases where evacuation was recommended, which was in 43.2% of consultations, and helped avoid unnecessary evacuations in 17.3% of consultations.

While these prior studies were able to demonstrate that telemedicine is useful in a select set of circumstances, such as facilitating care for patients at remote locations where an oculoplastic specialist is not readily available, they do not address the use of telemedicine in routine oculoplastic practice. The limited use of telemedicine in oculoplastics in the past may be in part because much of oculoplastic care is elective or semi-elective, so many patients can wait to access care without suffering significant morbidity or mortality.

CURRENT STATE OF OCULOPLASTICS TELEHEALTH

Due to the COVID-19 crisis, oculoplastics, like many medical specialties, has seen a rapid increase in the utilization of telehealth to safely perform patient visits. A survey of eye care providers found that there was a substantial increase in the proportion of visits performed via telemedicine; from 3% prior to the onset of the COVID-19 related shutdown to 57% during the height of the pandemic.[4] Additionally, among oculoplastic surgeons, prior to the pandemic, only 12.8% had incorporated telemedicine into their practice, compared with 70.5% during.[5] The massive increase in telehealth utilization appears to have been driven by several factors: a desire to avoid the infection risk posed by in-person encounters, the temporary closure of some medical offices, prohibitions against performing nonessential activities, and, within the United States, the increase in reimbursement for synchronous telehealth visits by Medicare and other insurers.

In order to guide their members, a number of the ophthalmic and plastic reconstructive surgery societies worldwide issued recommendations for the management of patients early in the COVID-19 crisis. A review article of the information provided by these societies found that all nine societies with published guidelines agree that any urgent procedures should not be delayed, while all elective services should be postponed.[6] However, the specificity regarding what types of clinical concerns met criteria for urgent evaluation and treatment varied between societies. While all of the nine societies with published guidelines recommended postponing nonurgent examinations and procedures, only four of them highlighted local shelter in place recommendations. There was only one society, the Asociación Colombiana de Cirugía Plastica Ocular, which recommended that surgeons perform their initial patient assessment via teleconsultation when possible. This may be due to limited familiarity with the use of telemedicine in oculoplastics practice at the time the guidelines were published.

Since these society guidelines came out, there has been an increase in the number of publications regarding the use of telemedicine in oculoplastics practice. There have been a variety of applications of telehealth in oculofacial plastic surgery during the pandemic. It has been used to screen new patients, allowing physicians to determine which patients need to come in for urgent or emergent evaluation and to postpone those patients whose appointments can be delayed safely. Surgeons have found that patients with eyelid conditions, such as ptosis, dermatochalasis, ectropion, entropion, eyelid retraction, and congenital deformities can be screened readily with telemedicine.[7] This practice reduced the number of patients who needed to be seen in person during the pandemic, without impacting their ultimate outcome.

In some areas, telehealth has also been used for consultation with physicians at remote locations, to minimize the need for transfer to academic centers where specialists are more likely to be present.[7] It has been proposed that specialists using telehealth methods could, in conjunction with emergency department physicians and local ophthalmologists, safely collaborate to manage patients with nonsurgical conditions, including nonsurgical subperiosteal abscesses and noninfectious orbital inflammatory disease.[7] Many physicians have also used telemedicine for monitoring of post-operative patients who had surgery prior to or during the pandemic, assuming the use of absorbable sutures, in order to minimize the number of in-person visits associated with surgery.[7-9] The implementation of these various telehealth applications varies significantly in different locations.

At one institution in the United Kingdom, a group of oculoplastics consultants prospectively evaluated video visits for patients over the course of a month during the pandemic.[10] Video visits were scheduled in place of in-person visits that had been canceled due to the pandemic, and included both new referrals and return visits, with a mix of routine and urgent appointments. Ninety-one percent of visits were follow-ups. Clinicians participating in the study found that video consults were particularly useful to see post-operative and other follow-up patients, and as a method for ensuring appropriate triage of new referrals. They also reported that resolution of the video during consults was sufficient to assess a number of exam findings, including eyelid position and movement, periocular swelling and hue, chemosis, ocular motility, diplopia, facial asymmetry, and to perform an assessment of larger orbital and lid tumors. In a number of cases, it was even found that video consultation in conjunction with referral information including imaging was adequate to determine the need for urgent surgical intervention. In these cases, the study authors would book the surgery remotely and then perform a final in-person exam on the day of surgery. This likely reduced time to surgery and certainly reduced the number of visits prior to surgery. Although telemedicine visits were found effective for evaluating a variety of conditions, they were judged less useful in the evaluation of new orbital patients. In addition to including clinician perceptions of telemedicine, this study also found acceptable rates of patient satisfaction with the video visits, with 94% finding visits easy to join and 62% preferring video to in-person visits.

In the United Kingdom, Jamison et al.[9] evaluated their use of synchronous video visits for both new and return oculoplastics patients, with the aim of determining whether specific patients or presenting concerns were better suited to video visits. Out of the patients evaluated over the course of the study, only 14.6% of new patients and 12.2% of return patients had to be booked for an in-person encounter because they were unable to be adequately assessed during a video visit. According to the study authors, oculoplastic conditions best suited to video visits as a new patient are ectropion, entropion, and dermatochalasis. Patients referred with these conditions were either able to be signed up for surgery without the need for an in-person visit prior or they were able to be discharged. It was felt that patients being evaluated for epiphora, lid lesions, and conjunctival lesions were less likely to benefit from telemedicine consultation.

In addition to the recently published data on the use of telemedicine in functional oculoplastics, there was a study performed in the United States prior to the pandemic looking at the use of Skype to perform initial home-based video visits with cosmetic oculoplastic patients in a single practice. This was found to be an efficient modality to increase patient flow and expand the patient base in a cosmetic practice.[11] This practice could continue to be useful even after the pandemic, particularly as patients may be less able or willing to take time off from work or to travel for cosmetic evaluations compared to functional ones.

Current usage of telemedicine in oculoplastics is predominantly synchronous, one-on-one home-based visits with the patient. Video is preferred as it allows the provider to perform a visual assessment of the patient and at least some portions of the exam. Asynchronous telehealth appears to be less commonly used, but it is sometimes used in the setting of providers sending photos or recorded video to oculoplastic surgeons for consultation regarding a clinical question. Informal usage of asynchronous telehealth, such as when a patient sends a photo to an oculoplastic surgeon they already have a relationship with (i.e., post-op question) or when a provider sends a photo or video to an oculoplastic surgeon as a "curbside" consult querying if they need subspecialist care, may be underrepresented in the literature.

BEST PRACTICES: PATIENT SELECTION AND TELEHEALTH INFRASTRUCTURE

Among all ophthalmic subspecialties, oculoplastics is uniquely well situated to the use of in-home synchronous video telehealth due to the external nature of many ocular adnexal diseases, the ability to review imaging such as MRI and CT scans from outside providers electronically, and the limited necessity for examination tools that can often only be used in-person, such as the slit lamp. Additionally, patients are frequently referred by other eye care providers, so visual acuity and other standard ocular exam findings are often already present in the referral notes. Furthermore, access may be especially challenging in this field, given that oculoplastic surgery is a small subspecialty that may be underrepresented in rural communities.

At this time, there are no clearly defined guidelines regarding best practices for telemedicine usage in oculoplastics due to the limited number of studies regarding its use. In the following subsections, the authors will review different telehealth modalities and their applications to oculofacial care, as well as postulate best practices for their use.

Synchronous Visits

Based on the current literature, synchronous home-based video visits are the most popular modality for the evaluation of oculoplastic patients. The authors propose that low-risk, post-op follow-up visits, provided no suture removal is needed, and discussion-based follow-up visits may be the best suited to telehealth visits (Table 3.1 and Table 3.2).

For example, if a patient has been examined by the surgeon and referred for imaging, and needs to then discuss the results with the surgeon, synchronous home-based telehealth (i.e., via video) follow-up is ideal.

Other visit types can be considered "moderately" appropriate for synchronous telehealth assessment. Telehealth may be used for these visit types in settings where access to an oculoplastic surgeon is challenging, such as in a rural area or during a public health emergency. This includes referrals for eyelid malpositions such as ptosis, dermatochalasis, ectropion, entropion, and eyelid retraction. These patients may even be able to be signed up for surgery with the final pre-operative exam occurring in-person on the day of the procedure. This would decrease the number of visits needed prior to surgery, and be especially helpful to those with poor access to transportation. The ability to sign patients up for surgery without an in-person visit, however, may be limited by the insurance or payment structure in place in the region—many United States health insurers require high-quality clinic photographs prior to the approval of ptosis and other oculoplastic surgeries, and this is challenging to obtain remotely. Eyelid lesion evaluations could also be categorized as "moderately appropriate" for synchronous video visits or asynchronous telehealth using photos, as long as potentially neoplastic lesions (including poorly visualized ones) can be scheduled for biopsy promptly. Aesthetic visits may also be considered moderately appropriate for telehealth—this patient population may especially appreciate the convenience of a telehealth visit, though the use of telehealth precludes same-day injection (e.g., botulinum toxin or fillers) and may limit close evaluation of skin (for the planning of facial lasers or peels).

Patients with potentially vision-threatening conditions, such as moderate to severe thyroid eye disease or certain orbital lesions, should be seen in-person for their initial consultation in order to facilitate accurate and rapid initiation of treatment. In a trial by Li et al.[12] looking at the use of tele-ophthalmology for screening and recurrence monitoring in neovascular age-related macular degeneration (AMD), it was found that when screening for recurrence of wet AMD, patients screened via telehealth had longer wait times until resumption of treatment, suggesting that for diseases where prompt treatment may be required (ex. optic neuropathy in thyroid eye disease) that there may be a delay in treatment when compared to an in-person visit.

Other diagnoses that would be inappropriate to assess via telehealth due to inadequate exam include epiphora, as lacrimal probing and irrigation are critical to the epiphora workup, and trichiasis, as abnormal lashes would be challenging to visualize. Neither of these diagnoses are urgent, and while an initial screening telehealth visit would not be harmful, it is also unlikely to be adequate.

While little data is available about synchronous visits using a telehealth facilitator, such as in a clinic-based telehealth encounter in oculoplastics, this is a promising model. It is especially relevant in areas where a skilled examiner—such as a comprehensive ophthalmologist, optometrist, or specially trained nurse or technician—is readily available but an oculoplastic surgeon is not, e.g., rural areas. The patient may visit

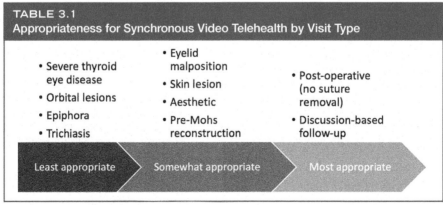

TABLE 3.1
Appropriateness for Synchronous Video Telehealth by Visit Type

- Severe thyroid eye disease
- Orbital lesions
- Epiphora
- Trichiasis

- Eyelid malposition
- Skin lesion
- Aesthetic
- Pre-Mohs reconstruction

- Post-operative (no suture removal)
- Discussion-based follow-up

Least appropriate > Somewhat appropriate > Most appropriate

Suzanne van Landingham, MD.

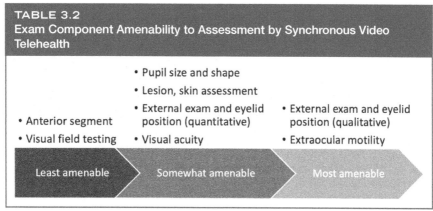

TABLE 3.2
Exam Component Amenability to Assessment by Synchronous Video Telehealth

Least amenable	Somewhat amenable	Most amenable
• Anterior segment • Visual field testing	• Pupil size and shape • Lesion, skin assessment • External exam and eyelid position (quantitative) • Visual acuity	• External exam and eyelid position (qualitative) • Extraocular motility

Suzanne van Landingham, MD.

a clinic with high-quality video set up to be examined with a distant oculoplastic surgeon observing and directing exam components. This technique could be used for the same indications as described above in order to overcome home technology limitations, and could additionally incorporate some examination techniques that are more challenging to examine without a presenter (for example, use of a Hertel exophthalmometer or measurement of eyelid excursion). The presenter could also take high-quality clinical photographs using a slit lamp camera or dermatoscope, a specially designed camera that dermatologists use to photograph skin lesions, which may be useful for surgical planning and submission to payors.

Asynchronous Visits

There is limited use of asynchronous telehealth in the oculoplastics literature. It has been used by the United States Army[3] and as the first stage of evaluation by physicians in India for triage of patients in remote areas.[2] Additionally, it has been demonstrated that evaluation of standardized smartphone photography may be comparable to in-office examination of post-operative eyelid surgery complications.[13] While this technology has been underused and understudied in the past, the authors believe it has promise in the domains of post-operative triage, triage of trauma or other emergencies, eyelid lesion evaluations, or for screening of eyelid malpositions in areas with poor access to care.

Asynchronous technology may be more commonly used than the literature would suggest. For example, post-operative patients often submit photos to their surgeon with questions regarding wound healing. This

may be accomplished through the electronic medical record, such as EPIC's MyChart, which allows patients to submit photographs in a secure, HIPAA-compliant manner, and facilitates saving the photographs for later review. It may also be accomplished less formally via email or text messaging.

Asynchronous photographic telehealth may also be useful for referring providers to inquire if subspecialist consultation is needed. For example, an emergency room provider in a rural hospital may send a photograph of an eyelid laceration to determine if it involves critical structures that require an oculoplastic specialist and therefore transfer (Fig. 3.1).

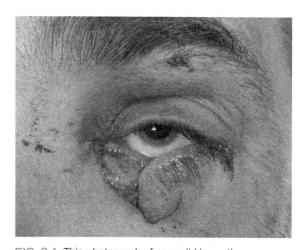

FIG. 3.1 This photograph of an eyelid laceration showing clear punctal involvement, which would need an oculoplastic surgeon for repair, may be sent as part of an asynchronous telehealth consultation. (Credit: Suzanne van Landingham, MD.)

With a high-quality image, the surgeon and consulting provider can determine with confidence whether the patient needs to be transferred or continue their care locally, potentially avoiding costly unnecessary transfers.

Asynchronous telehealth may be particularly useful for screening eyelid lesions, for example, a high-quality photo is sent to an oculoplastic surgeon to assess the urgency and need for assessment of the lesion. While there have been no studies published regarding this application within oculoplastics, in the dermatology literature, there is evidence that stored and forwarded photographs can be successfully used for the evaluation of skin cancer. In one study based in Switzerland,[14] patients were evaluated by taking photos of lesions that were then sent for remote review by dermatology. Out of 195 skin lesions that were evaluated, seven cases of skin cancer were present, all of which were ruled-in with tele-dermatology. This suggests that imaging of lid lesions could be used as a screening tool to evaluate which lesions might require biopsy. In the event of a lesion that appeared to be benign, patients could then be spared the necessity of traveling for an in-person consultation.

Asynchronous review of patient images could also be useful as a screening tool for patients in remote areas where video conferencing/synchronous telehealth technology may be challenging or unavailable due to lack of bandwidth. Additionally, asynchronous provider-to-provider communication with images may represent a useful avenue for triaging referrals. In order for any of these applications of asynchronous telehealth to be successful, they would require the use of a secure system with a rapid review of imaging so that there are no harmful delays in care.

TECHNIQUES FOR OCULOPLASTIC TELEMEDICINE VISITS

In order to have successful telemedicine visits, patients need to have access to a number of technological resources. The first and most critical is a reliable, high bandwidth connection to allow for video visits. Patients also need appropriate lighting to facilitate examination. Video conferencing lighting such as LED rings is now widely available online and patients who do a lot of video conferencing for personal or professional reasons may already have them. For remotely located patients who do not have an appropriate teleconferencing set up at home, video visits could be facilitated at the clinic through a local medical or optometry office. A critical component of any telehealth set up is access to appropriate and prompt in-person care as a backup in the event of technology failure, or if an issue needing urgent medical attention is identified.

Exam Components

Given the visual nature of the oculoplastics exam, there are many components of the exam that are amenable to assessment via video. However, there are a number of components that are more challenging to assess or may need to be judged qualitatively rather than quantitatively when seen via video.

Exam components that may be amenable to assessment via synchronous telehealth to the home include:

1. Pupillary exam: pupil size and shape can be noted; however, afferent pupillary defects cannot be detected.
2. Extraocular motility: this can be assessed by directing the patient on where to look for cardinal gaze positions. This was also the most likely component to be assessed in an as yet unpublished survey of American Society of Ophthalmic Plastic and Reconstructive Surgery (ASOPRS) members, with 67% performing this component of the exam during telehealth visits (Suzanne van Landingham, M.D., email communication, February 7, 2021).
3. Lesions: examination of lesions is variable depending on the video quality and size of the lesion. It is most likely to be beneficial in the case of relatively clear-cut diagnoses such as skin tags, large chalazia, cystic lesions, or a large/ulcerated malignancy.
4. External exam and eyelid position: This portion of the exam is quite amenable to qualitative evaluation via video, such as for noting the presence of ptosis, entropion, or lagophthalmos, though numerical measurements such as levator function are more challenging to obtain without a skilled telehealth presenter. Patients can be requested to hold a ruler up next to their eyes, allowing more quantitative assessment of items like lagophthalmos, marginal reflex distance, palpebral fissure height, and levator function. These measurements may be limited by the patient's ability to manipulate the ruler, as well as to perform maneuvers such as immobilizing their own brow during the examination, which is important for obtaining the most accurate results (Fig. 3.2).

Relevant oculoplastic exam components that are less amenable to video telehealth health are as follows:

1. Anterior segment exam: It may be possible to note the appearance of conjunctival injection, chemosis, and corneal opacity, however, nuanced evaluation is not possible given limits of magnification.

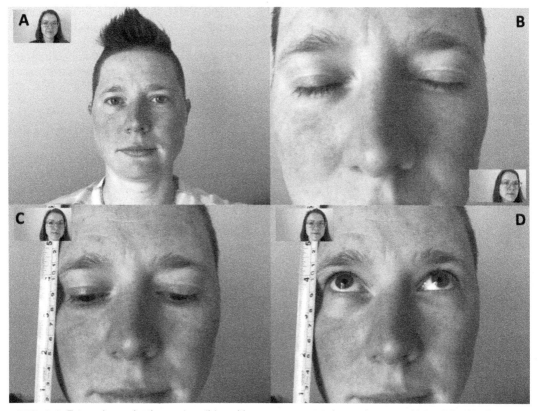

FIG. 3.2 External examination and eyelid position measurement via synchronous video telehealth. These screenshots from an iPhone FaceTime call show maneuvers for assessing (A) facial skin, gross eyelid and brow position; (B) eyelid skin, lashes, and lagophthalmos (none in this patient); (C) and (D) levator excursion. (Credit: The "patient" is a volunteer model with no prior training in medicine or telehealth, who has granted permission for use of their facial photograph in this publication).

2. Visual acuity: Use of a handheld Snellen chart that can be printed at home by the patient or even the use of newsprint can give an estimate of the patient's reading ability. It is difficult, though, to ensure proper occlusion of the contralateral eye and that the material is held at an appropriate distance. A presenter would be helpful for obtaining a more precise measurement. Methods to check visual acuity including apps are discussed in Chapters 2 and 13.

3. Visual field: It is not possible to obtain formal visual field testing, (required by many U.S. insurers for approval of ptosis repair surgery), via synchronous telehealth video to the home. If this is required, it would best be obtained through a clinic-based telehealth encounter with the information sent via asynchronous telehealth for review.

4. Clinical photography: High-quality clinical photography is useful for documentation of exam findings,

comparing findings from a visit to visit, and, in some cases, justifying functional surgeries to insurers.

Fortunately, as many patients are referred for oculoplastic consultation by other eye care providers, many of the above exam components that are more challenging to obtain via teleconsultation, such as visual acuity, may already be documented in the referral notes. For more precise measurements, it may be appropriate to have the video visit done in a clinic with a telehealth presenter who can facilitate the exam, such as at local optometry or primary care office.

High-tech solutions might also be useful in well-resourced settings. For example, Souverein et al.[15] performed a study in which a physician assistant, using video-capable glasses, recorded videos of pediatric patients referred for blepharoptosis in various gazes while a ruler was held next to their eyes. These videos were then reviewed by an oculoplastic surgeon to record the marginal reflex distance and levator function. With these measurements, the surgeon then determined whether the patient would benefit from surgery and, if necessary, which procedure would be performed. These same parameters were then recorded during an in-person visit with the surgeon and the results were compared, with a high correlation found between the video and in-person visits; 94.8% for marginal reflex distance 1 measurements and 98.3% for levator function. However, for many patients and video set ups, only an estimated measurement may be possible, and more detailed measurement may need to be done in-person as needed based on the screening exam.

OCULOPLASTICS TELEHEALTH: FUTURE DIRECTIONS

Recently, there have been widespread increases in the use of telehealth across many medical specialties. However, there are still only a limited number of studies evaluating telehealth usage in oculoplastics. The majority of these are from within the last year, describing the use of telehealth during the COVID-19 pandemic. Current work includes an ongoing clinical trial, which aims to demonstrate the utility of telemedicine in the first post-operative follow-up of patients following low-risk oculoplastic procedures, and includes assessment of patient satisfaction.[16] There is also the ongoing survey of American Society of Ophthalmic Plastic and Reconstructive Surgery (ASOPRS) members being conducted about the current usage of telehealth (Suzanne van Landingham, M.D., email communication, February 7, 2021).

To the authors' knowledge, most usage of telehealth in oculoplastics is synchronous, one-on-one home-based communication, via telephone or video. In addition to this, either asynchronous telehealth or synchronous telehealth visits with a presenter may be useful in some settings. Asynchronous telehealth applications may include taking a photo of an eyelid lesion and sending it to an oculoplastic surgeon to review. This may be underutilized, especially for rural or resource-poor areas, where access to an oculoplastic surgeon and/or to the technology necessary for a successful video visit may be quite limited. Improvement in billing and legal structures to support this type of care would be helpful to allow this to grow. Chapters 14 and 15 discuss reimbursement and legal/ethical issues with telehealth. Synchronous telehealth with presenter, again, may be useful for rural or resource-poor areas, such as the use of optometrists to screen patients in rural India.[2] However, there is a digital divide between urban and rural areas. Since rural areas potentially lack adequate high-speed internet, this divide needs to be addressed as it presents a major hurdle for the expansion of telehealth. In these settings, entirely asynchronous telehealth using photos may be the best option.

CONCLUSION

In summary, the use of telehealth within oculoplastics is rapidly expanding. As it continues to be used, and more data becomes available, it will be helpful to establish evidence-based best practices for its use within the field. Studies regarding physician and patient satisfaction with telehealth visits, as well as how this compares to satisfaction with in-person consultation will also be needed to guide its further development.

REFERENCES

1. Rayner S, Beaconsfield M, Kennedy C, Collin R, Taylor P, Murdoch I. Subspecialty adnexal ophthalmological examination using telemedicine. *J Telemed Telecare*. 2001;7(Suppl. 1):29–31. https://doi.org/10.1177/135763 3X010070S112.
2. Verma M, Raman R, Mohan RE. Application of teleophthalmology in remote diagnosis and management of adnexal and orbital diseases. *Indian J Ophthalmol*. 2009;57(5):381–384. https://doi.org/10.4103/0301-4738. 55078.
3. Mines MJ, Bower KS, Lappan CM, Mazzoli RA, Poropatich RK. The United States Army Ocular Teleconsultation program 2004 through 2009. *Am J Ophthalmol*. 2011;152(1):126–132.e2. https://doi.org/10.1016/j.ajo.2011.01.028.
4. Liu Y, Ruan MZC, Haq Z, Hwang DG. Eyecare provider attitudes toward and adoption of telehealth during the COVID-19 pandemic. *J Cataract Refract Surg*. 2021;47(4):549–551. https://doi.org/10.1097/j.jcrs.0000000000000398.
5. Assayag E, Tsessler M, Wasser LM, et al. Telemedicine comes of age during coronavirus disease 2019 (COVID-19): an international survey of oculoplastic surgeons. *Eur J Ophthalmol*. 2020. https://doi.org/10.1177/1120672120965471. Published online October 17. 1120672120965471.
6. Nguyen AX, Gervasio KA, Wu AY. COVID-19 recommendations from ophthalmic and plastic reconstructive surgery societies worldwide. *Ophthal Plast Reconstr Surg*. 2020;36(4):334–345. https://doi.org/10.1097/IOP.0000000000001776.
7. Langer PD, Bernardini FP. Oculofacial plastic surgery and the COVID-19 pandemic: current reactions and implications for the future. *Ophthalmology*. 2020;127(9):e70–e71. https://doi.org/10.1016/j.ophtha.2020.04.035.
8. Patel S, Hamdan S, Donahue S. Optimising telemedicine in ophthalmology during the COVID-19

pandemic. *J Telemed Telecare.* 2020. https://doi.org/10.1177/1357633X20949796. Published online August 16. 1357633X20949796.

9. Jamison A, Diaper C, Drummond S, et al. Telemedicine in oculoplastics: the real-life application of video consultation clinics. *Ophthalmic Plast Reconstr Surg.* 2021;37(3S):S104–S108. https://doi.org/10.1097/IOP.0000000000001852.

10. Kang S, Thomas PBM, Sim DA, Parker RT, Daniel C, Uddin JM. Oculoplastic video-based telemedicine consultations: Covid-19 and beyond. *Eye.* 2020;34:1–3. https://doi.org/10.1038/s41433-020-0953-6. Published online May 12.

11. Hwang CJ, Eftekhari K, Schwarcz RM, Massry GG. The aesthetic oculoplastic surgery video teleconference consult. *Aesthet Surg J.* 2019;39(7):714–718. https://doi.org/10.1093/asj/sjz058.

12. Li B, Powell A-M, Hooper PL, Sheidow TG. Prospective evaluation of teleophthalmology in screening and recurrence monitoring of neovascular age-related macular degeneration: a randomized clinical trial. *JAMA Ophthalmol.* 2015;

133(3):276–282. https://doi.org/10.1001/jamaophthalmol.2014.5014.

13. Sink J, Blatt S, Yoo D, et al. A novel telemedicine technique for evaluation of ocular exam findings via smartphone images. *J Telemed Telecare.* 2020. https://doi.org/10.1177/1357633X20926819. Published online June 6. 1357633X20926819.

14. Markun S, Scherz N, Rosemann T, Tandjung R, Braun RP. Mobile teledermatology for skin cancer screening: a diagnostic accuracy study. *Medicine (Baltimore).* 2017;96(10). https://doi.org/10.1097/MD.0000000000006278, e6278.

15. Souverein EA, Kim JW, Loudin NN, et al. Feasibility of asynchronous video-based telemedicine in the diagnosis and management of paediatric blepharoptosis. *J Telemed Telecare.* 2021. https://doi.org/10.1177/1357633X20985394. Published online January 20. 1357633X20985394.

16. U.S. National Library of Medicine: ClinicalTrials.gov. *Telemedicine Follow-Up for Routine, Low-Risk Oculoplastic Surgery.* ClinicalTrials.gov Identifier: NCT04235803. Available at: https://clinicaltrials.gov/ct2/show/NCT04235803.

CHAPTER 4

Cornea, Anterior Segment, and External Disease Telehealth

XIAOQIN ALEXA LU, MD

INTRODUCTION

Ocular telehealth for cornea and external diseases is in its infancy, especially when compared to other more established ocular telehealth programs, such as diabetic retinopathy screening. The goals of using telemedicine for cornea and external disease are to (1) safely and accurately detect or follow anterior segment (AS) diseases; (2) determine the urgency of the condition, and (3) commence initial treatment and provide appropriate referral. One of the main reasons AS disease telehealth is challenging is because accurate diagnosis and subsequent management often require slit lamp biomicroscopy. The slit lamp provides advanced magnification and stereopsis necessary to properly visualize the detail and depth of AS structures. Unfortunately, despite the importance of the slit lamp exam, the use of a slit lamp routinely in AS telehealth (even to take still images) is limited by the cost of the equipment and operator availability. A slit lamp, especially those capable of transmitting video and photos, can be twice the cost of a nonmydriatic fundus camera. In addition, in order to operate a slit lamp competently, it takes an experienced telehealth facilitator. All these conditions pose limitations on remote ocular telehealth visits for AS diseases.

Despite these challenges, a significant amount of innovation is occurring in this eye subspecialty area. Ongoing research is specifically advancing anterior segment technology; developing more portable and easier-to-use equipment that may eventually be able to substitute for an in-person slit lamp exam. Furthermore, there is continued interest to develop cornea and external disease telehealth programs, especially because AS diseases are the most common complaints presenting to primary care, urgent care, and emergency room settings—ideal locations for ocular telehealth because an eye provider is unlikely to be physically present.

This chapter will begin by discussing slit lamp vs external photography imaging modalities, and equipment used to take these photographs. Then, each anterior segment structure and telehealth use cases in the literature are reviewed, and finally, future directions of AS telehealth are highlighted.

Ocular Telehealth. https://doi.org/10.1016/B978-0-323-83204-5.00004-4

SECTION I: INITIAL ANTERIOR SEGMENT TELEHEALTH ASSESSMENT

Most ocular complaints presenting to primary care offices and emergency departments are caused by AS diseases. They could range from the relatively benign, such as dry eye syndrome, to much more serious conditions like corneal ulcers.[1] A significant number of AS diseases could cause permanent morbidity if not detected accurately and treated appropriately. Since the initial presenting locations are often remote from an eye care provider, being able to use a telehealth modality of care to bring the remote eye provider's expertise directly to the patient is incredibly appealing.

During the COVID-19 pandemic, telehealth visits were encouraged since social distancing and reduced in-person care were desired. For AS ocular telehealth, while a slit lamp exam is often necessary, the first step of an AS ocular telehealth triage visit might not require slit lamp images or video. A study by Woodward et al. used an anterior segment questionnaire to determine the urgency of the patient's complaint and to determine the need for an in-person visit (Fig. 4.1). The questionnaire used the symptoms of pain, burning, itching, grittiness, redness, glare, light sensitivity, blurry vision, and headaches. The questionnaire showed that certain symptoms: eye pain, glare, redness, and blurry vision, showed a high sensitivity to detect AS diseases (83%) and urgent AS diseases (92%).[2] This could be a helpful initial tool to screen a patient to determine whether an in-person versus a clinic-based telehealth encounter should be the patient's next visit. This questionnaire could also be administered to a patient during a home-based telehealth visit conducted either by telephone or by synchronous video. If the remote eye provider used a synchronous video it would provide the additional benefit to the eye provider who can actually visualize the patient's eyes, albeit via 2D video.

SECTION II: ANTERIOR SEGMENT IMAGING AND EXAMINATION MODALITIES

If the patient goes to a clinic for clinic-based telehealth, then a telehealth presenter has the opportunity to take images and videos of the anterior segment during a synchronous, asynchronous, or hybrid telehealth visit. Many modalities of AS imaging for telehealth visits have been studied in recent years. Most of these can be organized into two main groups: images obtained through a slit lamp, and images obtained without a slit lamp (external photograph). There are varying pros and cons for each type of imaging modality for anterior segment telehealth. When comparing slit lamp images to external photographs, the pros of taking slit lamp images are that images are usually higher quality with better magnification and lighting. However, one drawback for slit lamp based images is that few primary care facilities or emergency rooms have this expensive equipment and, perhaps more important, often lack trained operators. On the other hand, one pro of taking an external photo (images obtained without a slit lamp) is that these external photos are much easier to capture and require less training. They can even be taken by the patient him/herself and be transmitted electronically to the provider. Unfortunately, cons to external photographs include the lower quality of these images, lack of magnification, and lack of detail, all factors that may limit the ability to adequately diagnose certain AS conditions. In addition, external photographs are missing the slit beam which can provide helpful stereoscopic cues.[3]

The remainder of this section will focus on the technology used to take slit lamp images or video and then transition to discussing equipment available to take external photographs and the literature supporting accuracy of diagnoses with these external images. Chapter 13 also discusses slit lamp and anterior segment technology in greater detail.

Slit Lamp Photography With Smartphone Cameras

In the last few decades, smartphone technology has spread globally. In some countries, internet and telephone access are nearly ubiquitous; easier to obtain than other resources. The International Telecommunication Union reported that 95.5% of the world's population were mobile subscribers in 2014.[4] In low and middle-income countries, there was an estimate that there is greater than one electronic device with internet connection per person in 2013.[5] Smartphones can capture slit lamp images by two methods: freehand—the individual holds the smartphone camera up to the slit lamp ocular,- or second, assisted, mounting the smartphone to the slit lamp with an adapter. A few studies have compared different adapters for their ease of use and image quality.[6] Surprisingly, one study found a smartphone (iPhone 6) attached to a slit lamp with an adapter produced poorer quality photos than freehand. However, this study was based on subjective grading by the readers on the acceptability of image quality for evaluating the anterior segment structures and reader confidence in clinically managing post-operative patients, not for AS disease detection.[7] Other studies will be discussed in later sections of this chapter.

KELLOGG EYE CENTER
for eHEALTH
UNIVERSITY OF MICHIGAN
HEALTH SYSTEM

EYE PROBLEMS

Please answer the following questions for the **RIGHT EYE and LEFT EYE**. Answer the questions thinking of your vision as it is when corrected by any glasses or contact lenses that you usually use.

1. **In the last 7 days**, how much <u>pain or discomfort</u> have you had in & around your eye (ex: burning, itching, or aching)?

LEFT EYE	**RIGHT EYE**
o None	o None
o Mild	o Mild
o Moderate	o Moderate
o Severe	o Severe
o Very severe	o Very severe

1a. If you answered **yes** in Question 1, <u>how often</u> did you have the pain/discomfort?

LEFT EYE	**RIGHT EYE**
o Not Applicable	o Not Applicable
o Rarely	o Rarely
o Sometimes	o Sometimes
o Always	o Always

2. In the last 7 days, how much of a problem did you have with a <u>burning or stinging</u> eye?

LEFT EYE	**RIGHT EYE**
o No problem at all	o No problem at all
o A little bit of a problem	o A little bit of a problem
o Somewhat of a problem	o Somewhat of a problem
o Very much of a problem	o Very much of a problem

3. In the last 7 days, how much of a problem did you have with <u>itching</u> in or around your eye?

LEFT EYE	**RIGHT EYE**
o No problem at all	o No problem at all
o A little bit of a problem	o A little bit of a problem
o Somewhat of a problem	o Somewhat of a problem
o Very much of a problem	o Very much of a problem

FIG. 4.1 Anterior segment triage questionnaire. (Credit: used with permission from Kellogg Eye Center, Maria Woodward, MD.)

Slit Lamp Images With Portable Digital Cameras

Commercially available digital cameras can be used to capture slit lamp photographs with adapters. One study, published in 2018, found the quality of photographs was comparable between a cheaper portable compact camera attached to slit lamp versus a built-in slit lamp camera in viewing posterior capsule opacity. This study will be discussed more in the lens section.[8] One point of consideration with regard to slit lamp images is that the majority of transmitted slit lamp images are 2D, without the benefit of the reader seeing dynamic changes or stereopsis, which clearly differs from an in-person slit lamp examination. The use of the slit beam, ability to vary the focus depth, and videography can improve stereo cues for the reader, therefore, one innovation has been developed to recreate the slit lamp stereopsis by taking anterior segment photos using digital stereo-cameras. An abstract was presented during the 2020 Association for Research in Vision in

Ophthalmology (ARVO) meeting, which showcased a trial using a 3D stereoscopic digital camera (Fujifilm FinePix Real 3D W3 Digital Camera), with each camera aperture mounted to each slit lamp ocular with a universal adapter Snapzoom (http://snapzooms.com/). Binocular stereoscopic external, anterior segment and posterior segment 3D slit lamp videos were captured in all 13 eyes. Stereopsis effect was recreated with Google cardboard virtual reality viewer and in interlaced format viewed on FujiFilm FinePix Real 3D V1 Viewer (Fig. 4.2).

One drawback of this abstract was that the authors did not mention what type of pathology was examined.[9] It would be exciting to see further studies with a larger enrollment of patients, as 3D stereo photography or video would address the lack of stereopsis in 2D images. The practical use of this camera in ocular tele-

health might still be limited by the expertise to set up the 3D camera to the slit lamp and the remote eye provider owning a 3D viewer or a virtual reality headset.[3]

Remote-Controlled Slit Lamp Examination

Another innovation that allows for stereopsis and more closely approximates a true in-person slit lamp examination is the development of a remotely controlled slit lamp, which allows for a synchronous telehealth exam. This stereoscopic robotized drone slit lamp can be remotely controlled and allows the examiner to view the real-time images with a stereo viewer while simultaneously controlling the slit beam (intensity, height, width, and angle), biomicroscope motion, and image magnification. While using this slit lamp, the examiner and patient do not need to be in the same room. There is also audio communication capability

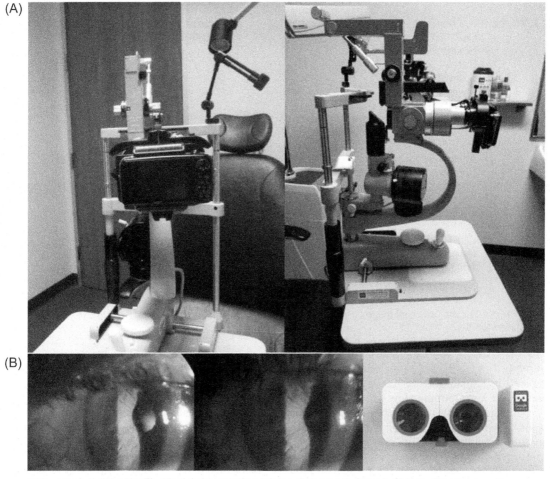

FIG. 4.2 A. Fujifilm FinePix 3D digital camera and Zeiss slit lamps B. Sample Side by Side Photo with Google Image Viewer. (Data from M. Ahmad et al.)

with the patient and other colleagues who can also co-control the drone slit lamp.[10] The study that validated the use of this slit lamp will be further discussed in the anterior chamber section. While the drone slit lamp is not currently available on the general market, the authors do have future plans to place them in remote Canadian clinic locations with limited access to ophthalmic care.[11]

External Photography With Smartphone Cameras

Given the near-ubiquitous nature of smartphones with high-resolution cameras built-in, there has been significant focus on using a smartphone to take external photographs as a substitute for a slit lamp photo or slit lamp exam. Smartphone AS telehealth is particularly appealing in countries where there are few eye care specialists and very limited access to care because of travel, cost, and distance. If smartphone cameras could be used to quickly and easily capture/ transmit images to remote specialists, it would immediately mean large-scale portability and flexibility in patient screening for cornea and external disease conditions.[12] Busy cornea subspecialists all over the world would then be able to screen more patients efficiently and provide more specialized care.[13] However, these images may not result in an accurate diagnosis of AS disease. The telehealth eye provider has to keep in mind the inadequacies of smartphone external photography. As mentioned earlier, aside from the lack of magnification and stereopsis, another limitation is the autofocus and color filters present on the smartphone camera. Images of the same eye, taken from different brands of smartphones, may display differently as a result of these focus and filter parameters.[3] In turn, this may affect diagnosis, especially if the area of concern has a particular color, or if color is important to diagnostic accuracy.

Earlier it was mentioned that one pro of external photographs is how easy it can be to take these photos, even by the patient him/herself. Patients often use their smartphones to take eye photographs to help the doctor visualize their areas of complaint. Studies have been done by the Kellogg Eye Center in Ann Arbor MI to help educate patients (and their family members) on how to capture adequate anterior segment pictures. The Kellogg Eye Center developed an easy-to-follow instruction sheet on eye photography with a smartphone for patients participating in telehealth visits. This tip sheet showed the patients how to get the best focus, lighting, and resolution to check for AS pathology (Fig. 4.3).

External Imaging With Smartphone Camera Attachments

In order to improve upon the external photos taken with smartphones, various attachments were made to improve visualization and magnification. These include clip-on macroscopic lenses and mounting devices for 20D lens on smartphones. Most of these attachments have not been individually validated by clinical trials. One study did compare one of the attachments, Easy Macro Lens (Sommerville, MA), a small $5 magnifying lens held within a rubber band that fits around an iPhone 5 (Apple, Cupertino, CA), to one without an attachment. Fifty-four patients had anterior segment imaging performed by using both apparatuses at the Floating Doctors' mobile clinic sites in Panama. Images were sent to California and graded by two board-certified ophthalmologists. Results showed the iPhone was significantly superior in imaging of the conjunctiva, whereas the Easy Macro Lens was superior in regards to the anterior chamber and iris.[14]

A study in Nepal compared anterior segment and fundus photos and videos taken using a smartphone-based ophthalmic camera system, the Paxos Scope (Verana Health, San Francisco, CA), to examination by trained technicians with direct ophthalmoscopy. The Paxos Scope is an inexpensive, portable, smartphone-based ophthalmic imaging adapter that enables any iPod or iPhone camera to produce high-quality magnified anterior and posterior segment photographs and videos. The results of the study showed the highest agreement for cataracts but a much lower agreement for posterior segment diseases.[15] This study's results will be discussed more in the lens section.

From a patient self-use perspective, the main limitation of cell phone attachments for AS telehealth is the lack of patient access. Patients are not likely to own an attachment to place on their phone correctly to take photos to send to their doctors. Some attachments also block the use of flash and autofocus on smartphone cameras. These attachments could be bought, however, for use by a telehealth presenter in an AS telehealth program, but again, providers have to understand the limitations and potential inaccuracy of external photographs to diagnose anterior segment disease (see Chapter 17, Ocular Triage, for more details).

External Photography With Digital Cameras

Commercially available anterior segment cameras and digital cameras, including single-lens reflex (SLR) cameras and the point-and-shoot compact cameras, have been used in ophthalmology to record clinical findings, and are mostly used with asynchronous ocular

- If possible, ask someone else to take the photo for you.
- Use a timer on the camera if you are alone.
- Hold the camera in a position where it's not casting a shadow on the face.
- Keep the camera as still as possible – use your elbows as a tripod or use a tripod!
- Keep the patient's head very still, maybe even with head in hands to keep stable.
- Use "burst mode" on the camera to take as many pictures as possible. Send as many as you think may help!
- Point the lens at the area of interest and get as close as the camera will allow while maintaining focus.
- Try to have your eye facing a strong, but not direct, light source. You are trying to get catch-light reflections in the patient's eyes (*arrows show the catch-light below*).
    - During the day, go outside and sit at the edge of the shaded area.
    - If inside, sit facing a sunny, but shaded window (aka looking out the window with the light coming into your eye). You can sit at an angle so the sun shines in your eye as much as possible for the person taking the photo. (*see angles below*).

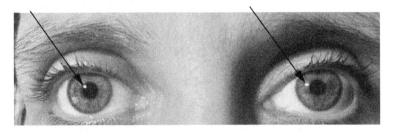

- Avoid taking the photo in direct sunlight.
- Add extra light if possible, for example, tape a white piece of paper on in front of the flashlight on your phone, and then point it towards the eye.
- If you can adjust the resolution of the photo, set it on high.

GREAT EXAMPLES

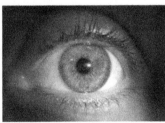 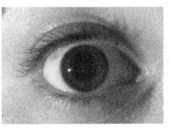 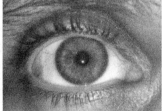

| Great photo of eye taken with iPhone while the flashlight is illuminating the eye | Can see the catch-light reflection | Great photo of eye taken with iPhone with the flash on |

NOT-SO-GREAT EXAMPLES

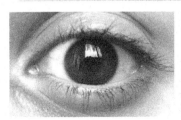 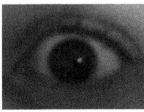 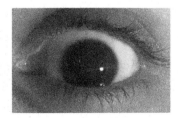

| Too much glare | Too dark, cannot see detail of eyeball | Out of focus- eyelashes are in focus but eyeball is not |

FIG. 4.3 Smartphone eye photography tip sheet. (Credit: used with permission from Kellogg Eye Center, Maria Woodward, MD.)

telehealth care. Recent studies have compared external AS photographs taken with SLR cameras versus photographs taken with smartphones.[16–18] These study results will be discussed in later sections of this chapter. Images from portable digital cameras were also compared to the gold standard slit lamp examination. At the Wills Eye Emergency Room, 76 eyes from 38 patients were photographed bilaterally for AS and nonmydriatic fundus photography with the portable Volk Pictor (Volk Optical Inc., Mentor, OH). The images were transmitted to 3 masked graders. The gold standard was slit lamp and binocular indirect ophthalmoscopic examination. The sensitivity rates of camera images were higher for posterior segment photos (96%) than AS photos (89%). Detection of all critical anterior segment findings demonstrated greater than 80% agreement with slit lamp examination, except for superficial punctate keratitis (68%) and cataract (59%).[19] This camera was likely limited by lack of high magnification to visualize the finer details on the surface of the cornea and lack of depth of focus to assess lenticular opacity. This portable camera is also relatively expensive ($6000 at the time of publication). The inherent high cost of digital cameras and the need for trained photography may limit their general use in ocular telehealth.[3]

Future Anterior Segment Imaging Technology

Many new technologies are being invented to address the constraints of the current modalities. However, these devices have not yet been validated with clinical trials. One example is the "eyeSmart Cyclops" for the iBall Slide Tablet, which allows the tablet to be connected to the slit lamp for slit lamp photographs and real-time video of the slit lamp exam.[20]

The Anterior View Attachment for the Horus Scope from JedMed is another technology currently available for anterior segment telehealth. This attachment plugs into a telehealth cart and allows for both synchronous and asynchronous telehealth. The device can capture both external photographs and slit lamp photos and videos. There are different settings for focal range, magnification, and the illumination can be used as a slit beam. The images and videos could be sent to a remote viewer for assessment. To this author's knowledge, the JedMed equipment also has not been officially studied for accuracy compared to an in-person slit lamp exam in the literature. Further studies are needed to validate these new technologies and compare them to the gold standard in-person slit lamp examination. Refer to Chapter 13 for additional information about anterior segment technology.

SECTION III: ANTERIOR SEGMENT STRUCTURES

The British Diabetic Association determined that any telehealth modality needed to be at least 80% sensitive in identifying diagnoses to be considered comparable to in-person eye care.[21] Therefore, 80% sensitivity is widely accepted as the "clinically safe" threshold utilized when interpreting the results of literature on new technology or novel telehealth programs. The gold standard for AS disease detection should be a slit lamp examination with an eye doctor. The rest of this chapter will discuss the latest studies using different telehealth modalities on parts of the AS not covered by other chapters in this book: conjunctiva, cornea, iris, anterior chamber, and lens.

Conjunctiva

Ocular telehealth has been used to detect and follow conjunctival diseases. Studies utilize either slit lamp photos or external photographs, though the majority are found to use external photographs taken with different camera types. In 1999, Threlkeld et al compared a synchronous, remote slit lamp video transmission with an in-person eye clinic examination. The slit lamp video examination was conducted by a telehealth facilitator a noneye provider. The video was then transmitted in real-time as a monocular view to a remote ophthalmologist reader for diagnosis. There was good sensitivity in detecting conjunctival pigmentation (100%); less sensitive in detecting pinguecula (70%); and poor sensitivity in detecting conjunctival follicles and papillae (0%).[22] In 2012, Bhosai et al investigated the use of external photographs, using the iPhone 4 compared to the more expensive and more complicated single-lens reflex (SLR) camera, for trachoma surveillance in Niger. The gold standard of clinical examination was performed by a certified examiner with 2.5× magnifying loupe and a flashlight. They found moderate reliability, but not always high accuracy when using iPhone 4 technology (sensitivity of 41%) when compared to SLR photographs (sensitivity of 88%) for monitoring clinically active trachoma.[17] Another study in 2017 by Woodward et al. showed that conjunctival lesions can be seen with increased ease with improved technology. A corneal specialist provided the gold standard diagnosis of the patient by slit lamp examination. External images of both eyes of the patient were obtained using two different types of cameras (an iTouch 5S, similar to a smartphone, and NidekVersaCam camera, an SLR camera) in multiple gazes and interpreted by three cornea specialists for the presence of AS pathology. They found that the diagnosis of pterygium using both cameras had high sensitivity (average sensitivity: iTouch 93% and Nidek 96%).[18] Nesemann et al. published a study in 2020 with the gold standard of in-person conjunctival examination of 412 children. External conjunctival photographs were taken with SLR camera and a smartphone coupled to a 3D-printed magnifying attachment. Three masked graders assessed the conjunctival photographs for inflammatory follicles in trachoma. SLR photo-grading was 95.0% sensitive and 93.6% specific, and smartphone photo-grading was 84.1% sensitive and 97.6% specific.[16] As the technology improves, some conjunctival lesions and disease findings seem adequately diagnosed by external photographs captured by SLR and smartphone cameras. SLR cameras operated by a trained photographer appear to have higher sensitivity in AS disease detection than smartphones.

Cornea

The cornea, with its transparent nature, small size, and 3D shape, is difficult to fully inspect without a slit lamp. An early study in 1999 by Kumar et al. showed digital camera external photographs had sensitivities ranging from 0% to 88% in detecting cornea diseases. The most sensitive was corneal graft (88%); the least sensitive were epithelial defect (0%), epitheliopathy (0%), keratic precipitate (0%), and cornea bullae (0%).[23] Even with improvement in camera technology and lighting, corneal diseases could be challenging to diagnose with external 2D images. The previously mentioned Woodward et al. study showed that the cornea was difficult to examine with external photography. Between the three readers, the sensitivity of diagnosing corneal scar was 29%–57%; and corneal abrasion 70%–92%. With both cameras (iTouch and Nidek), the sensitivity of diagnosing a cornea ulcer was 82.4%–94.1%. This was more reassuring as a cornea ulcer is a more urgent condition.[18] Interestingly, the quality of photographs did not improve the diagnosis sensitivity. Even though the photos were graded as lower quality on the iTouch device, the sensitivity to detect corneal issues did not increase significantly with the quality of photos on the Nidek camera. The overall sensitivity to detect any AS pathology ranged from 54% to 71% for iTouch and 66% to 75% for Nidek; specificity ranged from 82% to 96% for iTouch and 91% to 98% for Nidek. Neither portable camera met the suggested standard of 80% sensitivity established by the diabetic tele-retina studies for any AS diagnosis. This study cautioned eye care professionals that these cameras were not sensitive enough to pick up most corneal diseases, as many doctors received curbside or real consults with light diffused photos.[24]

Since the accuracy of AS disease imaging is variable, other literature has illustrated ways to improve the sensitivity of corneal disease detection. In 2014, Maamari et al. compared corneal external photographs taken with an iPhone 4S with +25D lens and white LED light; then the same iPhone with +25D lens and blue LED after staining with fluorescein. When the white-light and fluorescein photographs were assessed as a pair, the sensitivity of photographic diagnosis of an epithelial defect improved from 83% to 88.9%. However, the specificity decreased from 97% to 90.9%.[25] This study is more applicable in situations where the photographs are taken by a trained screener with access to fluorescein and iPhone attachments.

In 2017, another study by Woodward et al. evaluated patients in an ophthalmic consultation service examined by ophthalmologists and external photographs taken with portable cameras. The accuracy of diagnoses made based only on external photographs was compared to the diagnoses made based on the same photographs with the addition of visual acuity, a short summary of demographics (age, race, gender), and chief complaint. Graders detected AS pathology with 62%–81% sensitivity based only on photographs. The sensitivity increased to 87%–88% sensitivity based on photographs plus brief chief complaints and history. The conclusion was a reminder that ophthalmologists could detect ocular pathology on photographs more accurately if they were provided with relevant clinical information.[12]

Given the high variability in sensitivity and accuracy of detecting corneal disease with external photographs, the logical next step in AS telehealth for the cornea is to mimic slit lamp biomicroscopy with portable devices operated by a trained telehealth facilitator.[22,26,27] The previously mentioned study by Threlkeld, et al. showed that the sensitivity of a synchronous slit lamp video is only 56% for detecting corneal scars, and 0% for keratitis, compared to an in-person slit lamp examination.[22] However, this study was done in 1999 and the video was transmitted as a monocular view to the reader. Therefore, the technology limitations at that time could explain the results. Further validation of current slit-lamp–based technologies, like the 3D slit lamp camera, remotely controlled drone slit lamp, and portable slit lamp video camera on cornea clinical findings are needed.

In summary, the results of the above studies demonstrate that current technology might not be sufficiently sensitive in diagnosing corneal diseases. This is especially true during home-based telehealth visits where the portable camera is operated by a nonprofessional with inadequate lighting and poor magnification. The results did show that portable camera images might have high specificity to screen patients. By adding a chief complaint, brief history, visual acuity, along with fluorescein stained external photographs, increased magnification with an attachment, the sensitivity of detection could be improved. However, in order to add these elements, there would need to be trained personnel who could take the history and operate the camera.

Anterior Chamber

Any examination of a patient with a red eye or a painful eye is incomplete without evaluating the anterior chamber, which is very difficult to photograph or video. It is a normally clear, fluid-filled space that is located between two other optically clear structures: the cornea and the lens. High magnification and depth of focus are very important and necessitate the use of a slit lamp. The study in Panama, which compared external photographs taken by an iPhone 5 and the same phone with the Easy Macro Lens attachment, showed that the Easy Macro Lens captured better images of the anterior chamber and iris. The study did not mention the anterior chamber findings that were detected. The group also acknowledged that one of the study limitations is the lack of a slit lamp examination as the gold standard.[14] Recently, Luna et al. showed that a mechanized remotely operated stereoscopic drone slit lamp could assess the anterior chamber in post-operative patients and patients with uveitis, comparable to conventional slit lamp. Two remote ophthalmologists examined 48 eyes of 42 participants for anterior chamber depth and presence or absence of cells and flare using the drone slit lamp, then followed by conventional slit lamp. There were no significant inter-examiner differences in AC depth or cell detection. There was a substantial agreement when assessing AC cell and flare and moderate agreement when assessing AC depth. The drone slit lamp compared with conventional slit lamp had 98.3% sensitivity and 100% specificity for detecting AC cells; and 100% sensitivity and 88.2% specificity for detecting AC flare.[11] This device seems to be excellent in assessing a difficult part of AS anatomy using synchronous ocular telehealth. The implementation cost and availability were not mentioned in the study. Both of these factors can influence how these slit lamps will be used in the future.

Iris

Several studies have test different modalities of ocular telehealth to monitor iris conditions. In 1999, Threlkeld et al. showed good sensitivity in using synchronous slit lamp video transmission, in the detection of posterior synechiae (100%) and iridotomy (83%); less sensitivity with regard to an iris lesion (75%).[22] In 2018, Lapere et al. showed that with AS external photography, they were able to reliably detect growth in patients with iris nevi. The sensitivity was 100% with a specificity of 92% in all of the patients. These studies support the use of both slit lamp and external photography to accurately examine and monitor iris conditions using telemedicine.[28]

Lens

The final area of focus in this chapter is on cataracts, which is the most common cause of reversible blindness. According to the World Health Organization Report in 2000, cataracts caused 50% of the decreased vision worldwide.[29] Numerous studies and techniques were developed to detect visually significant cataracts through portable cameras. Most of these programs utilize 2D external photos and rely upon indirect methods of detection, such as the red reflex and/or vision. Two studies both reported higher sensitivity picking up cortical opacity compared to nuclear sclerosis.[22,23] This is not surprising as cortical opacity causes a more obvious obscuration of the red reflex. One of the most established studies was the Portable Eye Examination Kit (PEEK), developed and validated in a cohort study in Kenya.[30] Bastawrous et al. claimed that a photo taken on a smartphone with the PEEK app in a dark room in natural mydriasis was similar to using the direct ophthalmoscope. A remote eye care reader could examine the pictures of the red reflex and determine if there was any significant opacity in the optical pathway and the severity of the cataract. This information, along with the visual acuity could lead to a referral for an in-person exam. This technique was also utilized in neonates, infants, and children.[31,32] In a paper published in 2013, congenital cataract causes blindness in approximately 1.4 million children under age 15. Early detection and treatment could prevent blindness in half of these cases.[33]

In 2020, Coller et al. compared smartphone external photography and videography with Paxos Scope attachment to examination by a trained technician with a direct ophthalmoscope. About 140 patients over 18 years of age presenting to remote screening camps in Nepal with best-corrected visual acuity ≤ 20/60 in one or both eyes were enrolled. After an in-person examination with a technician with a direct ophthalmoscope, the patients had photos and videos taken with the Paxos Scope attachment. These were examined and diagnosed by remote ophthalmologists. The results showed that diagnosis agreement was highest for cataract and recommendation for cataract extraction.[15] A major limitation of this study was that the gold standard was not a slit lamp examination. In addition, the Paxos Scope is not available for sale.

In established ocular telehealth programs, such as Technology-based Eye Care Services (TECS), the external images are taken with nonmydriatic fundus camera by a skilled technician at a remote site, and then viewed by an ophthalmologist or optometrist reader asynchronously. In 2020, Maa et al. found that there was substantial agreement in cataract diagnosis between two remote TECS readers and the gold standard of in-person slit lamp exam.[34]

Another study investigated the use of telehealth for posterior capsule opacification (PCO). Oliphant et al. compared a commercially available slit lamp camera (Haag Streit, Germany) and a digital compact camera (Nikon Coolpix, Nikon, Japan), which was mounted on a regular clinic slit lamp (Haag Streit, Germany) using an adaptor, KJ-A1 Nikon Camera Adaptor (Suzhou Kangjie Medical Inc., Jiangsu, China). The patients were examined in-person and referred for YAG laser capsulotomy. Out of these patients, 72 patients were recruited. A trained technician took retro illumination slit lamp photos of the PCO. Two ophthalmologists then independently graded the PCO. The results showed there was no significant difference between mean scores when comparing slit lamp cameras vs portable digital cameras mounted on slit lamps.[8]

In summary, external photographs with smartphones have already been used internationally to detect visually significant cataracts in patients. The sensitivities can be improved by adding a measurement of vision. Sensitivity is also improved with smartphone attachments which can further visualize the red reflex. In circumstances where the equipment is available, anterior segment cameras and slit lamp mounted cameras can assess the lens under higher magnification.

FUTURE DIRECTIONS OF ANTERIOR SEGMENT TELEHEALTH

While at this time there are limited telehealth programs dedicated to the anterior segment, the future of AS telehealth looks very promising. Multiple studies suggest that the use of external photography, taken either with smartphones or digital cameras, can be used to detect and monitor conditions of the conjunctivae, cornea, iris, and lens.[12, 14–18] Slit lamp photos and videos, taken with a slit lamp camera or with a camera mounted to the slit lamp, are best for cornea and anterior chamber diseases.[11, 22, 26, 27] However, multiple areas in the technology need improvement, including increased portability, better stereopsis, and more magnification, before anterior segment telemedicine programs go into widespread use.

Current smartphone cameras are not designed to fully capture clear images of all anterior ocular structures needed to detect AS diseases with high sensitivity and accuracy. With future generations of smartphones, the cameras could further improve. Moreover, as technology advances, patient-owned electronic devices will have better cameras and become more affordable. This would potentially enable patients themselves to acquire better photographs of their eyes to send to their doctors in asynchronous visits. In developing countries, better technology would mean an inexpensive and easier way to screen patients for vision-threatening AS diseases.

Other avenues of improvement would be more studies to validate slit lamp videography and development of other devices that more closely mimic slit lamp biomicroscopy. More research is needed to validate anterior segment telehealth protocols with the gold standard in-person slit lamp examination. Nevertheless, with these upcoming future advancements, anterior segment ocular telehealth could deliver expert cornea subspecialty eye care to millions of patients in need, while saving valuable travel costs and time.

REFERENCES

1. Channa R, Zafar SN, Canner JK, Haring RS, Schneider EB, Friedman DS. Epidemiology of eye-related emergency department visits. *JAMA Ophthalmol.* 2016;134(3):312–319.
2. Woodward MA, Valikodath NG, Newman-Casey PA, Niziol LM, Musch DC, Lee PP. Eye symptom questionnaire to evaluate anterior eye health. *Eye Contact Lens.* 2018;44(6):384–389.
3. Armstrong GW, Kalra G, De Assirgunaga S, Friedman DS, Lorch AC. Anterior segment imaging devices in ophthalmic telemedicine. *Semin Ophthalmol.* 2021;36:149–156. Published online 3/3/2021.
4. Union IT. *ICT Facts and Figures; The World in 2014.* International Telecommunication Union Geneva, Switzerland; 2014.
5. Bastawrous A, Hennig BD, Livingstone IA. mHealth possibilities in a changing world. Distribution of global cell phone subscriptions. *J Mob Technol Med.* 2013;2:22–25.
6. Hudson A. Assessment of the usability of slit lamp adapters in conjunction with smartphones to capture anterior segment images. *Invest Ophthalmol Vis Sci.* 2017;58:4839.
7. Sanguansak T, Morley K, Morley M, et al. Comparing smartphone camera adapters in imaging post-operative cataract patients. *J Telemed Telecare.* 2017;23(1):36–43.

8. Oliphant H, Kennedy A, Camyn O, Spalton DJ, Nanavaty MA. Commercial slit lamp ANTERIOR segment photography versus digital compact camera mounted on a standard slit lamp with an adapter. *Curr Eye Res.* 2018;43(10):1290–1294.

9. Ahmad M, Solyman O, Arora K, Henderson AD. Stereoscopic three-dimensional (3D) slit lamp photography and videography using compact 3D digital camera. *Invest Ophthalmol Vis Sci.* 2020;61:499.

10. Nankivil D, Gonzalez A, Rowaan C, Lee W, Aguilar MC, Parel J. Robotic remote controlled stereo slit lamp. *Trans Vis Sci Tech.* 2018;7(4):1.

11. Luna GL, Parel J-M, Gonzalez A, et al. Validating the use of a stereoscopic robotized teleophthalmic drone slit lamp. *Can J Ophthalmol.* 2021;56:191–196.

12. Woodward MA, Bavinger JC, Amin S, et al. Telemedicine for ophthalmic consultation services: use of a portable device and layering information for graders. *J Telemed Telecare.* 2017;23(2):365–370.

13. Bastawrous A. Increasing access to eye care.. there's an app for that. Peek: smartphone technology for eye health. *Int J Epidemiol.* 2016;45(4):1040–1043.

14. Bhatter P, Cao L, Crochetiere A. Using a macro lens for anterior segment imaging in rural panama. *Telemed J E Health.* 2020;26(11):1414–1418.

15. Collon S, Chang D, Tabin G, Hong K, Myung D. Utility and feasibility of teleophthalmology using a smartphone-based ophthalmic camera in screening camps in Nepal. *Asia Pac J Ophthalmol.* 2020;9(1):54–58.

16. Nesemann JM, Seider MI, Snyder BM. Comparison of smartphone photography, single-lens reflex photography, and field-grading for trachoma. *Am J Trop Med Hyg.* 2020;103(6):2488–2491.

17. Bhosai SJ, Amza A, Beido N, et al. Application of smartphone cameras for detecting clinically active trachoma. *Br J Ophthalmol.* 2012;96(10):1350–1351.

18. Woodward MA, Musch DC, Hood CT, et al. Teleophthalmic approach for detection of corneal diseases: accuracy and reliability. *Cornea.* 2017;36(10):1159–1165.

19. Sieber M, Shahlaee A, Adam MK, Cohen M, Federman JL. Quality and utility of a portable anterior segment and non-mydriatic fundus camera linked to a smartphone-based virual consultation platform. *Invest Ophthalmol Vis Sci.* 2017;58:4840.

20. Loomba A, Vempati S, Davara N, et al. Use of a tablet attachment in teleophthalmology for real-time video transmission from rural vision centers in three-tier eye care network in India: eyeSmart Cyclops. *Int J Telemed Appl.* 2019;2019:1–9.

21. British Diabetic Association. *Retinal Photography Screening for Diabetic Eye Disease.* London: British Diabetic Association; 1997.

22. Threlkeld AB, Fahd T, Camp M, Johnson MH. Telemedical evaluation of ocular adnexa and anterior segment. *Am J Ophthalmol.* 1999;127:464–466.

23. Kumar S, Yogesan K, Constable IJ. Telemedical diagnosis of anterior segment eye diseases: validation of digital slit-lamp still images. *Eye.* 2009;23:652–660.

24. Woodward MA, Ple-Plakon P, Blachley T, et al. Eye care providers' attitudes towards tele-ophthalmology. *Telemed J E Health.* 2015;21:271–273.

25. Maamari RN, Ausayakhun S, Margolis TP, Fletcher DA, Keenan JD. Novel telemedicine device for diagnosis of corneal abrasions and ulcers in resource-poor settings. *JAMA Ophthalmol.* 2014;132(7):894–895.

26. Shimmura S, Shinozaki N, Fukagawa K, Shimazaki J, Tsubota K. Real-time telemedicine in the clinical assessment of the ocular surface. *Am J Ophthalmol.* 1998;125:388–390.

27. Barsam A, Bhogal M, Morris S, et al. Anterior segment slitlamp photography using the iPhone. *J Cataract Refract Surg.* 2001;36:1240–1241.

28. Lapere S, Weis E. Tele-ophthalmology for the monitoring of choroidal and iris nevi: a pilot study. *Can J Ophthalmol.* 2018;53(5):471–473.

29. World Health Organization. Prevention of blindness and deafness. In: *Global Initiative for the Eleimatino of Avoidable Blindness.* Geneva: WHO; 2000.

30. Bastawrous A, Mathenge W, Peto T. The Nakuru eye disease conhort study: methodology and rationale. *BMC Ophthalmol.* 2014;14:60.

31. Litmanovitz I, Dolfin T. Red reflex examination in neonates: the need for early screeening. *Isr Med Assoc J.* 2010;12(5):301–302.

32. American Academy of Paediatrics. Red reflex examination in neonates, infants, and children. *Pediatrics.* 2008;122(6):1401–1404.

33. World Health Organization. *Universal Eye Health: A Global Action Plan 2014–2019.* Geneva: World Health Organization; 2013.

34. Maa AY, Medert CM, Lu X, et al. Diagnostic accuracy of technology-based eye care services: the technology-based eye care services compare trial part I. *Ophthalmology.* 2020;127(1):38–44.

CHAPTER 5

Glaucoma Telehealth

ANNETTE L. GIANGIACOMO, MD • YAO LIU, MD, MS

INTRODUCTION

Background on Glaucoma and the Need to Expand Access to Care

Prevalence

Glaucoma is the leading cause of irreversible blindness worldwide and it is estimated that at least half of patients with this disease are unaware that they have it.[1] In addition, there are significant disparities in the distribution of ophthalmologists throughout the world. Two-thirds of the worlds' ophthalmologists reside in <10% of all countries, leaving many regions with a significant shortage of ophthalmologists per capita.[2] In the United States, 2.7 million individuals over 40 years of age have glaucoma[3] and it is predicted that the supply of ophthalmologists will not keep pace with the demand for glaucoma care in the aging population.[4] Thus, there is an urgent need to identify strategies to increase access to detecting, diagnosing, and managing patients with glaucoma.

Telehealth for glaucoma

Given glaucoma's relatively asymptomatic nature, it is typically first identified on a screening eye exam. Important exam findings include elevated intraocular pressure (IOP), increased cup-to-disc ratio, optic nerve rim thinning, abnormal retinal nerve fiber layer thickness, and visual field defects. Since all of this information can be measured and transmitted using telecommunications technology, glaucoma is amenable to several telehealth models which this chapter will collectively refer to as "tele-glaucoma."

Improved access to care and cost-effectiveness of tele-glaucoma

Tele-glaucoma can improve access to care in underserved rural and urban communities. In both settings, tele-glaucoma can also reduce travel times and increase patient convenience. In addition, tele-glaucoma can reduce wait times for appointments due to the shortage of eye care providers and provide care at a lower cost.[5,6] In a study from Canada, "access time" was defined as the amount of time between glaucoma referral and evaluation. "Cycle time" was defined as the amount of time between check-in and departure on the day of evaluation. Compared to in-person evaluation, access and cycle times were both significantly shorter for the tele-glaucoma visits (45 vs 88 days, and 78 vs 115 min, respectively).[7] In addition, the cost of a tele-glaucoma exam was $872 per patient or 80% of the cost of an in-person exam.[6] These reductions in travel time and costs are significant since

Ocular Telehealth. https://doi.org/10.1016/B978-0-323-83204-5.00005-6

glaucoma is a chronic disease that requires regular visits over a patient's lifetime. Furthermore, some patients may require family or friends to transport and accompany them to appointments so reductions in travel times substantially benefit those individuals as well. More research remains to be done to comprehensively evaluate impact on access to care and cost-effectiveness of various types of tele-glaucoma programs.

Validation of tele-glaucoma as a screening tool

Multiple studies in the literature support the safety and validity of using tele-glaucoma compared to an in-person exam for glaucoma screening. A meta-analysis of tele-glaucoma screening programs showed high sensitivity in detecting glaucoma.[8] However, compared to an in-person exam, tele-glaucoma had lower sensitivity but higher specificity.

Several studies comparing remote tele-glaucoma screening to in-person examination have found that ocular data was comparable between these two examination approaches. One study reviewed 107 patients who underwent tele-glaucoma evaluations consisting of auto-refraction, noncontact ("air-puff") tonometry, nonmydriatic fundus photography, and optical coherence tomography (OCT). Strong correlations were found between tele-glaucoma and in-person exams for IOP, cup-to-disc ratio, and glaucoma diagnosis (i.e., glaucoma, glaucoma suspect, or no glaucoma).[9] High correlation between ocular findings detected on telemedicine eye screening and in-person exam were also found in the Philadelphia telemedicine glaucoma detection and follow-up study.[10]

Another study assessed 309 patients who were evaluated in-person by a comprehensive ophthalmologist and using tele-glaucoma review of diagnostic testing by a glaucoma specialist. The authors found a high correlation between in-person and tele-glaucoma assessments of cup-to-disc ratio, as well as a positive predictive value of 77.5% and a negative predictive value of 82.2% for glaucoma diagnosis, using the results from the in-person evaluation as a reference standard.[11] Tele-glaucoma allows accurate assessment for glaucoma screening while reducing the need for in-person evaluation and increasing the efficiency of glaucoma care. Therefore, tele-glaucoma has substantial potential to expand access to care and reduce the global burden of vision loss from glaucoma.

EXAM COMPONENTS OF A TELE-GLAUCOMA PROGRAM

Visual Acuity and Pupil Assessment

Visual acuity and pupil assessment are essential components of the ophthalmic exam for all subspecialties,

including glaucoma, and are necessary for any tele-glaucoma program. Please refer to Chapter 13: Technology for details regarding telehealth technology for assessing vision and pupils.

Pachymetry

The two main methods for measuring central corneal thickness are ultrasound and optical techniques. Ultrasound devices tend to be portable, easy to use, and cost-effective, however, they are position-sensitive and contact the cornea during measurement. The Pachmate 2 (DGH Technology, Inc.) is a handheld device that runs on 2 AAA batteries and captures measurements in less than a second. The Pachette 4 (DGH Technology, Inc.) is a desktop device that also runs on 2 AA batteries and takes measurements quickly. Optical devices are typically mounted on a biomicroscope and measure central corneal thickness through interferometry. Such devices include anterior segment OCT, which provides a noncontact approach to measuring central cornea thickness.

Tonometry

Given the central role of IOP in the diagnosis and management of glaucoma, accurately assessing IOP is crucial in a tele-glaucoma program. The gold standard measurement of IOP remains Goldmann applanation tonometry (GAT), but this technique requires a more highly skilled technician or telehealth facilitator. GAT may be accomplished with a slit-lamp–mounted tonometer or with handheld devices such as the Perkins or Kowa. Rebound (iCare, Helsinki, Finland) and handheld applanation (Tonopen, Reichert, Depew, New York, USA) tonometers are portable, have single-use tips, and are easier to use by less skilled technicians. There are some discrepancies in measurements between different devices, however, portable handheld devices remain commonly used in ocular telehealth programs.[12] Home tonometry is possible with the iCare HOME or a contact lens device containing a sensor (Sensimed Triggerfish CLS, Sensimed AG, Lausanne, Switzerland). However, the iCare HOME is expensive and not yet widely utilized, but new business models in which the device is loaned to patients for a limited period of time are promising. Sensimed Triggerfish has been under development for many years but is not yet commercially available.[12] Chapter 11 (In-home Monitoring) and Chapter 13 (Technology) discuss these technologies in greater detail.

Gonioscopy

Assessing angle anatomy with gonioscopy is an advanced ophthalmic skill typically only completed by optometrists or ophthalmologists. However, the angle anatomy is important when assessing glaucoma, and the limited ability to perform gonioscopy using tele-health remains a limitation of the scope of care that can be provided with tele-glaucoma. A commercially available gonioscope (GS-1, NIDEK Co, Gamagori, Japan) may improve the quality of care by allowing remote assessment of the angle. This device provides a magnified 360-degree view of the angle, however, it is not cleared for clinical use and initial studies show that further refinement of the device is needed.[13] Gonioscopy is an advanced skill that may be less important for tele-glaucoma screening programs, but having gonioscopy performed at least once remains an integral component for the long-term management of patients with glaucoma.

Angle anatomy can also be assessed with anterior segment OCT (AS-OCT) as it provides a cross-sectional view of the angle. AS-OCT units are widely available and common devices include the Visante, Cirrus, and Spectralis OCT units. Limitations of these devices include that they do not deeply penetrate the sclera so the image quality of the angle recess may be inadequate, and this technology is not able to assess fine details such as peripheral anterior synechiae and neovascularization. The Visante OCT uses a longer wavelength of light and therefore is able to provide better quality images through greater penetration of the angle. While there remains limited consensus on the precise criteria for distinguishing between open or narrow angles using these devices, comparing views taken with the room lights off and on can be helpful in identifying narrow angles that may be at risk for acute angle closure glaucoma.[14]

Perimetry

For any tele-glaucoma program, the ideal functional assessment for visual field defects would be quick, easy, inexpensive, and as accurate as the gold standard, standard automated perimetry. The technology chosen may depend upon the goal of the tele-glaucoma program. For instance, frequency doubling technology (FDT) is probably the most common screening visual field test, but its main limitation lies in its significant learning curve for patients.[12] Standard automated perimetry machines are expensive, large, and not easily mobile, so several other laptop, tablet, and smartphone-based options have been developed. Unfortunately, none have been shown to be neither as robust nor directly comparable to standard automated perimetry. Future studies are needed to enhance the usability, reliability, portability, and accessibility of more portable perimetry techniques for tele-glaucoma. The rest of this section discusses perimetry options that could be utilized

with tele-glaucoma in greater depth. Chapter 13 (Technology) also offers details on particular devices.

Standard automated perimetry—Humphrey/Octopus

Functional assessment of the impact of nerve damage by perimetry forms another pillar in the care of all patients with glaucoma. The gold standard test remains standard automated perimetry (SAP) and the mainstays for this type of testing are the Humphrey Visual Field (Carl Zeiss Meditec, Inc., Dublin, CA, USA) and Octopus (Haag-Streit USA Inc., Mason, OH, USA) devices. Strategies to improve test efficiency include Swedish interactive thresholding algorithm (SITA) standard (24-2), SITA Fast, and SITA Faster (24-2c) modules, yet they remain relatively time-consuming, require well-trained technicians, and can be challenging for patients to complete.

Frequency doubling technology

The stimulus in Frequency Doubling Technology preferentially tests a subset of retinal ganglion cells that have been hypothesized to be selectively damaged in early glaucoma. In patients with mild to moderate glaucoma, significant correlations of mean deviation (MD) and pattern standard deviation (PSD) were found between standard automated perimetry and frequency doubling technology. It is commonly used for glaucoma screening because of the shorter test duration and greater portability of the machine compared to standard automated perimetry. As noted earlier, it does have a significant learning curve for patients.[12,15]

Laptop-based options

Moorfields Motion Displacement Test (MMDT) is a software program for suprathreshold visual field assessment that runs on a laptop. The presentation of the stimuli corresponds with the test locations of the Humphrey Visual Field SITA Standard 24-2 testing algorithm. The test is completed one eye at a time, in a dimly lit room with the chin in a fixed chin/forehead rest 30 cm from the monitor. It takes approximately 5 min to test both eyes and can be completed without refractive correction. It also has a learning curve but has been shown to have a sensitivity of 88.5% and a specificity of 85% for distinguishing between glaucomatous and nonglaucomatous eyes.[16]

Tablet-based options

Melbourne Rapid Fields (MRF), (GLANCE Optical Pty Ltd., Melbourne, Australia) is an iPad-based application that allows visual field measurement in home or remote settings. The eyes are tested in a monocular fashion, in a dim room, with the device brightness at its maximum setting. The iPad is set 33 cm away and the individual's normal reading glasses are worn. Guidance is given to the patient throughout testing via tablet-generated voice commands. Mean and pattern deviations can be calculated and have been found to correlate with those of Humphrey Visual Field SITA Standard 24-2 testing algorithm. Further study is needed to verify its accuracy before being used widely.[16]

Visual Fields Easy (VFE) is another iPad-based method that provides a quick, easy, and portable test of visual function. It takes 3 min per eye to complete and the test shows high sensitivity (91%), specificity (100%), positive predictive value (100%), and negative predictive value (90%).[17] It has also been shown to be effective in detecting moderate and advanced visual field loss.[18] However, it is not currently in widespread use.

Smartphone-based options

Mobile Visual Perimetry Frequency Doubling Technology (MVP FDT) combines a smartphone-based app with a head-mounted display to allow for an extremely portable device for assessing visual function with results comparable to Humphrey Visual Field FDT.[19] Along with a Bluetooth-enabled remote, the FDT C-20 screening protocol can be run on the smartphone-based app. This device can be built at a low cost($150) and can be used by patients with physical limitations due to the head-mounted display.[20]

Virtual reality

There are several options available to test visual fields using virtual reality-based technology. The VisuALL S (Olleyes) Analyzer is a virtual reality visual function platform that is a mobile device for performing automated perimetry. This modality is an automated, wearable headset with ambient control to allow patients to be tested in any position and in any illumination. It has been shown to have results correlating with those from the Humphrey Field Analyzer, though further study is needed. [VisuALL S pamphlet] Vision Vivid Perimetry (VVP) is a head-mounted virtual reality platform to assess visual function based on oculo kinetic function. Preliminary studies show that appears to be accurate for use in both glaucoma patients and glaucoma suspects.[21] Finally, the nGoggle visual function system is a head-mounted, wireless electroencephalogram system that allows multifocal steady-state visual evoked potential signal acquisition. It is in the early stages of study but has been shown to have better accuracy in detecting glaucoma compared to global parameters of static automated perimetry. These virtual reality-based technologies provide a portable, more objective way of assessing visual function that could improve the future effectiveness of tele-glaucoma programs.[22]

Imaging

Photography of the posterior pole plays a key role in tele-glaucoma since it allows visualization of the retina and optic nerve for the purposes of screening and monitoring glaucoma progression. Traditional fundus cameras tend to be bulkier, more expensive, and require a skilled technician or ophthalmic photographer to use, which makes them less widely used in ocular telehealth programs. Due to these limitations, smaller tabletop and portable, handheld camera systems have emerged that overcome some of these limitations while still producing high-quality images.

Nonmydriatic fundus photography

Advances in imaging technology have resulted in an abundance of commercially available, high-quality tabletop nonmydriatic fundus cameras. Tele-glaucoma protocols for optic disc photography may include stereo disc photography along with images of the macula or anterior segment. A few notable units that allow stereo imaging include: (1) the Topcon NW8F plus which provides a 45-degree field of view, has autofocus for refractions of −13D to +12D, and has red-free images and fluorescein angiography; (2) the Zeiss VISUCAM 200 which can give 45- and 30-degree fields of view, has autofocus for −35D to +35D, provides red-free images, autofluorescence, as well as anterior segment imaging[23]; and the TRC-NW400 with touchscreen operation. Other less expensive and more portable handheld devices have emerged as well. These include the Volk PictorPlus, Volk PictorPrestige, and the RetinaVue700.[23] However, handheld cameras remain more limited with regards to their functionalities and the gradeability of nonmydriatic fundus images compared to tabletop models.

There have been exponential advancements in smartphone technology which have stimulated an interest in smartphone-based cameras for ocular telehealth. Given the global increase in telecommunications throughout the world (for example, growth of 600% in India in 5 years), smartphone-based technology has great potential for advancing access to high-quality care for patients around the world. In general, there are several limitations including beam alignment, intensity of the flash causing pupil constriction, and difficulty achieving adequate illumination.[23] An example of a smartphone-based camera is the Welch Allyn iExaminer, which is a handheld device that aligns the optical axes of the PanOptic ophthalmoscope with the visual axis of an iPhone to photograph the fundus and nerve.[23] More information regarding fundus cameras and retinal imaging can be found in Chapter 13.

Retinal nerve fiber layer and ganglion cell complex assessment with OCT

Retinal nerve fiber layer thickness is most commonly measured using Spectral-Domain Optical Coherence Tomography (SD-OCT) with commercially available units such as the Cirrus (Carl Zeiss Meditec, Inc., Dublin, CA, USA) and Spectralis (Heidelberg Engineering, Inc., Franklin, MA, USA) OCT. Since the macula contains a large number of retinal ganglion cells, its importance in glaucoma assessment is emerging towards becoming a standard component of glaucoma evaluation. The ganglion cell complex, consisting of the retinal nerve fiber layer, ganglion cell layer, and the inner plexiform layer, has shown to be of greater value than overall macular thickness for assessing glaucoma.[12] In addition to the retinal nerve fiber layer and the ganglion cell complex, OCT can be used to measure cup-to-disc ratio, disc area, and other parameters that can be helpful for diagnosing and monitoring patients with glaucoma.

Special consideration: Imaging of bleb morphology

High-quality imaging of post-operative blebs is needed to appropriately evaluate and manage complex glaucoma patients. There are many options for self-assembled and commercially available cell phone slit lamp adapters for evaluation of the anterior segment, however, reports are mixed regarding the utility of these options. With practice, one can align a cell phone camera freehand with the ocular, but this technique requires a high degree of skill and precision that may not be easily achieved by a telehealth facilitator. The Marco ION is a high-grade slit lamp adapter that holds an iPhone and attaches to a standard slit lamp. It utilizes a HIPAA-compliant, password-protected app to acquire, display, and upload photos. Another option is the Slit LED which is a remote-controlled slit lamp guided by a telehealth facilitator whose images can be sent for remote evaluation by a provider. The drawbacks of this device are that it requires a synchronous telehealth evaluation (and tele-glaucoma is mostly achieved asynchronously) and is not yet commercially available. Another promising technology is the telehealth cart anterior segment attachment by JedMed. While this is not a fully functional slit lamp, it may be capable of

providing a sufficiently high-quality anterior segment exam in a tele-glaucoma program, including postoperative bleb evaluation. Anterior segment imaging technologies are also discussed in Chapters 4 and 13.

MODELS OF TELE-GLAUCOMA CARE

The majority of tele-glaucoma programs are asynchronous, wherein information is gathered by a telehealth facilitator and interpreted remotely at a later time by an eye care provider. There may also be a hybrid component, in which the provider may choose to have a real-time video or phone-based visit with the patient after reviewing the testing to provide patient education and counseling on the next steps.

Glaucoma Screening

Glaucoma screening programs seek to identify patients with or at risk of developing glaucoma with the aim of achieving earlier detection to reduce disease burden. Risk factors for developing glaucoma include race, family history, and a history of ocular trauma or steroid use. These risk factors can be quickly assessed with a questionnaire that is either self-administered or administered with the help of a telehealth facilitator. The main exam elements for glaucoma screening include evaluation for elevated IOP and a large cup-to-disc ratio, thus tonometry and imaging of the optic nerve comprise important components of a tele-glaucoma screening protocol (Table 5.1). Visual field testing is prone to artifacts in the setting of screening, potentially resulting in high numbers of false positives, and thus low program effectiveness. The authors favor a parsimonious approach to visual field testing in tele-glaucoma screening programs due to the relatively low prevalence of glaucoma in the general population.

Targeting screening efforts in populations at high risk for glaucoma, such as older, nonwhite populations, and those with a first-degree family history of glaucoma, is more cost-effective than performing screening in the general population. This approach would result in a higher positive predictive value (i.e., a greater proportion of patients with abnormal screening results actually having glaucoma). Another approach to improve the cost-effectiveness of tele-glaucoma screening programs is to embed glaucoma screening within an existing clinical program such as primary care-based teleretinal screening programs for diabetic retinopathy.

There are a variety of settings in which tele-glaucoma screening may be performed, including community- and clinic-based programs. A community-based tele-glaucoma study targeting high-risk individuals in

TABLE 5.1
Recommended Components for Tele-Glaucoma Care Models

Care Model	Recommended Components	Personnel for Acquiring Patient Data
Basic screening	• Brief questionnaire/history • Tonometry • Optic nerve imaging (nerve photos, maybe OCT)	• Patient self-report (questionnaire only) • Telehealth facilitator
Glaucoma consultation or follow-up care	• Detailed questionnaire/history • Visual acuity (may include refraction) • Assessment for relative afferent pupillary defect • Visual field testing • Tonometry • Pachymetry • Anterior segment photography • Optical coherence tomography • Optic nerve and retinal photography	• Telehealth facilitator (ophthalmic technician)
Post-operative management	All of the above, plus: • Slit lamp photography or videography	• Licensed eye provider, performing elements based on scope and clinical training

New York City showed a high prevalence of glaucoma. Of 8547 individuals screened, 54% were Hispanic and 16% were African American. One quarter of patients were referred for further glaucoma evaluation while 60% were recommended to have routine evaluation. The strongest predictors of glaucoma suspect were elevated IOP and cup-to-disc ratio > 0.5.[24] Similarly, a shared-care tele-ophthalmology collaboration between the Rotterdam Eye Hospital and 10 commercial optometrists showed success in detecting glaucoma using nerve fiber analyzer images, with high levels of agreement on image interpretation(81%) between optometrists and trained technicians at the hospital. Further testing was required in 27% of individuals, and ophthalmology consultation was needed in only 11%.[25]

A clinic-based screening model in the Philadelphia area targeted high-risk individuals from underserved primary care clinics. They included individuals who were Black/African American, Hispanic/Latino, or Asian over 40 years of age, Caucasians over 65 years of age, and those with a family history of glaucoma or diabetes. Two-field, nonmydriatic photography was obtained by a technician who took one photograph centered on the optic nerve and the other on the macula. IOP was measured with iCare rebound tonometry. Data was transmitted through an electronic health record and reviewed by a glaucoma fellowship-trained ophthalmologist and a certified reader. A detailed in-person follow-up protocol was employed and the study found a high correlation between the asynchronous and

synchronous glaucoma evaluations. The time needed to complete the tele-glaucoma visits was less than half of that needed to complete the in-person visit, with an approximately 80% reduction in the cost of screening per participant. Participants reported high satisfaction for both asynchronous and in-person visits.[10] A similar clinic-based program in Alabama utilizing iCare rebound tonometry (iCare USA, Inc., Raleigh, NC) for IOP measurement, Maestro2 OCT (Topcon USA, Inc., Paramus, NJ) for retinal nerve fiber layer imaging and Humphrey Visual Field SITA-FAST (Carl Zeiss Meditec USA, Inc. Pleasanton, CA) for visual field testing is currently underway.[26]

Glaucoma Consultation

Tele-glaucoma programs providing initial glaucoma consultation are intended to provide in-depth evaluation of patients with a diagnosis of glaucoma or glaucoma suspect. These consults require additional testing capabilities and greater eye care provider expertise beyond that of a tele-glaucoma screening program. A detailed questionnaire can assess glaucoma risk factors as described previously for glaucoma screening, with additional questions added related to current and past glaucoma treatments (i.e., medication use, medication intolerances, laser treatments, or surgeries). Visual acuity remains important, and if possible, refraction can detect uncorrected refractive error. Pachymetry is essential to aid in glaucoma risk stratification and determination of target IOP. As with glaucoma screening programs, tonometry and optic nerve imaging remain important exam elements for glaucoma consultation. Visual field testing protocols should be comprehensive (e.g., Humphrey Visual Field SITA Faster 24-2c, Humphrey Visual Field SITA Standard 24-2, etc.).For patients diagnosed with glaucoma, it is essential to assess for progression using these visual field testing modalities. Gonioscopy should ideally be assessed at least once in a tele-glaucoma program, however, this would need to be completed by a trained optometrist or ophthalmologist, as currently there are no validated automated or photographic methods to predict angle-closure risk.

There are several examples of tele-glaucoma consultation programs that have been conducted in the U.S. and internationally. Eye care quality and accessibility improvement in the community (EQUALITY) is a community–academic collaboration between optometrists at Walmart Vision Centers and glaucoma specialists at a reading center based at the University of Alabama. In this program, dilated comprehensive eye exams and glaucoma testing and preliminary management are completed by the optometrists. Then, the glaucoma specialists, in an asynchronous manner, provide feedback after reviewing the patients' exam and diagnostic information.[27] Patients also received education about ocular health and glaucoma. The results regarding agreement between providers on diagnosis, management, impact of education on adherence to in-person clinic follow-up, patient satisfaction, and costs are pending.

Tele-glaucoma consultation programs have been most well-established in Canada. A remote program in underserved areas of Alberta uses a "hub and spoke" model in which comprehensive ophthalmologists and optometrists act as "spokes" that send standardized data to the "hub" where glaucoma specialists interpret the data and send recommendations for management of the patient. This store-and-forward program has a turn-around time of 10 days and allows for a variety of follow-up options including teleconsultation with the optometrist or an in-person examination with the glaucoma specialist.[28]

Another program in Edmonton, Canada is a partnership between an academic center and a private glaucoma practice. Patients referred for glaucoma evaluation are reviewed by a tele-glaucoma coordinator to see if a tele-glaucoma visit could be appropriate based on a standardized set of criteria. Patients meeting the criteria are offered a tele-glaucoma option within-person evaluation with an ophthalmic technician or nurse who collects a standardized set of data based on the protocol. Glaucoma specialists then asynchronously interpret the data. The typical interval from referral to consult report is 1 month (compared to the typical 3–4 month interval for an in-person glaucoma consultation).[28]

Finally, a program in Western Australia provides imaging at a primary care or medical clinic. Those images are then reviewed in an asynchronous manner by an ophthalmologist who then videoconferences with the patient and primary care provider to discuss their findings and provide recommendations for further glaucoma management.[28]

Long-Term Management/Glaucoma Follow-Up Care

Since glaucoma is a life-long condition and there is a relative shortage of eye care providers, many glaucoma specialists accumulate large patient populations over time, which can result in very busy clinics. Tele-glaucoma could play an increasingly important role towards more efficiently managing the long-term care of glaucoma patients, focusing on the detection and management of glaucoma progression. A simulated tele-glaucoma program that utilized readers, that were either glaucoma specialists or optometrists experienced in glaucoma management, showed similar levels of agreement in detecting progression between readers (62%–69%) as well as low intra-reader variability between in-person and tele-glaucoma evaluations(65%).[29] In another study evaluating the use of tele-glaucoma among established glaucoma clinic patients, trained technicians gathered data as requested from the previously scheduled in-person visit, including visual acuity and field measurements, tonometry, and optic disc imaging, and completed a standard patient questionnaire. Disagreement regarding possible glaucoma progression between in-person and tele-glaucoma evaluations occurred in 3.4% of patients, with misclassification occurring in fewer than 2% of patients. Inter-observer agreement was fair with 75% sensitivity and 89% specificity.[30] Long-term glaucoma management studies using tele-glaucoma models are needed to determine best practices for optimizing clinical outcomes and patient safety.

At the Veterans Administration, a tele-glaucoma program has been developed within a comprehensive screening ocular telehealth program, Technology-based Eye Care Services (TECS) (see Chapter 2 for details on the TECS program). In this program, patient data is collected using the standard TECS protocol, but there is additional guidance on glaucoma management for various scenarios, including elevated IOP, possible progression on OCT, or visual field testing. The tele-glaucoma management protocol provides consistency, but also allows eye care providers to tailor their decisions because glaucoma management remains one of the most complex part in eye care. Studies regarding clinical outcomes, patient satisfaction, and cost-effectiveness of this tele-glaucoma program are pending.

Post-Op Management

Monitoring of glaucoma patients during both the early and late post-operative periods is an emerging area of ocular telehealth. These programs require high-resolution slit beam imaging, obtained by a highly skilled telehealth facilitator, such as a comprehensive ophthalmologist or an optometrist. An eye provider near to the patient could tele-present the post-op patient to a remote glaucoma specialist using either asynchronous, synchronous, or a hybrid model. In the early post-operative period, it would be essential to have the in-person provider comfortable and skilled in performing post-operative assessments such as evaluation for bleb leaks and wound healing. It may also be essential for the in-person provider to be licensed and proficient in post-operative manipulations such as bleb massage or argon laser suture lysis when indicated (Table 5.1). These imaging and exam skills would be helpful for long-term monitoring of blebs from trabeculectomies and glaucoma drainage devices.

New imaging technologies could be useful for post-operative tele-glaucoma evaluation. One study compared real-time remote-controlled slit lamp examination with standard two-dimensional slit lamp photography of the anterior segment in eyes following trabeculectomy. The results showed that the remote-controlled slit lamp exam provided superior accuracy with regards to anterior chamber depth and bleb morphology compared to the two-dimensional photos.[31] In addition, the real-time remote-controlled slit lamp examination yielded similar results to those obtained through an in-person slit lamp examination. There is also early evidence that newer generations of smartphones (i.e., iPhone X) produce superior photos of bleb morphology compared to an older model (i.e., iPhone 6S).[32] A major area of need for tele-glaucoma and ocular telehealth in general (see Chapters 4 and 17) is improved imaging of the anterior segment. Continued advancements in anterior segment imaging could be useful for telehealth monitoring and post-operative evaluation following glaucoma surgery.

Virtual Care in the Setting of the COVID-19 Pandemic

During the COVID-19 pandemic that began in March 2020, virtual eye care expanded tremendously due to safety concerns regarding in-person clinic visits. Novel approaches to providing patient care were developed including for glaucoma. One particularly unique approach was the "drive-through IOP check" wherein a patient would have their IOP checked while in their car by a provider or technician using a handheld device. The IOP check was then followed by a telehealth visit via either a secure message, phone call, or video visit. Additionally, the pandemic increased interest in adoption of home-based monitoring of glaucoma, including IOP measurements and visual field testing.

ARTIFICIAL INTELLIGENCE AND FUTURE DIRECTIONS

Artificial intelligence (AI) is a field that has grown exponentially with great potential for increasing the throughput of data interpretation, as well as providing predictive modeling and clinical decision support for tele-glaucoma. A few examples include the ability to predict future visual field loss based on existing visual fields,[33] the ability to assess cup-to-disc ratio comparably to assessments by a glaucoma specialist,[34] and the ability to detect the future onset of glaucoma from fundus photography with high accuracy.[35] Further details regarding the role of AI can be found in Chapter 18.

CONCLUSION

Ongoing technological innovations continue to contribute toward the ability to provide increasingly sophisticated tele-glaucoma care. Telehealth approaches for glaucoma screening, diagnosis, and ongoing management have the potential to increase access to glaucoma specialty care, reduce travel for many patients, and improve clinical outcomes.

REFERENCES

1. Shaikh Y, Yu F, Coleman A. Burden of undetected and untreated glaucoma in the United States. *Am J Ophthalmol.* 2014;158(6):1121–1129.e1.
2. Resnikoff S, Lansingh VC, Washburn L, et al. Estimated number of ophthalmologists worldwide (International Council of Ophthalmology update): will we meet the needs? *Br J Ophthalmol.* 2019;104:588–592.
3. https://www.nei.nih.gov/eyedata/glaucoma.
4. Parke DW. *The Ophthalmology Workforce.* Eyenet Magazine; 2020:16–17.

5. Quigley HA. 21st century glaucoma care. *Eye.* 2019;33(2):254–260.

6. Thomas S, et al. The cost-effectiveness analysis of teleglaucoma screening device. *PLoS One.* 2015;10(9):e0137913.

7. Arora S, Rudnisky CJ, Damji KF. Improved access and cycle time with an 'in-house' patient-centered teleglaucoma program versus traditional in-person assessment. *Telemed J E Health.* 2014;20(5):439–445.

8. Thomas SM, Jeyaraman MM, Hodge WG, et al. The effectiveness of tele-glaucoma versus in-patient examination for glaucoma screening: a systematic review and meta-analysis. *PLoS One.* 2014;9(12), e113779.

9. Chandrasekaran S, Kass W, Thangamathesvaran L, et al. Tele-glaucoma versus clinical evaluation: the New Jersey health foundation prospective clinical study. *J Telemed Telecare.* 2020;26(9):536–544.

10. Hark L, et al. Philadelphia telemedicine glaucoma detection and follow-up study: confirmation between eye screening and comprehensive eye examination diagnosis. *Br J Ophthalmol.* 2019;103(12):1820–1826.

11. Kiage D, Kherani IN, Gichuhi S, et al. The Muranga teleophthalmology study: comparison of virtual(teleglaucoma) with in-person clinical assessment to diagnose glaucoma. *Middle East Afr J Ophthalmol.* 2013;20(2):150–157.

12. Strouthidis NG, Chandrasekharan G, Diamond JP, et al. Teleglaucoma: ready to go? *Br J Ophthalmol.* 2014;98(12):1605–1611.

13. Teixeira F, Sousa DC, Leal I, Barata A, Neves CM, Pinto LA. Automated gonioscopy photography for iridocorneal angle grading. *Eur J Ophthalmol.* 2020;30(1):112–118.

14. Kent C. Making the most of anterior segment OCT. *Rev Ophthalmol.* 2011;18(4):39–46.

15. Wadood AC, Azuara-Blanco A, Aspinall P, et al. Sensitivity and specificity of frequency-doubling technology, tendency-oriented perimetry, and humphrey swedish interactive threshold algorithm-fast perimetry in a glaucoma practice. *Am J Ophthalmol.* 2002;133:327–332.

16. Hamzah JC, Daka Q, Azuara-Blanco A. Home monitoring for glaucoma. *Eye.* 2020;34(1):155–160.

17. Santos AS, Morabe ES. "VisualFields easy": an iPad application as a simple tool for detecting visual field defects. *Philipp J Ophthalmol.* 2016;41:22–26.

18. Johnson CA, Thapa S, Xiang Y, et al. Performance of an iPad application to detect moderate and advanced visual field loss in Nepal. *Am J Ophthalmol.* 2017;182:147–154.

19. Alawa KA, Nolan RP, Han E, et al. Low-cost, smartphone-based frequency doubling technology visual field testing using a head-mounted display. *Br J Ophthalmol.* 2021;105(3):440–444.

20. Taylor R, et al. *Perimetry Goes High-Tech and Mobile.* Eyenet Magazine; 2020:33–34.

21. Greenfield A, Deiner NA, et al. *Measurement Reproducibility Using Vivid Vision Perimetry: A Virtual Reality-Based Mobile Platform.* ARVO poster; 2020. https://eventpilot.us/web/page.php?page=IntHtml&project=ARVO20&id=3366488.

22. Wu Z, Medeiros FA. Recent developments in visual field testing for glaucoma. *Curr Opin Ophthalmol.* 2018;29(2):141–146.

23. Panwar N, et al. Fundus photography in the 21st century—a review of recent technological advances and their implications for worldwide healthcare. *Telemed J E-Health.* 2016;22(3):198–208.

24. Al-Aswad LA, Joiner DB, Wang X, et al. Screening for glaucoma in populations at high risk: the eye screening New York project. *Cogent Med.* 2017;4:1367059.

25. Mul D, et al. Improving the quality of eye care with tele-ophthalmology: shared-care glaucoma screening. *J Telemed Telecare.* 2004;10(6):331–336.

26. Rhodes LA, Register S, Asif I, et al. Alabama screening and intervention for glaucoma and eye health through telemedicine (AL-SIGHT): study design and methodology. *J Glaucoma.* 2021;30(5):371–379.

27. Owsley C, Rhodes LA, McGwin Jr G, et al. Eye care quality and accessibility improvement in the community (EQUALITY) for adults at risk for glaucoma: a study rationale and design. *Int J Equity Health.* 2015;14:135.

28. Kassam F, Yogesan K, Sogbesan E, et al. Teleglaucoma: improving access and efficiency for glaucoma care. *Middle East Afr J Ophthalmol.* 2013;20(2):142–149.

29. Odden JL, Khanna CL, Choo CM, et al. Telemedicine in long-term care of glaucoma patients. *J Telemed Telecare.* 2020;26(1–2):92–99.

30. Clarke J, Puertal R, Kotecha A, et al. Virtual clinics in glaucoma care: face-to-face versus remote decision-making. *Br J Ophthalmol.* 2017;101:892–895.

31. Kashawagi K, et al. Comparison of a remote operating slit-lamp microscope system with a conventional slit-lamp microscope system for examination of trabeculectomy eyes. *J Glaucoma.* 2013;22(4):278–283.

32. Kalra G, Ichhpujani P, Thakur S, et al. A pilot study for smarthone photography to assess bleb morphology and vasculature post-trabeculectomy. *Int Ophthalmol.* 2021;41(2):483–490.

33. Wen JC, Lee CS, Keane PA, et al. Forecasting future Humphrey visual fields using deep learning. *PLoS One.* 2019;14(4), e0214875.

34. Khouri AS, Szirth BC, Shahid KS, Fechtner RD. Software-assisted optic nerve assessment for glaucoma tele-screening. *Telemed J E Health.* 2008;14(3):261–265.

35. Thakur A, Goldbaum M, Yousefi S. Predicting glaucoma before onset using deep learning. *Ophthalmol Glaucoma.* 2020;3(4):262–268.

CHAPTER 6

Retina, Uveitis, Ocular Oncology Telehealth

STEPHANIE J. WEISS, DO • AKSHAR ABBOTT, MD

INTRODUCTION

The growing need for retinal screening examinations related to high rates of diabetes mellitus (DM) coupled with significant strides in retinal imaging due to technological advances has led to a rapidly growing demand for accurate and cost-effective telehealth programs for the posterior segment. For the past two decades, the role of telemedicine in eye care, particularly retinal subspecialty care, has become progressively more sophisticated with improved effectiveness. In fact, the most widespread use of ocular telehealth in the world focuses on retinal disease: diabetic retinopathy (DR). The infrastructure of DR screening via telehealth models provides the foundation for several other ocular specialties, such as comprehensive eye screening, anterior segment telehealth, and glaucoma telehealth among others.

The nature of retina, in general with pathologies largely diagnosed by clear pattern recognition, makes it an ideal subspecialty to safely be done with telehealth, which, in the ophthalmic field, relies heavily upon image-based diagnosis. For example, DR is diagnosed based on the appearance of retinal hemorrhage, exudate and vascular changes, findings easily detected with imaging, which made DR a perfect target for early adopters of telehealth in eye care. As teleretinal screening examinations have become more widespread, more robust quality control standards have been established, and fundus imaging technology has improved, the role of telemedicine in retinal subspecialty care has grown far beyond the boundaries of diabetic retinopathy. Indications for teleretinal examinations have grown, for example, to include macular degeneration.

Telemedicine has also been used to implement remote retinal subspecialty consultation services designed to improve patient access to a higher level of care. Retina telehealth programs are typically asynchronous or hybrid, with the patient presenting to a clinic or other healthcare setting to receive testing, with an option to discuss results with the provider via phone or video. Telehealth can also help to ease the burden of in-person ophthalmic examinations, thereby expanding access to in-person expert care.[1] As the rapid development of teleretinal services continues, the field will likely see expanding indications for teleretinal screening and monitoring, thus allowing for in-person retina clinics to focus on pathology and in-person interventions.

DIABETIC RETINOPATHY

Diabetic retinopathy (DR) is the most common cause of blindness in working-age adults in the United States.[2] While there are excellent treatment options available to prevent vision loss related to DR, the ability to appropriately treat DR is limited by patient compliance, socioeconomic factors, and access to regular screening examinations to diagnose pathology.[2,3] DR is commonly asymptomatic in early stages, which likely contributes to poor compliance with the annual retinal screening examinations recommended by many professional societies including the American Academy of Ophthalmology.[3] An estimated 40%–50% of adults in the United States with DM do not undergo the recommended ophthalmic screenings.[3] Moreover, it has been estimated that 26% of patients with type 1 DM and 36% of patients with type 2 DM in the United States have never had their eyes examined.[4] Older age, lower education level, residence in a rural location, and recent DM diagnosis have been linked to poor compliance with retinal screening examinations.[4] Early detection of DR can improve outcomes, underscoring the importance of developing effective screening programs. The development of teleretinal screening programs has had a significant positive impact on the face of diabetic retinal screening over the past two decades. Mounting evidence supporting the utility of telemedicine in diabetic retinal screening examinations has encouraged the continued development of such programs, with more and more sites embracing telehealth as part of retinal care (Fig. 6.1).

History and Development of Diabetic Screening Programs

The landmark Early Treatment Diabetic Retinopathy Study (ETDRS) study established the use of fundus photography in the diagnosis of diabetic retinopathy.[5]

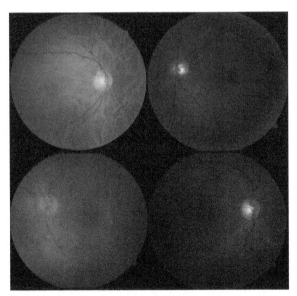

FIG. 6.1 Single mydriatic 45-degree fundus photo of mild (*top left*) moderate (*top right*), and severe (*bottom left*) nonproliferative diabetic retinopathy, mixed hypertensive and severe nonproliferative diabetic retinopathy (*bottom right*) detected via a teleretinal diabetic retinopathy screening program. (Credit: Photo by Stephanie J. Weiss, DO; Rhonda Ziegler, COA).

This study developed a gold standard for retinal imaging, consisting of a 7-field imaging protocol to capture a significant portion of the retina with stereoscopic color fundus photographs.[5] The study was able to accurately detect retinal hemorrhages, microaneurysms, hard exudates, new vessel and fibrous proliferation, and macular edema with a high degree of interreader agreeability suggesting a high level of accuracy in diagnosing and grading diabetic retinopathy with fundus photographs alone.[5]

While not initially designed for a telemedicine program, the ETDRS protocol became the gold standard against which future telemedicine programs would be compared to, in order to demonstrate an acceptable level of accuracy and reliability, especially when compared to the traditional in-person dilated fundus examination. In 2002, Lin et al. described a DR screening program that demonstrated a high level of agreement in the grading of retinopathy between a single digital fundus photo and the standard ETDRS 7-field fundus photography.[6] Moreover, this same study determined that a single digital fundus image was actually more sensitive than a dilated fundus examination, with early retinopathy being most commonly missed with an in-person exam.[6] Starting in

2001, the Joslin Vision Network became a mainstay in the establishment of successful teleretinal screening programs for DR.[7] This protocol, initially based on digital fundus photos from a nonmydriatic fundus camera, demonstrated a high level of agreement between these photos and the ETDRS 7-field fundus photography.[7] The same protocol also demonstrated a high level of agreement when compared to an in-person dilated fundus examination from a retina specialist, with agreement on the exact stage of DR in 72.5% of eyes and agreement within one stage of DR in 89.3% of eyes.[8] As the development of this network continued, ultra-widefield fundus imaging was incorporated with the use of an Optos device to capture a single 200-degree fundus image. In comparing ultra-widefield imaging to traditional fundus imaging, the ultra-widefield protocol was found to be superior in terms of reduced rate of ungradable images and increased identification of DR.[9]

Within the Veterans Affairs (VA) network of hospitals and clinics in the United States, the Joslin Vision Network protocol was adopted to improve diabetic teleretinal screening for military veterans.[10] In 2005, Cavallerano et al. described a program within a VA medical center in which the Joslin Vision Network protocol was successfully implemented. The images were captured at the VA and then transferred to the Joslin Vision Network for interpretation, ultimately resulting in a large, VA enterprise-wide program to remotely detect and grade DR and diabetic macular edema (DME). The VA teleretinal imaging program was so successful that others began to innovate based on the same infrastructure, leading to the development of more ocular telehealth services for Veterans, including Technology-based Eye Care Services (TECS). The TECS program performs diabetic screenings along with comprehensive eye care screening examinations and refractions within the VA system.[11] This national program, initially launched in 2015, includes refraction, intraocular pressure determination, external photographs, and three 45-degree field fundus images taken typically after mydriasis on a nonmydriatic tabletop digital fundus camera.[11] TECS was designed to reach veterans located in rural communities with limited access to medical care and homeless veterans.[11] Once established, the program improved access to care with more than 98% of veterans attending an appointment within 30 days of scheduling. This program also demonstrated significant cost savings with an average of $148.00 savings per visit to the VA medical center and $52.00 savings per visit to the veteran in travel cost reductions.[11] Perhaps most importantly, this program was shown to have a high level of accuracy with substantial agreement compared to in-person visits when detecting and grading DR.[12]

Diabetic Teleretinal Screening Program Standards and Quality Control

As various DR screening programs continued to develop across the United States and the world, the need for a well-defined set of standards for quality control became apparent. The American Telehealth Association (ATA) sought to create four distinct categories to stratify teleretinal DR screening programs based on their ability to detect DR relative to the gold standards of retinal evaluation.[2] In their most recent guidelines from 2011, they describe category 1 as a system that can divide patients into two groups, those who have no retinopathy or minimal nonproliferative diabetic retinopathy (NPDR) and those who have more than minimal NPDR.[2] Examples of category 1 programs include the EyePACS program in California, USA,[13] and the DigiScope program in Baltimore Maryland, USA.[14] Category 2 describes a system that can determine if sight-threatening DR is present (based on presence of diabetic macular edema (DME), severe NPDR, or proliferative diabetic retinopathy (PDR)).[2] This category allows for prompt referral for in-person management.[2] An example of a category 2 program is the National Health Services (NHS) Diabetic Eye Screening program in the United Kingdom.[1,15] The NHS program, founded in 2003, employs two 45-degree field fundus photos captured with pupillary dilation.[15] Category 3 is defined as a system that can identify every stage of DR as defined by ETDRS including mild, moderate, and severe NPDR, early and high-risk PDR, and DME. This type of program must be able to accurately determine the follow-up and treatment strategies equivalent to recommendations that would be provided during a clinical retina examination with dilated fundus examination.[2] The Joslin Vision Network in the United States[7] is an example of a category 3 program. Category 4 includes systems that are capable of matching or exceeding the ETDRS standard in staging DR and detecting DME.[2] This would indicate a program would be able to serve as a replacement for an ETDRS protocol in any clinical or research setting.[2] This standard has yet to be met by a well-established tele-eye program.[1]

In 2019, Bodnar et al.[16] published findings from the Ophthalmic Digital Health workshop, supported by the American Academy of Ophthalmology (AAO), the American Society of Cataract and Refractive Surgeons (ASCRS), the American Society of Retina Specialists (ASRS) along with a number of other professional societies, and the US Food and Drug Administration. These findings recommended the use of a fundus camera with resolution sufficient to detect small microaneurysms and noted the risk of DME going undetected on teleretinal examinations without supplemental optical coherence tomography (OCT) imaging.[16] They also found that widefield or ultra-widefield imaging may reduce the incidence of ungradable images.[16]

Accuracy of Diabetic Teleretinal Screening Programs

Teleretinal programs aim to provide diagnostic information comparable to the gold standard in-person dilated fundus examination or ETDRS standard. As such, many programs have sought to establish the accuracy, sensitivity, and specificity of DR screening programs and other telemedicine programs based on fundus imaging. Shi et al.[17] performed a meta-analysis to determine the overall sensitivity and specificity of previously studied teleretinal programs for DR screening, finding a pooled sensitivity of at least 80% in detecting the absence of DR or the presence of low- or high-risk DR.[17] The pooled sensitivity in detecting mild or moderate NPDR or DME exceeded 70% and the pooled sensitivity in detecting severe NPDR was 53%.[17] The pooled specificity was at least 90% in all DR conditions except mild NPDR which was found to have a specificity of 89%.[17] In 2020, cumulative data from Ullah et al. showed that ophthalmic telehealth programs are very sensitive and specific for establishing the absence of retinopathy.[18] However, they found a less consistent sensitivity and specificity in detecting and grading retinopathy.[18]

Effect of Imaging Modality in Diabetic Teleretinal Screening Programs

To maximize the efficacy of ocular telehealth programs, careful consideration when choosing the best imaging modality is paramount. Fundus image acquisition after mydriasis has been shown to yield superior diagnostic accuracy when compared to nonmydriatic images.[17] However, pupil dilation can limit patient compliance and nonmydriatic fundus imaging has also been shown to be effective in screening for DR.[19,20] With the advent of widefield and ultra-widefield fundus imaging, one must also weigh the utility of this modality against the standard field of view (Figs. 6.2 and 6.3). Many successful programs have utilized fundus imaging with a standard 30-degree or 45-degree field of view to screen for and diagnose DR. The Canadian Retina Research Network program has shown success with a protocol utilizing two 45-degree fundus photos.[21] However, they also found success with ultra-widefield fundus imaging.[21] Comparisons between a standard ETDRS 7-field

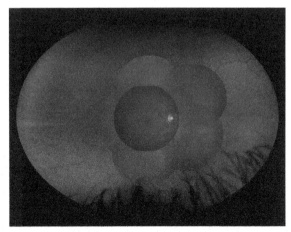

FIG. 6.2 Mydriatic ultra-widefield fundus photo (Optos) with overlay of a 7-field ETDRS montage fundus photo and single field 45-degree fundus photo (Zeiss Visucam). (Credit: Photo by Stephanie J. Weiss, DO; Jennifer Minnick, OD; Harjas Aulakh, OD; Heidi Tedrick, CRA).

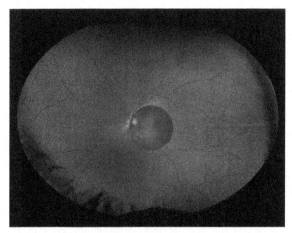

FIG. 6.3 Nonmydriatic ultra-widefield fundus photo (Optos) with overlay of a single 30-degree small pupil mode fundus photo (Zeiss Visucam). (Credit: Photo by Stephanie J. Weiss, DO; Jennifer Minnick, OD; Harjas Aulakh, OD).

fundus imaging protocol and a single ultra-widefield fundus image have demonstrated a high degree of agreement in the diagnosis of DR.[22,23] In fact, the use of wide-angle fundus imaging (100 degree–200 degree field of view) has been shown to have the highest level of diagnostic accuracy when compared to mydriatic and nonmydriatic standard field of view imaging.[17] Widefield images are capable of detecting peripheral pathology that can be missed even with the 7-field ETDRS imaging protocol and have been shown to be very effective in DR screening.[23,24] Afshar et al. developed a program utilizing an ultra-widefield camera mounted in a mobile van capable of traveling around major urban cities in the United States to reach an indigent patient population that would otherwise have been likely to go without eye care.[25]

The role of optical coherence tomography (OCT) in diabetic screenings

The conversation regarding the utility of OCT as part of a teleretinal program has largely centered around its ability to accurately diagnose DME during a DR screening examination. Overall, recent studies found the pooled sensitivity in detecting DME to be 59%–70% with a pooled specificity exceeding 90%.[17,18] Several programs have found an improvement in DME detection with the addition of OCT.[21,26–28] Weng et al. compared fundus photography to OCT in diagnosing DME and found that a significant percentage of eyes appearing to have DME on fundus photos did not actually have DME on OCT and that a significant percentage of eyes not appearing to have DME on fundus photos actually did have DME on OCT, thus suggesting fundus photos alone can be inaccurate in detecting DME.[26] Similarly, Felfeli et al. found that 38% of patients with DME required the addition of OCT to make the correct diagnosis.[28] However, similar comparative studies have conversely shown no benefit of OCT in detecting DME or other retinal pathology.[29,30] Given the lack of consensus on this issue, further evaluation is necessary to determine the true utility of OCT in teleretinal programs. More detailed information regarding imaging modality considerations can be found in Chapter 13: Technology Considerations.

Placement of Diabetic Teleretinal Screening Programs in Primary Care Offices

Another advantage of DR screening telemedicine programs is the ability to place screening cameras within primary care and endocrinology offices managing DM. The benefits to a program utilizing primary care or endocrinology offices include alleviation of barriers to care such as specialist availability, socioeconomic and geographic factors, and limitations to compliance.[19] A number of telemedicine programs have established the effectiveness of primary care and endocrinology-based telemedicine DR screening programs in improving compliance with screening recommendations and access to care.[19,31–36] Bastos de Carvalho et al. found that while 88% of diabetic patients visit their primary care office at least once per year, only 29.9% of diabetic patients had an annual eye examination.[19] This

highlights not only the discrepancy between systemic care and eye care but also the potential to reduce that gap through telehealth. The same group found that in a Kentucky state-wide safety net setting, the DR screening rates significantly increased to 47.7% of diabetic patients with the implementation of a program utilizing a nonmydriatic fundus camera in primary care offices and pre-existing clinic staff to perform the screenings.[19] A similar program in Los Angeles County, California found that DR eye screening compliance increased from 40.6% to 56.9% with the addition of a program utilizing mydriatic digital fundus cameras in primary care offices.[36] They also found an 89.2% reduction in wait time for DR screening exams (from 158 days to 17 days on average) and a reduced burden on in-person clinics with only 32.2% of patients screened requiring an in-person exam.[36]

Reaching Rural and Underserved Populations for Diabetic Teleretinal Screening

In addition to the placement of telemedicine DR screening programs in primary care offices, the advantages of placing them in rural or underserved regions have also been well established over the past several years.[37–41] As previously mentioned, this has been shown to be successful in the United States within state-wide safety net clinics.[19,36,39] On average, 60% of patients in the US with DM have an annual eye exam.[36] However, in a safety net patient population that rate can be lower than 25%, making this a particularly important population to reach.[36] The telemedicine model has also worked well within the Veterans Health Administration serving underserved and rural veterans in the United States. Worldwide, this model has proven to be particularly useful in underdeveloped regions within Kenya,[37] Chile,[38] Brazil,[40] and Sub-Saharan Africa.[41] Utilizing a smartphone-based DR screening platform targeting the Brazilian Xavante Indian population, Korn Malerbi et al. demonstrated a higher rate of DR than previously reported, thus highlighting the heightened importance of performing these screenings in such vulnerable populations.[40] In their study, 22.9% of patients had some level of DR, and 9.7% of patients were found to have sight-threatening DR.[40]

Compliance Rates and Conversion to In-Person Examinations for Diabetic Retinopathy

Telemedicine screening programs have been proven to significantly increase compliance with annual diabetic eye screening examinations for all types of patients.[19,28,31,36,42] In addition to improved screening rates, an important outcome of teleretinal screening programs is the enhanced ability to capture in-person referrals. It is important to note that telemedicine programs do not decrease rates of in-person visits, but rather increase rates of more relevant referrals for patients with true pathology.[43] Stebbins et al.[31] found high rates of compliance with referrals, noting that 56.3% of referred patients had an in-person exam within 3 months and 75.5% of patients had an examination within 1 year. Joseph et al.[42] found that when compared to a policy of universal referral for in-person examination, teleretinal screening followed by targeted referrals only when necessary yielded an 18.8% increase in compliance (37.5% of patients universally referred for in-person exam were compliant while 56.3% of patients referred following telemedicine screening were compliant). A similar study found 81.9% of patients deemed to have sight-threatening retinopathy on screening examination were seen for an in-person examination to undergo further evaluation and treatment when necessary—a capture rate much higher than would be expected without the first level of remote screening.[33]

MACULAR DEGENERATION

While diabetic retinopathy has dominated the field of ocular telehealth, the growth and continued development of such programs has led to a significant expansion in indications for retinal examinations. Among the conditions leading in tele-eye advancement of recent years has been age-related macular degeneration (AMD). Several telemedicine programs have found success in screening for AMD and others have successfully implemented protocols able to monitor non-neovascular (also known as dry or nonexudative) AMD.[12,34,44] Most commonly, pre-existing DR screening programs have been found to also be effective in screening for AMD.[12,34] Duchin et al.[44] described a program by which a nonmydriatic digital fundus camera was used to screen for referable AMD via the same pathway already developed to screen for referable DR. When compared to a traditional in-person exam, the telemedicine protocol was comparable, with high levels of sensitivity and specificity in detecting referable AMD.[44] Maa et al.[12] also described similar success in detecting AMD with acceptable sensitivity and specificity utilizing only digital fundus imaging via the previously established DR screening program within the VA system known as TECS. Both of these programs are examples of successful telehealth AMD screening programs that utilize only fundus imaging.

The Role of Optical Coherence Tomography (OCT) in Tele-Macular Degeneration Management

As OCT began to integrate into teleretinal screening programs more and more, the potential to monitor and even manage AMD remotely became possible. Existing DR screening programs began to integrate AMD screening into their protocols, and new programs began to specifically target AMD care. The addition of OCT allows for enhanced detection of subtle retinal pathology including early development of choroidal neovascular membrane and early signs of intraretinal and subretinal fluid that would be imperative in identifying the need for prompt referral and treatment to assure adequate monitoring of non-neovascular and/or neovascular (also known as wet or exudative) AMD. Li et al.[45] described a telemedicine program in Canada designed to screen for AMD and monitor neovascular AMD. In this prospective study, they describe two protocols, one being a screening protocol designed to evaluate eyes referred to retina subspecialty care for suspected neovascular AMD, and the other a monitoring protocol designed to monitor stable inactive neovascular AMD.[45] Both arms found a slightly longer interval between identification of treatment requirement and initiation of treatment in the telemedicine arms, likely owing to the added step of a telemedicine screening visit prior to an in-person treatment visit. However, neither group resulted in a significant decline in visual acuity outcomes or any other adverse outcomes.[45] Andonegui et al.[46] described a similar program utilizing telemedicine with fundus photography and OCT to monitor patients with a history of previously treated neovascular AMD, with the goal of monitoring and determining the need for additional treatment. They found the telemedicine platform not only to be highly sensitive and specific but also to be highly efficient.[46] While not necessary in programs designed to screen for AMD, OCT can provide significant advantages in the evaluation of higher risk cases, making the evaluation and monitoring of AMD possible.

OTHER RETINAL PATHOLOGY

Although diabetic retinopathy and AMD are by far the most prevalent retinal conditions screened for and evaluated via a telemedicine platform, a number of other retinal pathologies have been identified via teleretinal programs.[47]

Hypertensive Retinopathy, Myopic Degeneration, and Epiretinal Membranes

In many cases, other retinal pathologies have been identified incidentally during diabetic retinopathy screening examinations. Hypertensive retinopathy has been identified as one such pathology, with Mastropasqua et al. estimating hypertensive retinopathy to be present in 34.3% of all teleretinal examinations.[34,48] Mastropasqua et al.[48] also estimated evidence of myopic degeneration to be present in 2.5% of all diabetic screening examinations. Epiretinal membrane has also been described as an incidental finding identified during teleretinal DR screenings (Fig. 6.4).[34]

Acute Retinal Pathology

Ocular telehealth is not typically utilized in acute eye care. More details on this topic can be found in Chapter 17, Ocular Triage. Despite this, several reports

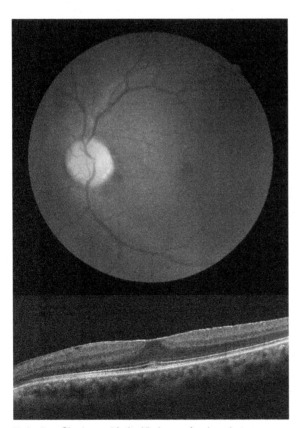

FIG. 6.4 Single mydriatic 45-degree fundus photo depicting epiretinal membrane (*top*) diagnosed via an ocular telehealth screening program and confirmed via in-person examination with OCT (*bottom*). (Credit: Photo by Stephanie J. Weiss, DO; Rhonda Ziegler, COA).

have suggested the potential of utilizing a telemedicine platform in acute care settings when in-person care might not be possible. McCord et al.[49] described a small series of retinal detachments that were diagnosed via the TECS platform initially designed to provide comprehensive and DR screening examinations. In these cases, the patients were triaged by primary care providers to require non-urgent eye care referrals, but the telemedicine program revealed acute retinal pathology requiring urgent management.[49] This suggests the potential benefit of teleretinal examinations to bridge the gap in providing acute care in rural and underserved settings where access to immediate in-person eye care might not be possible.[49] Similarly, Schallhorn et al.[50] described a case of a patient aboard a US Navy aircraft carrier being unable to receive in-person care who was diagnosed with syphilitic uveitis and acutely managed remotely via a modified telemedicine platform.

Choroidal Nevus

While choroidal nevi have been described as an incidental finding via pre-existing screening programs,[34] a telemedicine program specifically designed to monitor iris and choroidal nevi has also been described.[51] Given the obvious malignant potential associated with nevi, special care must be taken to ensure such programs are designed with all necessary diagnostic equipment and trained subspecialists to safely and effectively monitor high-risk or malignant features. Lapere et al.[51] described a tele-ocular oncology consultation service that included a trained ultrasound technician performing a- and b-scan ultrasounds, ultrasound biomicroscopy, along with standard fundus photography and OCT for a trained ocular oncologist to interpret the images. The program included monitoring of low-, medium- and high-risk iris and choroidal nevi and found 100% sensitivity and negative predictive value in evaluating such lesions.[51] While this type of program requires significantly more resources than most telemedicine programs in ophthalmology, this platform has the potential to provide critical subspecialty care to a population that might otherwise have limited access to highly subspecialized ophthalmologist providers (Fig. 6.5).[51]

CMV

As diabetic teleretinal screening clinics have been installed in primary care and endocrinology offices where systemic diabetic care is occurring, teleretinal cytomegalovirus (CMV) screening clinics have also been established in infectious disease (ID) clinics providing systemic human immunodeficiency virus (HIV) care. Jirawison et al.[52] described this type of program but

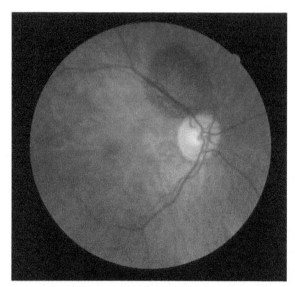

FIG. 6.5 Single mydriatic 45-degree fundus photo of a peripapillary choroidal nevus diagnosed via an ocular telehealth screening program. (Credit: Photo by Stephanie J. Weiss, DO; Rhonda Ziegler, COA).

found limited sensitivity in detecting the presence of CMV when utilizing 45-degree fundus photos montaged to cover an 85-degree field of view. In this case, the limited detection of CMV was attributed to small peripheral CMV lesions not captured on fundus images alone.[52] However, it was suggested that these types of screening programs can be beneficial in detecting immediately vision-threatening disease.[52] While there is likely some utility with a CMV teleretinal screening program for risk stratification and to determine the need for urgent referral, current evidence suggests telemedicine may be inadequate to replace in-person screening examinations entirely for this indication. Ultra-widefield images able to capture substantially more retina in a single image have the potential to significantly improve the sensitivity of these types of screening programs.

VIRTUAL MEDICAL RETINA CLINICS

As ocular telehealth programs have become more sophisticated, teleretinal programs have progressed from screening to platforms that allow for remote management of retinal pathology. This type of program typically relies on a trained retina specialist to evaluate and/or manage patients remotely in an asynchronous manner and utilizes fundus images and OCT. In some cases, remotely acquired images are reviewed by a retina specialist to evaluate for pathology and determine the most appropriate time frame for in-person referral, if necessary.[53–55] As with other telemedicine programs, this leads to increased compliance for resultant in-person examinations, reduces travel burden for patients, and improves access to retina specialists by increasing the number of in-person examination appointments.[53] Azzolini et al.[54] also demonstrated improved visual outcomes when patients with AMD were screened in a remote medical retina clinic prior to an in-person examination, likely secondary to improved efficiency in referring patients for in-person exam quickly when indicated.

Development of medical retina clinics via telemedicine has advanced significantly within the United Kingdom (UK).[55–57] Moorfields Eye Hospital has played a significant role in the continued innovation and implementation of virtual medical retina clinics.[56,57] Starting in 2016, Moorfields Eye Hospital sought to improve access to retina care via telemedicine and effectively allocate resources to patients requiring in-person care.[56,57] These virtual clinics use asynchronous telehealth methods, consisting of visual acuity measurements along with fundus imaging and OCT.[57] Patients were initially referred to participate in the virtual medical retina clinic from pre-existing in-person medical retina clinics or as new patients from the national diabetic retinopathy screening services (DRSS) program that was already well established in the UK.[57] After implementation, 70% of patients were considered appropriate for further virtual follow-up care, 15% of patients were discharged from the retina clinic, and only 15% of patients were referred for in-person care.[56] This underscores the potential for telemedicine to reduce the burden on in-person clinics and better provide access to patients requiring in-person management.

While most telemedicine medical retina clinics allow for retina specialists to remotely evaluate retinal pathology, programs have also been designed to allow retina specialists to work in conjunction with local ophthalmologists to manage patients remotely.[58] Starr et al. developed a program by which patients were initially seen by retina specialists for an in-person consultation.[58] After the initial visit, patients were managed by local ophthalmologists within the same network with the remote guidance of retina specialists via an asynchronous telemedicine platform by which retina specialists remotely reviewed imaging following each exam and made recommendations for the following visit.[58]

EXPANSION OF TELEHEALTH IN RETINA CARE IN THE ERA OF COVID-19

The effects of the COVID-19 pandemic have been felt throughout the medical field, with telemedicine playing an important role in providing access to care since there are limitations to in-person examinations. While the field of eye care has been an early adopter of telemedicine in general, the lack of readily available home monitoring equipment and the difficulty for patients to perform self-examinations prevented many retina specialists from utilizing home-based synchronous telehealth during the pandemic.[59] The success of most retina telehealth programs relies on imaging equipment capable of adequately capturing the fundus and a telehealth facilitator to perform this task. Without this capability, retinal telehealth programs are severely limited as diagnosis and management are so dependent on imaging.[60] In fact, ophthalmologists were found to be significantly less likely to adopt telemedicine visits than other surgical providers, with retina specialists being the least likely among all ophthalmologists.[59] However, telemedicine visits did increase during the COVID-19 pandemic, particularly at the beginning of the pandemic.[60] Aweidah et al. described their experience after their entire retina service was forced to quarantine for 2 weeks secondary to a COVID-19 exposure. During this time, retina specialists remotely reviewed OCT images and successfully directed non-retina ophthalmologists in the management of a variety of conditions including AMD, DME, and retinal vein occlusions.[61] While at home retinal care was limited, a survey of retina specialists during the pandemic revealed the use of home monitoring and teleretinal care (including remote history taking and triaging, virtual consultations or clinics, electronic referrals, and automated image analysis or decision making) had increased significantly, suggesting the potential for continued expansion within the field of teleretinal care even in a post-pandemic era.[62]

FUTURE DIRECTIONS OF TELEHEALTH IN RETINA CARE

The role of telemedicine in retinal care has expanded dramatically over the past two decades. As the indications for retina telehealth programs continue to grow to include a broader range of pathology, the utility of telemedicine will continue to progress. The integration of artificial intelligence (AI) with increasingly more sophisticated algorithms will allow for even better care going forward. More information regarding the development of AI in retina telehealthcare can be found in Chapter 18.

REFERENCES

1. Chee R-I, Darwish D, Fernandez-Vega A, et al. Retinal telemedicine. *Curr Ophthalmol Rep*. 2018;6(1):36–45. https://doi.org/10.1007/s40135-018-0161-8.
2. Li HK, Horton M, Bursell S-E, et al. Telehealth practice recommendations for diabetic retinopathy, second edition. *Telemed J E Health*. 2011;17(10):814–837. https://doi.org/10.1089/tmj.2011.0075.
3. Health Care Accreditation, Health Plan Accreditation Organization—NCQA. *NCQA*. Accessed 22.02.21 https://www.ncqa.org/.
4. Witkin SR, Klein R. Ophthalmologic care for persons with diabetes. *JAMA*. 1984;251(19):2534–2537.
5. Grading diabetic retinopathy from stereoscopic color fundus photographs—an extension of the modified Airlie House classification. ETDRS report number 10. Early treatment diabetic retinopathy study research group. *Ophthalmology*. 1991;98(5 Suppl):786–806.
6. Lin DY, Blumenkranz MS, Brothers RJ, Grosvenor DM. The sensitivity and specificity of single-field nonmydriatic monochromatic digital fundus photography with remote image interpretation for diabetic retinopathy screening: a comparison with ophthalmoscopy and standardized mydriatic color photography. *Am J Ophthalmol*. 2002;134(2):204–213. https://doi.org/10.1016/s0002-9394(02)01522-2.
7. Sanchez CR, Silva PS, Cavallerano JD, Aiello LP, Aiello LM. Ocular telemedicine for diabetic retinopathy and the Joslin Vision Network. *Semin Ophthalmol*. 2010;25(5–6):218–224. https://doi.org/10.3109/08820538.2010.518893.
8. Cavallerano AA, Cavallerano JD, Katalinic P, et al. Use of Joslin Vision Network digital-video nonmydriatic retinal imaging to assess diabetic retinopathy in a clinical program. *Retina*. 2003;23(2):215–223. https://doi.org/10.1097/00006982-200304000-00013.
9. Silva PS, Horton MB, Clary D, et al. Identification of diabetic retinopathy and ungradable image rate with ultrawide field imaging in a national teleophthalmology program. *Ophthalmology*. 2016;123(6):1360–1367. https://doi.org/10.1016/j.ophtha.2016.01.043.
10. Kirkizlar E, Serban N, Sisson JA, Swann JL, Barnes CS, Williams MD. Evaluation of telemedicine for screening of diabetic retinopathy in the Veterans Health Administration. *Ophthalmology*. 2013;120(12):2604–2610. https://doi.org/10.1016/j.ophtha.2013.06.029.
11. Maa AY, Wojciechowski B, Hunt K, Dismuke C, Janjua R, Lynch MG. Remote eye care screening for rural veterans with technology-based eye care services: a quality improvement project. *Rural Remote Health*. 2017;17(1):4045. https://doi.org/10.22605/rrh4045.
12. Maa AY, Medert CM, Lu X, et al. Diagnostic accuracy of technology-based eye care services: the technology-based eye care services compare trial part I. *Ophthalmology*. 2020;127(1):38–44. https://doi.org/10.1016/j.ophtha.2019.07.026.
13. Cuadros J, Bresnick G. EyePACS: an adaptable telemedicine system for diabetic retinopathy screening. *J Diabetes Sci Technol*. 2009;3(3):509–516. https://doi.org/10.1177/193229680900300315.

14. Zimmer-Galler I, Zeimer R. Results of implementation of the DigiScope for diabetic retinopathy assessment in the primary care environment. *Telemed J E Health*. 2006;12(2):89–98. https://doi.org/10.1089/tmj.2006.12.89.

15. Scanlon PH. The English National Screening Programme for diabetic retinopathy 2003–2016. *Acta Diabetol*. 2017;54(6):515–525. https://doi.org/10.1007/s00592-017-0974-1.

16. Bodnar ZM, Schuchard R, Myung D, et al. Evaluating New Ophthalmic Digital Devices for Safety and Effectiveness in the Context of Rapid Technological Development. *JAMA Ophthalmol*. 2019;137(8):939–944. https://doi.org/10.1001/jamaophthalmol.2019.1576.

17. Shi L, Wu H, Dong J, Jiang K, Lu X, Shi J. Telemedicine for detecting diabetic retinopathy: a systematic review and meta-analysis. *Br J Ophthalmol*. 2015;99(6):823–831. https://doi.org/10.1136/bjophthalmol-2014-305631.

18. Ullah W, Pathan SK, Panchal A, et al. Cost-effectiveness and diagnostic accuracy of telemedicine in macular disease and diabetic retinopathy: a systematic review and meta-analysis. *Medicine (Baltimore)*. 2020;99(25): e20306. https://doi.org/10.1097/MD.0000000000020306.

19. Bastos de Carvalho A, Ware SL, Lei F, Bush HM, Sprang R, Higgins EB. Implementation and sustainment of a statewide telemedicine diabetic retinopathy screening network for federally designated safety-net clinics. *PLoS One*. 2020;15(11): e0241767. https://doi.org/10.1371/journal.pone.0241767.

20. Yaslam M, Al Adel F, Al-Rubeaan K, et al. Non-mydriatic fundus camera screening with diagnosis by telemedicine for diabetic retinopathy patients with type 1 and type 2 diabetes: a hospital-based cross-sectional study. *Ann Saudi Med*. 2019;39(5):328–336. https://doi.org/10.5144/0256-4947.2019.328.

21. Boucher MC, Qian J, Brent MH, et al. Evidence-based Canadian guidelines for tele-retina screening for diabetic retinopathy: recommendations from the Canadian Retina Research Network (CR2N) Tele-Retina Steering Committee. *Can J Ophthalmol*. 2020;55(1 Suppl. 1):14–24. https://doi.org/10.1016/j.jcjo.2020.01.001.

22. Soliman AZ, Silva PS, Aiello LP, Sun JK. Ultra-wide field retinal imaging in detection, classification, and management of diabetic retinopathy. *Semin Ophthalmol*. 2012;27(5–6):221–227. https://doi.org/10.3109/08820538.2012.708812.

23. Kernt M, Hadi I, Pinter F, et al. Assessment of diabetic retinopathy using nonmydriatic ultra-widefield scanning laser ophthalmoscopy (Optomap) compared with ETDRS 7-field stereo photography. *Diabetes Care*. 2012;35(12):2459–2463. https://doi.org/10.2337/dc12-0346.

24. Hussain N, Edraki M, Tahhan R, et al. Telemedicine for diabetic retinopathy screening using an ultra-widefield fundus camera. *Clin Ophthalmol*. 2017;11:1477–1482. https://doi.org/10.2147/OPTH.S135287.

25. Afshar AR, Oldenburg CE, Stewart JM. A novel hybrid fixed and mobile ultra-widefield imaging program for diabetic teleretinopathy screening. *Ophthalmol Retina*. 2019;3(7):576–579. https://doi.org/10.1016/j.oret.2019.03.007.

26. Wang YT, Tadarati M, Wolfson Y, Bressler SB, Bressler NM. Comparison of prevalence of diabetic macular edema based on monocular fundus photography vs optical coherence tomography. *JAMA Ophthalmol*. 2016;134(2):222–228. https://doi.org/10.1001/jamaophthalmol.2015.5332.

27. Sanborn GE, Wroblewski JJ. Evaluation of a combination digital retinal camera with spectral-domain optical coherence tomography (SD-OCT) that might be used for the screening of diabetic retinopathy with telemedicine: a pilot study. *J Diabetes Complicat*. 2018;32(11):1046–1050. https://doi.org/10.1016/j.jdiacomp.2018.08.010.

28. Felfeli T, Alon R, Merritt R, Brent MH. Toronto tele-retinal screening program for detection of diabetic retinopathy and macular edema. *Can J Ophthalmol*. 2019;54(2):203–211. https://doi.org/10.1016/j.jcjo.2018.07.004.

29. Maa AY, McCord S, Lu X, et al. The impact of OCT on diagnostic accuracy of the technology-based eye care services protocol: part II of the technology-based eye care services compare trial. *Ophthalmology*. 2020;127(4):544–549. https://doi.org/10.1016/j.ophtha.2019.10.025.

30. O'Halloran RA, Turner AW. Evaluating the impact of optical coherence tomography in diabetic retinopathy screening for an Aboriginal population. *Clin Exp Ophthalmol*. 2018;46(2):116–121. https://doi.org/10.1111/ceo.13018.

31. Stebbins K, Kieltyka S, Chaum E. Follow-up compliance for patients diagnosed with diabetic retinopathy after teleretinal imaging in primary care. *Telemed J E Health*. Mar 2021;303–307. https://doi.org/10.1089/tmj.2019.0264. Published online June 15.

32. Bursell S-E, Fonda SJ, Lewis DG, Horton MB. Prevalence of diabetic retinopathy and diabetic macular edema in a primary care-based teleophthalmology program for American Indians and Alaskan Natives. *PLoS One*. 2018;13(6). https://doi.org/10.1371/journal.pone.0198551, e0198551.

33. Martinez JA, Parikh PD, Wong RW, et al. Telemedicine for diabetic retinopathy screening in an urban, insured population using fundus cameras in a primary care office setting. *Ophthalmic Surg Lasers Imaging Retina*. 2019;50(11):e274–e277. https://doi.org/10.3928/23258160-20191031-14.

34. Gao X, Park CH, Dedrick K, et al. Use of telehealth screening to detect diabetic retinopathy and other ocular findings in primary care settings. *Telemed J E Health*. 2019;25(9):802–807. https://doi.org/10.1089/tmj.2018.0016.

35. Choremis J, Chow DR. Use of telemedicine in screening for diabetic retinopathy. *Can J Ophthalmol*. 2003;38(7):575–579. https://doi.org/10.1016/s0008-4182(03)80111-4.

36. Daskivich LP, Vasquez C, Martinez C, Tseng C-H, Mangione CM. Implementation and evaluation of a large-scale teleretinal diabetic retinopathy screening program in the Los Angeles County Department of Health Services. *JAMA Intern Med*. 2017;177(5):642–649. https://doi.org/10.1001/jamainternmed.2017.0204.

37. Nanji K, Kherani IN, Damji KF, Nyenze M, Kiage D, Tennant MT. The muranga teleophthalmology study: a comparison of virtual (teleretina) assessment with in-person clinical examination to diagnose diabetic retinopathy and age-related macular degeneration in Kenya.

Middle East Afr J Ophthalmol. 2020;27(2):91–99. https://doi.org/10.4103/meajo.MEAJO_144_19.

38. Avendaño-Veloso A, Parada-Hernández F, González-Ramos R, Dougnac-Osses C, Carrasco-Sáez JL, Scanlon PH. Teleophthalmology: a strategy for timely diagnosis of sight-threatening diabetic retinopathy in primary care, Concepción, Chile. *Int J Ophthalmol.* 2019;12(9):1474–1478. https://doi.org/10.18240/ijo.2019.09.16.

39. Toy BC, Aguinaldo T, Eliason J, Egbert J. Non-mydriatic fundus camera screening for referral-warranted diabetic retinopathy in a Northern California safety-net setting. *Ophthalmic Surg Lasers Imaging Retina.* 2016;47(7):636–642. https://doi.org/10.3928/23258160-20160707-05.

40. Korn Malerbi F, Lelis Dal Fabbro A, Botelho Vieira Filho JP, Franco LJ. The feasibility of smartphone based retinal photography for diabetic retinopathy screening among Brazilian Xavante Indians. *Diabetes Res Clin Pract.* 2020;168:108380. https://doi.org/10.1016/j.diabres.2020.108380.

41. Matimba A, Woodward R, Tambo E, Ramsay M, Gwanzura L, Guramatunhu S. Tele-ophthalmology: opportunities for improving diabetes eye care in resource- and specialist-limited Sub-Saharan African countries. *J Telemed Telecare.* 2016;22(5):311–316. https://doi.org/10.1177/1357633X15604083.

42. Joseph S, Kim R, Ravindran RD, Fletcher AE, Ravilla TD. Effectiveness of teleretinal imaging-based hospital referral compared with universal referral in identifying diabetic retinopathy: a cluster randomized clinical trial. *JAMA Ophthalmol.* 2019;137(7):786–792. https://doi.org/10.1001/jamaophthalmol.2019.1070.

43. Chasan JE, Delaune B, Maa AY, Lynch MG. Effect of a teleretinal screening program on eye care use and resources. *JAMA Ophthalmol.* 2014;132(9):1045–1051. https://doi.org/10.1001/jamaophthalmol.2014.1051.

44. Duchin KS, Asefzadeh B, Poulaki V, Rett D, Marescalchi P, Cavallerano A. Teleretinal imaging for detection of referable macular degeneration. *Optom Vis Sci.* 2015;92(6):714–718. https://doi.org/10.1097/OPX.0000000000000598.

45. Li B, Powell A-M, Hooper PL, Sheidow TG. Prospective evaluation of teleophthalmology in screening and recurrence monitoring of neovascular age-related macular degeneration: a randomized clinical trial. *JAMA Ophthalmol.* 2015;133(3):276–282. https://doi.org/10.1001/jamaophthalmol.2014.5014.

46. Andonegui J, Aliseda D, Serrano L, et al. Evaluation of a telemedicine model to follow up patients with exudative age-related macular degeneration. *Retina.* 2016;36(2):279–284. https://doi.org/10.1097/IAE.0000000000000729.

47. Maa AY, Patel S, Chasan JE, Delaune W, Lynch MG. Retrospective evaluation of a teleretinal screening program in detecting multiple nondiabetic eye diseases. *Telemed J E Health.* 2017;23(1):41–48. https://doi.org/10.1089/tmj.2016.0039.

48. Mastropasqua L, Perilli R, D'Aloisio R, et al. Why miss the chance? incidental findings while telescreening for diabetic retinopathy. *Ophthalmic Epidemiol.* 2020;27(4):237–245. https://doi.org/10.1080/09286586.2020.1715450.

49. McCord SA, Lynch MG, Maa AY. Diagnosis of retinal detachments by a tele-ophthalmology screening program. *J Telemed Telecare.* 2019;25(3):190–192. https://doi.org/10.1177/1357633X18760418.

50. Schallhorn CS, Richmond CJ, Schallhorn JM. Military teleconsultation services facilitate prompt recognition and treatment of a case of syphilitic uveitis aboard a United States navy aircraft carrier at sea during combat operations without evacuation capability. *Telemed J E Health.* 2020;26(6):821–826. https://doi.org/10.1089/tmj.2019.0059.

51. Lapere S, Weis E. Tele-ophthalmology for the monitoring of choroidal and iris nevi: a pilot study. *Can J Ophthalmol.* 2018;53(5):471–473. https://doi.org/10.1016/j.jcjo.2017.11.021.

52. Jirawison C, Yen M, Leenasirimakul P, et al. Telemedicine screening for cytomegalovirus retinitis at the point of care for human immunodeficiency virus infection. *JAMA Ophthalmol.* 2015;133(2):198–205. https://doi.org/10.1001/jamaophthalmol.2014.4766.

53. Hanson C, Tennant MTS, Rudnisky CJ. Optometric referrals to retina specialists: evaluation and triage via teleophthalmology. *Telemed J E Health.* 2008;14(5):441–445. https://doi.org/10.1089/tmj.2007.0068.

54. Azzolini C, Torreggiani A, Eandi C, et al. A teleconsultation network improves the efficacy of anti-VEGF therapy in retinal diseases. *J Telemed Telecare.* 2013;19(8):437–442. https://doi.org/10.1177/1357633X13501760.

55. Amoaku W, Bailey C, Downey L, et al. Providing a safe and effective intravitreal treatment service: strategies for service delivery. *Clin Ophthalmol.* 2020;14:1315–1328. https://doi.org/10.2147/OPTH.S233061.

56. Kern C, Kortuem K, Hamilton R, et al. Clinical outcomes of a hospital-based teleophthalmology service: what happens to patients in a virtual clinic? *Ophthalmol Retina.* 2019;3(5):422–428. https://doi.org/10.1016/j.oret.2019.01.011.

57. Kortuem K, Fasler K, Charnley A, et al. Implementation of medical retina virtual clinics in a tertiary eye care referral centre. *Br J Ophthalmol.* 2018;102(10):1391–1395. https://doi.org/10.1136/bjophthalmol-2017-311494.

58. Starr MR, Barkmeier AJ, Engman SJ, Kitzmann A, Bakri SJ. Telemedicine in the management of exudative age-related macular degeneration within an integrated health care system. *Am J Ophthalmol.* 2019;208:206–210. https://doi.org/10.1016/j.ajo.2019.03.021.

59. Aguwa UT, Aguwa CJ, Repka M, et al. Teleophthalmology in the era of COVID-19: characteristics of early adopters at a large academic institution. *Telemed J E Health.* Jul 2021;739–746. https://doi.org/10.1089/tmj.2020.0372. Published online October 16.

60. Portney DS, Zhu Z, Chen EM, et al. COVID-19 and utilization of teleophthalmology: trends and diagnoses (CUT Group). *Ophthalmology.* 2021. https://doi.org/10.1016/j.ophtha.2021.02.010. Published online February 10.

61. Aweidah H, Safadi K, Jotkowitz A, Chowers I, Levy J. Hybrid telehealth medical retina clinic due to provider exposure and quarantine during COVID-19 pandemic. *Clin Ophthalmol.* 2020;14:3421–3426. https://doi.org/10.2147/OPTH.S276276.

62. Faes L, Rosenblatt A, Schwartz R, et al. Overcoming barriers of retinal care delivery during a pandemic-attitudes and drivers for the implementation of digital health: a global expert survey. *Br J Ophthalmol.* 2020. https://doi.org/10.1136/bjophthalmol-2020-316882. Published online October 16.

CHAPTER 7

Pediatric Ocular Telehealth

ANKOOR S. SHAH, MD, PHD • R.V. PAUL CHAN, MD, MSC, MBA

INTRODUCTION

Telehealth in pediatric ophthalmology has a long history, beginning with asynchronous retinopathy of prematurity screening programs.[1-6] Over time, the field has expanded to include synchronous videos and direct-to-home activities such as patient-to-provider visits,[7] which gained popularity during the initial phases of the novel coronavirus pandemic (COVID-19) that started in 2020.[8-11] This chapter reviews the various cases of ocular telehealth use in pediatric ophthalmology and gives the reader a point of reference for establishing similar programs.

PATIENT-TO-PROVIDER TELEHEALTH

Patient-to-provider telehealth in pediatric ophthalmology may be subcategorized into three distinct entities as mentioned in Chapter 1: synchronous, hybrid, and asynchronous telehealth visits.

Synchronous Telehealth Visit Structure

Synchronous telehealth visits are conducted with real-time audio and video connections between a patient and a provider. In pediatric ophthalmology, the visit will include the patient, parents or guardians, and the provider. It may also include other professionals important for the child's care such as occupational and physical therapists, developmental specialists from early intervention programs, or a teacher for the visually impaired. Essentially, synchronous telehealth visits mimic the traditional in-person visits.

A synchronous telehealth visit in pediatric ophthalmology is structured similarly to an in-person encounter. Historical information, virtual examination, and time for counseling are key components, and the order of these components may vary based on the situation. For example, in cases where the child is young, performing an examination immediately after understanding the chief complaint may be preferred before the novelty of the virtual format wears off and the child becomes uncooperative.

In pediatric ophthalmology, the history of a patient in a synchronous telehealth visit is obtained in a manner similar to the traditional in-person visit. Parents or guardians are asked to offer their reasons for the visit, their observations, and their concerns in an open-ended format, followed by more focused questioning from the telehealth provider. Additional key players such as other professionals accompanying the visit may also provide key historical content. These elements of patient history are critical to record in the visit note as would be done for an in-person visit.

Ocular Telehealth. https://doi.org/10.1016/B978-0-323-83204-5.00007-X

Virtual examination in a synchronous telehealth visit in pediatric ophthalmology is the next key component of the encounter.[9] It begins with observation of the child, assessing age, stature, posture, and facial structure by inspection. Additionally, visual behavior may be ascertained by watching the child engage in the video screen, parents, guardians, siblings, pets, or toys in the environment. In older children, a virtual evaluation of the vision may be possible.[12–14] Various other aspects of the eye-focused physical examination may be elucidated using the guidance provided in Table 7.1.

The counseling portion of a synchronous telehealth visit in pediatric ophthalmology is the last component. As in an in-person visit, the telehealth provider will give a synopsis of the findings and how they relate to the chief complaint and historical elements. The provider should also suggest next steps, including urgent or non-urgent follow-up, testing, glasses, medications, and further medical or surgical therapy. Parental or guardian questions are also a part of this aspect of the synchronous telehealth visit.

TABLE 7.1

Maneuvers That May be Used to Conduct a Virtual Examination for a Synchronous Telehealth Visit Between a Patient and a Provider in Pediatric Ophthalmology

Element	Suggested Virtual Maneuver
Visual acuity	Infant/toddler
	Check fixate and follow with parent or sibling holding toys
	Screen share age-appropriate videos and observe the child's fixation behavior
	Observe differences in response to occlusion
	Verbal child
	Ask child to describe items around the room with both eyes and each eye individually
	Older child/teenager/adult
	Ask patient to read items across the room and give a report of their relative visual acuity
	Screen share a visual acuity chart and understand relative acuity between eyes
	Downloadable applications for checking visual acuity
Color vision	Ask the patient to do a subjective red desaturation
Confrontation visual field testing	Best when the patient is using a computer rather than a mobile phone for a wider display
	Attempt patient self-administration (subjective)
	Perform counting fingers or double simultaneous stimulation tasks
	Present an Amsler grid via video camera or screen share
Pupils	Observe
	Enhance with a flashlight if needed
	Relative afferent pupillary defect testing may be possible with an assistant
External examination	Observe under appropriate lighting
	Check for erythema, eyelid position and movement, margin-to-reflex distance, symmetry (or asymmetry) of skin folds, etc.
	Estimate proptosis via "worm's-eye" view
Eyelids and adnexa	Observe by bringing the eye close to the camera
	Ask the patient to lift the lids and look down to observe the lacrimal gland
	Ask the patient to evert the lower eyelids by pulling down and looking up

TABLE 7.1 Maneuvers That May be Used to Conduct a Virtual Examination for a Synchronous Telehealth Visit Between a Patient and a Provider in Pediatric Ophthalmology—cont'd	
Element	**Suggested Virtual Maneuver**
Anterior segment	Observe
	Enhance observation with external lighting if needed; light reflex testing can show health of the ocular surface
	Side illumination (as for Rizzuti sign in keratoconus) gives views into the anterior chamber and at the lens
Ocular motility	Utilize a parent or sibling to move a toy in the case of young children
	Ask the patient to look in all directions of gaze
	Observe doll's head maneuvers initiated by parents while by the child fixates on the screen or a movie via screen share
	Ask the patient to conduct smooth pursuit and saccadic eye movements
Eye alignment	Observe the corneal light reflex in different directions of gaze
	Ask the parent or the patient to assist with cover-uncover and cross-cover testing; estimate the deviation
	Ask the patient to describe the relative separation in diplopic images in directions of gaze

Adapted from with permission Bowe T, Hunter DG, Mantagos IS, et al. Virtual visits in ophthalmology: timely advice for implementation during the COVID-19 public health crisis. *Telemed J E Health*. 2020;26:1113–1117.

Synchronous Telehealth Visit Types

Synchronous telehealth visits may be conducted for new, return, preoperative, and postoperative visit types in pediatric ophthalmology.[7,8] For new visits, the substantial advantages of a synchronous telehealth visit include a detailed history, a quick virtual examination, and counseling focused on the next steps of care. For example, a newborn baby with a "tumor" on the surface of the eye may be determined quickly to have a limbal dermoid and scheduled for in-person evaluation within the next few weeks instead of an immediate evaluation. A new-onset esotropia in a 5-year-old child may confirm the presence of the esotropia and prompt an immediate in-person visit, and a new adult strabismus patient with a long history of prior surgery may be evaluated to review prior procedures and to understand the goal of further surgery for that patient. Each of these new-patient encounters represents using telehealth for appropriate triaging prior to in-person encounters (which are often difficult to access) and may allow for more streamlined subsequent visits.

Return synchronous telehealth visits may help understand the effect of treatment initiated during a previous visit or may serve as a check-in for a patient. For example, a child with anisometropic amblyopia-prescribed glasses and/or patching therapy may be evaluated via a synchronous telehealth visit to check whether adherence to the treatment plan is achieved. Moreover, if the child is old enough, a virtual evaluation of the vision may be possible using a variety of methods.[12–14] Even when not fully accurate, the testing of visual acuity in an amblyope may allow the telehealth provider to understand the difference between the two eyes, which in turn may gauge the progress of treatment. A return visit might also be considered for an acquired, accommodative esotropia patient for whom full-time glasses therapy has been prescribed. A quick check-in may ensure that the child has started wearing the glasses and has improvement in eye alignment.

Preoperative synchronous telehealth visits may be useful to reassess the child (or adult strabismus patient) prior to surgery and explain the surgical process to patients, parents, and guardians. The utility of this visit type often comes in the ability to allow the child to "go play" if the patient is at home, thereby allowing the parent or guardian to concentrate on the conversation. Images or a blank canvas upon which to draw may be displayed by the telehealth provider via screen share to augment the surgical counseling.

Finally, postoperative synchronous telehealth visits may serve as a useful check-in. Questions from patients and families about the healing process often arise, and these questions may be evaluated and answered by the telehealth provider. Additionally, the provider may be able to ascertain whether the patient is following the normal postoperative healing process quickly by a visualization of the eye(s) instead of an in-person encounter that takes more time for all parties.

Webside Manner

Webside manner is an important consideration in conducting a successful synchronous telehealth visit.[9,15–17] It begins with best practices for an optimal visit, which are outlined in Table 7.2,[9] and it proceeds with the typical aspects of an in-person encounter as follows:[17]

1. Establish a relationship
   a. Convey respect with a welcome and an introduction of all parties;
   b. Collaborate to set an agenda for the virtual visit;
   c. Introduce the features of the device and platform as necessary;
   d. Demonstrate empathy;
2. Develop the relationship
   a. Elicit the patient and parent/guardian history and concerns;
   b. Actively listen;
   c. Validate emotions;
3. Engage the relationship
   a. Offer diagnosis and treatment options;
   b. Contextualize the conversation from the patient's perspective;
   c. Engage the patient in the next steps.

Confidence on the part of the telehealth provider that the virtual encounter will be successful is also critical to convey to the patient. "Success" of the visit may vary

TABLE 7.2
Best Practices for a Successful Synchronous Telehealth Visit

Tip	Specifications and Reasoning
Position the device on a stable surface at eye level	Maximizes resolution
	Stabilization minimizes the number of pixels that need to refresh continuously
	Improves viewing angle and contrast
Have good lighting	Natural lighting on the face and eyes is ideal
	Accurately represents coloration and contrast of the skin and conjunctiva
	Maximizes resolution
	Indoor lighting and flashlights on mobile devices can be used as substitutes
	Avoid backlighting
Speak slowly and clearly	Transmission to patients and guardians will be most clear
Introduce everyone	Introduction of the provider and care team is critical to ensure transparency to the patient
	Introduction of the key patient-side participants allows the provider to understand the roles of each person involved in the care of the child
Positioning	Infant/toddler: Parent's lap or high chair
	Child: Lap, chair, or seat
	Teenager/adult: Table, chair, or couch
Use nonverbal cues	Alter facial expressions as you would during normal conversations
	Move closer and further from the video camera to mimic leaning in to listen or to examine
	Use intonations in voice to convey different feelings, such as active listening, empathy, and emphasis
	Make sure that hand gestures are made above the chest level to ensure that they are seen
Look at the camera when counseling	Gives the patient and guardian the impression that you are making eye contact

Modified from Bowe T, Hunter DG, Mantagos IS, et al. Virtual visits in ophthalmology: timely advice for implementation during the COVID-19 public health crisis. *Telemed J E Health*. 2020;26:1113–1117.

depending on the scenario; for example, a virtual visit that identifies a problem that needs an emergent or urgent follow-up in-person encounter may still be successful if the patient is examined in person in a timely manner. Patients also genuinely appreciate the dedicated time that the telehealth provider sets aside for their agenda.[18]

Diagnoses Amenable to a Synchronous Telehealth Encounter

Synchronous telehealth visits may be useful in a wide variety of diagnostic situations in pediatric ophthalmology. In some cases, these visits may be sufficient to reassure a patient and parent/guardian; in other cases, these visits may prompt an emergent, urgent, or routine follow-up in-person encounter. The key to keeping patients safe in using the synchronous telehealth encounter is to convert it to the traditional in-person visit when either the patient or the telehealth provider is uncomfortable with any aspect of the virtual visit.

Amblyopia and strabismus, the bread and butter of pediatric ophthalmology, are two diagnoses amenable to synchronous telehealth visits. For example, new patients failing a vision screening test at a pediatrician's office or at school may benefit from a near-immediate synchronous telehealth visit. This initial visit may be used to gather the history, review the failed vision screening document (which often contains the refraction data from a photoscreener), screen visual acuity,[12–14] obtain basic examination elements (Table 7.1), and discuss an appropriately timed in-person encounter. One might consider using these visits to direct patients appropriately toward optometric, orthoptic, or ophthalmologic appointments, and these near-immediate visits may alleviate anxiety among patients and referring providers, thereby improving quality of care.

Pediatric ophthalmology often also encompasses many comprehensive ophthalmological problems. Thus, synchronous telehealth encounters may be useful in diseases of the adnexa, orbit, anterior and posterior segments, and optic nerve as outlined in Table 7.3. Additionally, some real-world examples are shown in Fig. 7.1.

TABLE 7.3
Suggested Scenarios for Synchronous Telehealth Encounters in Pediatric Ophthalmology

Amblyopia and ocular motility

Failed vision screen	Triage, diagnose, and recommend the next steps in a child who failed vision screening
Amblyopia	Evaluate adherence to treatment plan (i.e., glasses and patching/atropine therapy)
	Evaluate response to therapy using virtual visual acuity measurement
Strabismus	Triage new patient with suspected strabismus
	Evaluate response to therapy glasses for an established patient with strabismus (i.e., intermittent exotropia or accommodative esotropia)
	Postoperative evaluation of eye alignment and healing
Cranial nerve palsy/Diplopia	Triage, diagnose, and initiate the next steps in treatment
	Evaluate whether prescribed prism therapy is working
	Understand recovery of muscle function after entrapment
Nystagmus	Triage, diagnose, and determine the next steps in evaluation and treatment

Ocular adnexa and orbit

Blepharitis	Triage, diagnose, and initiate therapy in a patient with eye irritation
	Evaluate response to therapy from prior in-person visit
Chalazion	Triage, diagnose, and initiate therapy
	Evaluate response to therapy from prior in-person visit
Eyelid lesion	Triage, diagnose, and initiate treatment
	Evaluate postsurgical healing, counsel, and review pathology

Continued

TABLE 7.3
Suggested Scenarios for Synchronous Telehealth Encounters in Pediatric Ophthalmology—cont'd

Ocular adnexa and orbit continued	
Ptosis	Triage, diagnose, and initiate treatment plan
	Evaluate postsurgical healing and counsel
Thyroid eye disease	Evaluate ocular motility, proptosis, visual acuity, and anterior segment appearance
Preseptal cellulitis	Triage, diagnose, and initiate therapy
	Evaluate treatment efficacy
Orbital cellulitis	Triage, diagnose, and initiate the next steps in treatment
	Evaluate treatment efficacy after medical or surgical management
Anterior segment	
Dry eye syndrome	Triage, diagnose, and initiate therapy in a patient with eye irritation
	Evaluate response to therapy from prior in-person visit
Subconjunctival hemorrhage	Triage, diagnose, and determine necessity for immediate evaluation
	Evaluate resolution of pain, redness, and irritation from prior visit
Allergic, viral, or bacterial conjunctivitis	Triage, diagnose, and initiate treatment
	Evaluate response to treatment
Corneal abrasion	Evaluate for corneal opacification that might signify infection
	Evaluate resolution of pain, redness, and irritation after initiation of treatment
	Evaluate corneal light reflex to check whether the reflex is sharp (and thus the abrasion healed)
Iritis (non-juvenile idiopathic arthritis related)	Evaluate response to therapy by inspecting for redness, pain, and photophobia
Posterior segment and optic nerve	
Idiopathic intracranial hypertension	Evaluate adherence to treatment plan and recurrence/worsening of symptoms
Optic neuropathy	Evaluate follow-up subjective and objective visual function, including acuity, color vision, and visual field
Anisocoria	Triage, diagnose, and initiate the next steps in evaluation

Many scenarios span various subspecialties in ophthalmology, and thus further information about the approach to those cases is available in the other chapters of this book. Moreover, none of the suggestions here supersede sound clinical judgment, and the synchronous telehealth encounter is NOT a replacement for in-person encounters but an adjunct.

Evidence for Efficacy of Care Delivery and for Patient Satisfaction

Early studies show that synchronous telehealth visits in pediatric ophthalmology are successful from both the provider and patient perspectives. For the provider, one study examined 57 synchronous telehealth encounters conducted prior to the COVID-19 pandemic.[7] Visits included 37 strabismus cases, 7 ocular surface conditions, and 13 orbital/periorbital-related concerns. An immediate postvisit survey asked the provider to rate the visit as "very effective," "somewhat effective," "somewhat ineffective," or "very ineffective." A total of 36 completed surveys (55% completion rate) were submitted,

and the providers rated these visits as effective in 91% of cases with 72% classified as "very effective" and 19% classified as "effective."

Patient-side evaluations of synchronous telehealth visits are equally good. In the aforementioned study, patients were also provided with a survey immediately after the visits. The median patient satisfaction with the appointment was 9 on a scale of 1 to 10, with 10 being excellent.[7] Patients noted convenience, efficiency, and improved access to care as the benefits of these types of visits, and all patients indicated that they would be likely to schedule another synchronous telehealth encounter. Similarly, a study of 219 synchronous

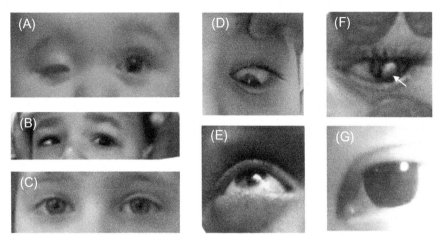

FIG. 7.1 Screen-capture images from synchronous telehealth visits, illustrating the various diagnoses amenable to care via this modality. (A) A 10-month-old child with right anophthalmia being treated with a hydrogel expander. Eyelid positioning and orbital expansion may be estimated by observation. (B) A 23-month-old child with a left sixth abducens nerve palsy demonstrated by a gentle doll's head maneuver performed by his mother. (C) A 5-year-old child at postoperative month 3 status post botulinum toxin injection for an acute sixth abducens nerve palsy caused by an ependymoma. Light reflex evaluation and parental cross-cover testing showed no misalignment in primary gaze. (D) An 11-year-old boy elevates his eyelid during evaluation of the superior limbus for a flare of vernal keratoconjunctivitis. (E) A 16-year-old, developmentally delayed, young man with tearing 3 weeks after cataract surgery. Oblique viewing and illumination highlights the anterior chamber, which appears free of gross hypopyon or significant fibrinous debris. There is also a reassuring lack of perilimbal injection. (F) A 9-month-old girl with a congenital cataract shows a maintained central red reflex. The parents used a smart phone with the flash illuminator constantly on (flashlight mode) to capture the image live, which indicated no significant progression of the lens opacity located inferior temporally (arrow) in comparison to the last office visit evaluation. (G) A 16-year-old young woman with eczema diagnosed with a central cataract in the setting of subacutely diminished vision. (Modified from Areaux RG, Jr., de Alba Campomanes AG, Indaram M, et al. Your eye doctor will virtually see you now: synchronous patient-to-provider virtual visits in pediatric tele-ophthalmology. *J AAPOS*. 2020;24(4):197–203.)

telehealth visits in pediatric ophthalmology during the COVID-19 pandemic showed 82% of patients were either satisfied or very satisfied with their visit.[19] These patients elaborated that the technology worked well and appreciated the convenience, and one commented, "A telehealth appointment is superior to no appointment at all," which highlights that patients value the ability to connect with a provider regardless of whether the provider can perform all of the detailed examinations of the in-person visits.

Hybrid Telehealth Visits

As mentioned in Chapter 1, hybrid telehealth visits combine asynchronous data capture with synchronous interactions between the patient and the provider. In pediatric ophthalmology, asynchronous data capture may include a technician visit to obtain visual acuity, stereoacuity, color vision, intraocular pressure, formal visual field, or anterior and posterior segment photo-graphic images. It may also involve an orthoptist visit to obtain a comprehensive sensorimotor evaluation or a prism fit for diplopia, and it may involve a radiology visit to obtain magnetic resonance imaging for neurological concerns or orbital evaluations. These clinical data are subsequently used in a synchronous meeting with the patient and care takers to discuss the results and to provide ongoing management. For example, visual acuity and stereoacuity may be helpful in managing amblyopia and determining whether previously initiated patching or atropine penalization therapy is working. Color vision, visual field testing, and posterior segment imaging of the optic nerve may be used to counsel patients subsequently in a synchronous visit about ongoing management of idiopathic intracranial hypertension or other potential optic neuropathies. Sensorimotor evaluations may be used to understand whether an intervention such as glasses therapy or prism fitting is working or whether strabismus surgery may be necessary. Essentially, many of the scenarios mentioned in Table 7.3 may be evaluated and managed through a hybrid approach.

Asynchronous Telehealth

Asynchronous telehealth in pediatric ophthalmology is yet another means of increasing patient access to eye-care providers. These communications are typically initiated by the patient as a message followed by a response from the provider, but the reverse scenario may also be useful in clinical practice. These communications may entail a text-based message alone or text and images together, and the communication should be based within a secure patient portal. The purpose of these encounters may be expansive, including questions about management, such as how many hours per day to perform patching therapy, an update on eye healing and alignment after strabismus surgery, an evaluation of allergic conjunctivitis or chalazion treatment, or a request for refill of chronic medication such as atropine. In strabismus specifically, numerous applications (9 gaze, See Vision, LLC; EyeTurn, EyePhone, LLC; StrabisPix, Boston Children's Hospital) for assessment and measurement of eye alignment are showing promise in clinical practice.[20-22] These applications guide patients through self-capture of eye images, ocular alignment, and motility. The prescribed capture technique has the advantage of standardizing the patient submission, thereby maximizing the utility of the images and then helping providers counsel patients on the next steps.

PROVIDER-TO-PROVIDER TELEHEALTH

Teleconsultations between non-ophthalmic and ophthalmic providers in the field of retinopathy of prematurity (ROP) are some of the earliest examples of ocular telehealth in pediatric ophthalmology.[5] These teleconsultations occur between a neonatologist and an ophthalmologist, but similar models between pediatric or emergency medicine physicians and an ophthalmologist might be useful given the paucity of education in ophthalmology in medical schools today.[23] In addition, teleconsultations among ophthalmologists may connect subspecialty pediatric ophthalmologists with comprehensive ophthalmologists or other ophthalmology specialists for certain cases.

Synchronous Non-ophthalmic Provider-to-Ophthalmic Provider Telehealth

Pediatricians, pediatric subspecialists (e.g., endocrinologists, neurologists, neurosurgeons), urgent-care providers, and emergency physicians might benefit from having real-time pediatric ophthalmology consultations. In telehealth consultations, the ophthalmologist would be remotely available on call to see a patient with the local provider. The pediatric ophthalmologist might provide advice based on the history and physical examination of the local provider, guide further history and examination in real time, and help manage next steps. Data on whether this type of model is useful, efficient, safe, and cost-effective is still in its early phases, but a proof of concept has been established with emergency eye care.[24,25]

Asynchronous Non-ophthalmic Provider-to-Ophthalmic Provider Telehealth Visits

Retinopathy of prematurity (ROP) is the primary asynchronous provider-to-provider telehealth in pediatric ophthalmology. These teleconsultations came about due to various necessities, including geographic barriers to providing appropriate neonatal screening,[26,27] lack of expertise and resources,[28-31] and need for more efficient care.[32] For approximately 20 years, effective ROP screening programs have been established both in resource-rich and resource-limited environments using store-and-forward systems.[5,28,29,32-37] In addition to the ROP-use case, asynchronous provider-to-provider communications with text alone or with text and images together are used routinely among primary providers such as pediatric nurse practitioners, pediatricians, urgent-care providers, and pediatric ophthalmologists. Much of these communications are not formalized but should be classified as asynchronous telehealth. For the remainder of this section, however, the ROP use case will be discussed in depth as a guidepost on how to establish a successful system of asynchronous provider-to-provider telehealth.

Premature infants within a neonatal intensive care unit (NICU) need several components at both the local and distant sites for successful asynchronous telehealth screening and treatment of ROP. On the local patient site, components include:
(a) NICU provider;
(b) Retinal imaging system;
(c) NICU screener; and
(d) Access to the internet.

At the distant ophthalmic provider site, components include:
(a) Access to the internet;
(b) Ophthalmologist with expertise in ROP;
(c) Reporting system to communicate back to the NICU provider; and
(d) Mechanism to provide in-person care.

In establishing an asynchronous program, all steps for the stakeholders must be delineated in written documents outlining the standard operating procedures to ensure the safety of the infants involved.

At the local site where the premature infant is admitted, the NICU providers are the first key components of the system. These NICU providers include intensivists, nurse practitioners, physician assistants, house officers, and nurses caring for the infant at hand. Referral for the asynchronous provider-to-provider telehealth program must be initiated by these stakeholders using appropriate screening guidelines. In high-income countries, the joint policy statement from the American Academy of Pediatrics Section on Ophthalmology, the American Academy of Ophthalmology, the American Association for Pediatric Ophthalmology and Strabismus, and the American Association of Certified Orthoptists guides screening.[38,39] In low- and middle-income countries, the referral guidelines may vary given the different circumstances afforded the premature infant.[28,31] Local NICU providers refer the infant for screening, provide appropriate clinical history, oversee the collection and transmission of data, receive the evaluation from the specialist, and implement the treatment plan.

The second key component at the local site is the imaging system to capture retinal images from the premature infant and the operator. Many early studies discussed using the RetCam II and III systems (Clarity Medical Systems Inc., Pleasanton, CA, USA; now from Natus Medical Incorporated, Pleasanton, CA, USA) for imaging of the retina;[6] however, less expensive imaging alternatives have also shown feasibility.[3] The NICU screener is intrinsically linked to the imaging system as this person captures the retinal images of the infant. In many early studies, this individual was a NICU nurse trained to use the imaging system and provide standardized images of the retina. More recently, studies have shown that trained, nonmedical professionals may also be excellent screeners,[40–42] which has the potential to drive down costs and improve access.

The third component at the local site is access to the internet along with a file management system capable of securely organizing and transmitting clinical history and images for each infant. Home-grown, secure email transmission of the data has been utilized,[6] and more formalized software systems for organizing the images and ensuring lossless transmission have also been described with TeleCare Software (i2i Telesolutions and Telemedicine Pvt. Ltd., Bangalore, India),[41] among others. For each system, a stable connection to the internet via wired, wireless, cellular, or satellite technology is needed with a minimum 20–30 kbps and tolerance of delayed transmission.[28]

At the distant site, a partner ophthalmologist with expertise in ROP will review the images and report back to the referring provider, giving guidance for the next steps, whether it be continued observation or an in-person intervention. The first component required at the distant site is access to an internet system capable of downloading and allowing secure reviews of the clinical history and imaging of the infant. The second component is the ophthalmologist with expertise in ROP and in evaluating ROP via telemedicine. The third component is the reporting system, allowing the ophthalmologist reader to document and to communicate findings securely and efficiently with the referring NICU provider.

Once screening and review are complete, a mechanism for implementation of further care for the premature infant might include subsequent imaging at a specified interval, an in-person examination at a specified interval, or medical and surgical treatment of ROP. If an in-person examination or treatment is needed from the ophthalmologist, a clear mechanism to implement the intervention is necessary and may involve bringing the ophthalmologist to the patient or the infant to the ophthalmologist. These arrangements need to be clearly defined at the outset with monitoring of adherence to ensure patient safety. Finally, numerous studies have shown that asynchronous provider-to-provider telehealth for retinopathy of prematurity improves the speed of diagnosis[4] while also decreasing cost[1,2,43,44] without sacrificing accuracy.[38]

Synchronous and Asynchronous Ophthalmic Provider-to-Ophthalmic Provider Telehealth Visits

Comprehensive ophthalmologists are tasked with being generalists for the eyes and may often encounter pediatric eye diseases such as strabismus, amblyopia, and congenital cataracts or glaucoma, which would benefit from real-time consultation with a pediatric ophthalmologist. In addition, on-call ophthalmologists might encounter an eye muscle laceration from trauma that requires treatment in the office, emergency room, or operating room. In each of these cases, synchronous communication between the ophthalmologist at the point of care and the pediatric ophthalmologist may facilitate patient care, and this often happens through audio-only or visual communication informally. Similarly, asynchronous communication between other ophthalmologists and pediatric ophthalmologists occurs routinely among individual practices, former colleagues (e.g., resident classmates), and formalized consultation agreements. For these telehealth encounters, the purpose is to further enhance the ophthalmic care of the patient by engaging a pediatric ophthalmologist. Appropriate documentation of the conversation should occur in the patient record.

CONCLUSIONS

Telehealth in pediatric ophthalmology involves both synchronous and asynchronous aspects, and it may involve direct patient-to-provider or provider-to-provider consultations. The field is rapidly evolving, and there is significant evidence that telehealth will be a large part of pediatric ophthalmology (and all of ophthalmology) in the future. Consideration for training and review of materials, such as this text, will be important for all ophthalmologists in the future.

REFERENCES

1. Castillo-Riquelme MC, Lord J, Moseley MJ, et al. Cost-effectiveness of digital photographic screening for retinopathy of prematurity in the United Kingdom. *Int J Technol Assess Health Care*. 2004;20(2):201–213.
2. Jackson KM, Scott KE, Graff Zivin J, et al. Cost-utility analysis of telemedicine and ophthalmoscopy for retinopathy of prematurity management. *Arch Ophthalmol*. 2008;126(4):493–499.
3. Skalet AH, Quinn GE, Ying GS, et al. Telemedicine screening for retinopathy of prematurity in developing countries using digital retinal images: a feasibility project. *J AAPOS*. 2008;12(3):252–258.
4. Richter GM, Sun G, Lee TC, et al. Speed of telemedicine vs ophthalmoscopy for retinopathy of prematurity diagnosis. *Am J Ophthalmol*. 2009;148(1):136–42 e2.
5. Richter GM, Williams SL, Starren J, et al. Telemedicine for retinopathy of prematurity diagnosis: evaluation and challenges. *Surv Ophthalmol*. 2009;54(6):671–685.
6. Wang SK, Callaway NF, Wallenstein MB, et al. SUNDROP: six years of screening for retinopathy of prematurity with telemedicine. *Can J Ophthalmol*. 2015;50(2):101–106.
7. Shah AS, Meyers H, Brown C, et al. Direct-to-consumer virtual visits: is this the next generation health-care delivery system for pediatric ophthalmology? *J AAPOS*. 2018;22(4):e14–e15.
8. Areaux Jr RG, de Alba Campomanes AG, Indaram M, et al. Your eye doctor will virtually see you now: synchronous patient-to-provider virtual visits in pediatric tele-ophthalmology. *J AAPOS*. 2020;24(4):197–203.
9. Bowe T, Hunter DG, Mantagos IS, et al. Virtual visits in ophthalmology: timely advice for implementation during the COVID-19 public health crisis. *Telemed J E Health*. 2020;26(9):1113–1117.
10. Kapoor S, Eldib A, Hiasat J, et al. Developing a pediatric ophthalmology telemedicine program in the COVID-19 crisis. *J AAPOS*. 2020;24(4):204–8 e2.
11. Nelson LB. Telemedicine in pediatric ophthalmology. *J Pediatr Ophthalmol Strabismus*. 2020;57(5):282.
12. Miller JM, Jang HS, Ramesh D, et al. Telemedicine distance and near visual acuity tests for adults and children. *J AAPOS*. 2020;24(4):235–236.
13. Samanta A, Mauntana S, Barsi Z, Yarlagadda B, Nelson PC. Is your vision blurry? A systematic review of home-based visual acuity for telemedicine. *J Telemed Telecare*. 2020 Nov 22:1357633X20970398. https://doi.org/10.1177/1357633X20970398. Epub ahead of print. PMID: 33222600.
14. Silverstein E, Williams JS, Brown JR, et al. Teleophthalmology: evaluation of phone-based visual acuity in a pediatric population. *Am J Ophthalmol*. 2021;221:199–206.
15. Finkelstein JB, Tremblay ES, Van Cain MS, et al. From Bedside to Webside: A Qualitative Study of Pediatric Clinicians' Use of Telemedicine. *JMIR Hum Factors* 2021, in press.
16. McConnochie KM. Webside manner: a key to high-quality primary care telemedicine for all. *Telemed J E Health*. 2019;25(11):1007–1011.
17. Modic MB, Neuendorf K, Windover AK. Enhancing your webside manner: optimizing opportunities for relationship-centered care in virtual visits. *J Patient Exp*. 2020;7(6):869–877.
18. Rosler G. Pediatric telehealth experiences: myths and truths about video visits from a parent. *J Patient Exp*. 2020;7(6):836–838.
19. Staffieri SE, Mathew AA, Sheth SJ, et al. Parent satisfaction and acceptability of telehealth consultations in pediatric ophthalmology: initial experience during the COVID-19 pandemic. *J AAPOS*. 2021;25(2):104–107.
20. Leite CA, Pereira TS, Chiang J, et al. Evaluation of ocular versions in graves' orbitopathy: correlation between the qualitative clinical method and the quantitative photographic method. *J Ophthalmol*. 2020;2020:9758153.
21. Phanphruk W, Liu Y, Morley K, et al. Validation of StrabisPIX, a mobile application for home measurement of ocular alignment. *Transl Vis Sci Technol*. 2019;8(2):9.
22. Pundlik S, Tomasi M, Liu R, et al. Development and preliminary evaluation of a smartphone app for measuring eye alignment. *Transl Vis Sci Technol*. 2019;8(1):19.
23. Shah M, Knoch D, Waxman E. The state of ophthalmology medical student education in the United States and Canada, 2012 through 2013. *Ophthalmology*. 2014;121(6):1160–1163.
24. Kumar S, Yogesan K, Hudson B, et al. Emergency eye care in rural Australia: role of internet. *Eye*. 2006;20(12):1342–1344.
25. Ribeiro AG, Rodrigues RA, Guerreiro AM, Regatieri CV. A teleophthalmology system for the diagnosis of ocular urgency in remote areas of Brazil. *Arq Bras Oftalmol*. 2014;77(4):214–218.
26. Weaver DT, Murdock TJ. Telemedicine detection of type 1 ROP in a distant neonatal intensive care unit. *J AAPOS*. 2012;16(3):229–233.

27. Begley BA, Martin J, Tufty GT, Suh DW. Evaluation of a remote telemedicine screening system for severe retinopathy of prematurity. *J Pediatr Ophthalmol Strabismus.* 2019;56(3):157–161.

28. Al-Khaled T, Valikodath NG, Patel SN, et al. Addressing the third epidemic of retinopathy of prematurity through telemedicine and technology: a systematic review. *J Pediatr Ophthalmol Strabismus.* 2021;58(4):261–269.

29. Ossandon D, Zanolli M, Stevenson R, et al. A national telemedicine network for retinopathy of prematurity screening. *J AAPOS.* 2018;22(2):124–127.

30. Valikodath N, Cole E, Chiang MF, et al. Imaging in retinopathy of prematurity. *Asia Pac J Ophthalmol (Phila).* 2019;8(2):178–186.

31. Bowe T, Nyamai L, Ademola-Popoola D, et al. The current state of retinopathy of prematurity in India, Kenya, Mexico, Nigeria, Philippines, Romania, Thailand, and Venezuela. *Digit J Ophthalmol.* 2019;25(4):49–58.

32. Moshfeghi DM. Systemic solutions in retinopathy of prematurity. *Am J Ophthalmol.* 2018;193:xiv–xviii.

33. Bowe T, Ung C, Campbell JP, Yonekawa Y. Telemedicine for retinopathy of prematurity in 2020. *J Vitreoretin Dis.* 2019;3(6):452–458.

34. Brady CJ, D'Amico S, Campbell JP. Telemedicine for retinopathy of prematurity. *Telemed J E Health.* 2020;26(4):556–564.

35. Thanos A, Yonekawa Y, Todorich B, et al. Screening and treatments using telemedicine in retinopathy of prematurity. *Eye Brain.* 2016;8:147–151.

36. Weaver DT. Telemedicine for retinopathy of prematurity. *Curr Opin Ophthalmol.* 2013;24(5):425–431.

37. Weaver DT. Use of telemedicine in retinopathy of prematurity. *Int Ophthalmol Clin.* 2014;54(3):9–20.

38. Fierson WM, Capone Jr A, American Academy of Pediatrics Section on O, American Academy of Ophthalmology AAoCO. Telemedicine for evaluation of retinopathy of prematurity. *Pediatrics.* 2015;135(1):e238–e254.

39. Fierson WM; American Academy of Pediatrics Section on Ophthalmology; American Academy of Ophthalmology; et al. Screening Examination of Premature Infants for Retinopathy of Prematurity. *Pediatrics.* 2018;142(6):e20183061. Pediatrics. 2019 Mar;143(3):e20183810. Erratum for: Pediatrics. 2018 Dec;142(6).

40. Murthy KR, Murthy PR, Shah DA, et al. Comparison of profile of retinopathy of prematurity in semiurban/rural and urban NICUs in Karnataka, India. *Br J Ophthalmol.* 2013;97(6):687–689.

41. Vinekar A, Gilbert C, Dogra M, et al. The KIDROP model of combining strategies for providing retinopathy of prematurity screening in underserved areas in India using wide-field imaging, tele-medicine, non-physician graders and smart phone reporting. *Indian J Ophthalmol.* 2014;62(1):41–49.

42. Quinn GE, Ying GS, Daniel E, et al. Validity of a telemedicine system for the evaluation of acute-phase retinopathy of prematurity. *JAMA Ophthalmol.* 2014;132(10):1178–1184.

43. Kelkar J, Kelkar A, Sharma S, Dewani J. A mobile team for screening of retinopathy of prematurity in India: cost—effectiveness, outcomes, and impact assessment. *Taiwan J Ophthalmol.* 2017;7(3):155–159.

44. Isaac M, Isaranuwatchai W, Tehrani N. Cost analysis of remote telemedicine screening for retinopathy of prematurity. *Can J Ophthalmol.* 2018;53(2):162–167.

CHAPTER 8

Tele-Neuro-Ophthalmology

MELISSA W. KO, MD • KEVIN E. LAI, MD

BACKGROUND

Prior to the COVID-19 pandemic, fewer than 15% of US physicians identified telehealth as part of their skillset[1] and fewer than 4% of neuro-ophthalmologists who are members of the North American Neuro-Ophthalmology Society (NANOS), the largest international organization of neuro-ophthalmologists in the world, utilized synchronous telehealth.[2] A survey of pre- and peri-COVID-19 telemedicine utilization in neuro-ophthalmology found that there was a 17-fold increase of synchronous telehealth visit adoption, such that an additional 64% of neuro-ophthalmologists began utilizing synchronous telehealth visits in the immediate period following the start of the pandemic. Respondents cited benefits including ensuring continuity of care, improving patient access to care, and patient convenience.[2] Respondents also increased the adoption of asynchronous telehealth models including remote interpretation of tests, second opinion record review, and interprofessional consultations. The main barriers to implementation cited by neuro-ophthalmology telehealth adopters and nonadopters include concerns about data/physical exam quality, reimbursement, medical liability, and sufficient infrastructure support for implementation.[2] In this chapter, examination components and validated applications that can aid the neuro-ophthalmic synchronous telehealth examination, are addressed.

The Case for Tele-Neuro-Ophthalmology

The value proposition supporting increased adoption of synchronous telehealth in neuro-ophthalmology includes improving existing workforce shortage, allowing patients with physical impairment, geographical and social distancing limitations access to care, expanding neuro-ophthalmic education and training, and harnessing the aspects of neuro-ophthalmology that are amenable to telehealth delivery.

Workforce/patient access to care

A 2019 NANOS US membership survey found that there are 1.63 million people per 1.0 clinical full-time

Ocular Telehealth. https://doi.org/10.1016/B978-0-323-83204-5.00008-1

equivalent (CFTE) neuro-ophthalmologist, with only 386 individuals in active practice (187 CFTE) in the nation, concentrated in metropolitan areas.[3] Prior to the COVID-19 pandemic, the median wait time for a new patient appointment was 6 weeks and over 20% of survey respondents reported greater than 3-month wait times.[3] With projections indicating that an additional 180 physicians (working 0.5 CFTE) are required to meet the metric of one neuro-ophthalmologist for every 1.2 million individuals, there is a sizable workforce shortage with low numbers of trainees entering the field coupled with physician retirements.[3–5] While pipeline efforts are underway within NANOS, there remains a sizable gap between sufficient numbers of neuro-ophthalmologists needed to service the globe. Telehealth adoption partially mitigates the workforce shortage by allowing a wider patient catchment area for each neuro-ophthalmologist. Additionally, based on data from the authors' Indiana synchronous telehealth in neuro-ophthalmology utilization study, it was observed that during the peri-COVID period, more established patients were seen via telemedicine while more new patients were seen in-person.[6] This triage effectively opened limited in-person slots to those patients who most needed an in-person eye examination and allowed established stable patients the opportunity for their most pressing concerns to be addressed and answered via a synchronous home-based telehealth visit.

Educational mission

Accredited Council of Graduate Medical Education (ACGME) program requirements for neurology and ophthalmology training programs state that "at each training program there must be sufficient faculty members with competence to instruct and supervise residents at that location and that faculty members must have subspecialty expertise" including neuro-ophthalmology.[7,8] Prior to the COVID-19 pandemic, neuro-ophthalmology workforce shortages required some US training programs to secure outside neuro-ophthalmology faculty. Projections suggest that this arrangement may increase in the future. In one example, a faculty member travels over 200 miles per month to train residents lacking an on-site neuro-ophthalmologist. This physician provides remote synchronous (through telecommunications) and asynchronous teaching (via their online neuro-ophthalmology curriculum) that has also been utilized by global learners (K. Golnik, personal communication, April 2, 2020). Additional tele-educational opportunities include the Neuro-ophthalmology Virtual Education Library (NOVEL) and the Eccles Health Sciences Library at the University of Utah with more than 14,000 users and 77,000-page views from 144 countries[8] (N. Lombardo, personal communication, April 24, 2020). NOVEL and NANOS developed the Illustrated Curriculum with content for basic, intermediate, and advanced learners to support residencies and fellowships, fill curriculum gaps, and increase the availability of neuro-ophthalmology resources.[9]

During the COVID-19 pandemic, many academic neuro-ophthalmologists rapidly implemented remote trainee education. In practical terms, all parties (the trainee, patient, and attending) are all in separate locations and on virtual platforms. The resident or fellow begins the synchronous telehealth visit by evaluating the patient. They then "leave" the virtual examination room to present to the attending who is geographically distant. From there, both the learner and attending virtually "enter" the patient's virtual room to evaluate the patient together. Given workforce shortages, neuro-ophthalmic synchronous and asynchronous telehealth curricula will benefit from continued development and expansion to introduce medical students to the subspecialty and then recruit, train, and retain residents.

Harnessing the neuro-ophthalmic exam using synchronous telehealth

While overall adoption of ocular telehealth following the start of COVID-19 is unavailable, sampling of several ophthalmology tertiary academic centers suggests that adoption has been relatively low, around 2% of all total ophthalmology visits during 2020.[10] However, within that single digit percentage adoption at those centers, neuro-ophthalmology visits comprised 22%–60% of all telehealth visits, suggesting that there are unique aspects of the neuro-ophthalmic examination that better translate into telehealth visits compared to other ophthalmic specialties.[10] A survey of patient and physician experiences of telemedicine evaluations within neuro-ophthalmology across three tertiary care US academic centers noted that 87% of neuro-ophthalmologist responses indicated that they felt the visit and examination provided enough information for decision-making.[11] Areas of the examination perceived by 50% or more of physician responses to be easy to conduct via telemedicine included: range of eye movements, visual acuity, Ishihara color plate assessment, Amsler grid testing, and red desaturation evaluation. The pupil exam and saccadic eye movement evaluation were considered moderately easy to perform via telemedicine.[11] There is a tremendous opportunity to harness the aspects of the neuro-ophthalmic examination that are most amenable to the delivery of telemedicine. Later in this chapter, the authors discuss the components of the neuro-ophthalmic examination that have validated applications and programs for use in telehealth.

MODELS OF TELE-NEURO-OPHTHALMOLOGY

While the discussion has focused on synchronous telehealth visits in the previous sections, it is helpful to consider telehealth models which blend both synchronous and asynchronous modalities, into the neuro-ophthalmic visit.

Combined Synchronous and Asynchronous Care

While there are neuro-ophthalmic exam components that readily translate into synchronous, home-based ocular telehealth, key examination challenges remain, including securing adequate fundoscopy, visual field testing, and optical coherence tomography (OCT). One model to address these important eye exam elements is utilizing clinic-based asynchronous telehealth to do testing and then having the physician conducting a separate synchronous home-based telehealth encounter with the patient. Specific to neuro-ophthalmology, patients can obtain fundus photography, computerized visual fields, and OCT imaging at a locally equipped eye provider or neuro-ophthalmologist's office and then have a separately scheduled appointment for the neuro-ophthalmic consultation.

Interprofessional Consultation (also Called E-Consult)

The *interprofessional consultation (IPC)* is where a referring provider requests a specialist opinion based solely through chart and data review, without the specialist formally seeing the patient. The specialist then renders their verbal and written or just written report back to the requesting provider. This is considered the 21st-century "curbside consultation." Compared to pre-pandemic practice, this modality of telehealth increased by nearly fivefold in adoption by neuro-ophthalmologists during the early peri-COVID period.[2] The benefits of IPC include that it is a provider to neuro-ophthalmologist interaction without requiring the patient to virtually or physically be seen by the specialist. Within the United States, this is also a billable and reimbursable form of care. Unlike the "curbside consultation," the liabilities are reduced because the necessary records and imaging studies are available for the consultant to review and there is formal documentation detailing communication between the referring provider and the consultant specialist.

IPCs are exceptionally robust when deployed across a healthcare system with an integrated electronic medical record. One neuro-ophthalmologist in a large private healthcare system reported that their practice is nearly 75% IPCs with the remaining 25% reserved for in-person visits.[12] This has provided exceptional empowerment and education for the general ophthalmologists employed within this large healthcare system and permits unprecedented and robust patient access to neuro-ophthalmic care for large underserved regions.

Remote Interpretation of Data

Remote Interpretation of Data is an asynchronous telehealth modality whereby a patient obtains testing (e.g., fundus photography, visual field, OCT analysis) in an encounter that is separate from a consultation with the neuro-ophthalmologist. The test is sent for interpretation only to the neuro-ophthalmologist, who generates a report to the requesting provider. In this scenario, the neuro-ophthalmologist is not providing management or treatment guidelines, but rather simply performing the test interpretation. Prior to the pandemic, approximately 27% of surveyed neuro-ophthalmologists provided this service, increasing to 32% during the early peri-COVID period.[2] This value does not fully reflect the growth of this modality, as in the immediate peri-COVID period surveyed, 22% had to discontinue its use due to the required shutdown of offices/practices. Interestingly, 15.6% of previous nonusers adopted this practice during the peri-COVID period.[2]

Other Available Modalities

Other forms of telehealth include the synchronous modalities of Virtual Check-In and Phone visits and asynchronous communication through Online Patient Portal Communication.

Virtual Check-Ins are brief communications via phone or video chat with an established patient who has initiated the communication. This type of encounter is used to determine whether or not the patient needs to be seen in the office for a new problem or change to an existing issue. Documentation should include the nature of the visit, the eye provider's medical decision-making (including whether or not the patient needs to be seen), and the total time spent on call.[13] Nonqualified calls include those related to follow-up of recent visit diagnoses (within the last 7 days) including test result updates or communication that results in scheduling an urgent evaluation (within 24 h or next available appointment). Use of the telephone for rendering care was the first and oldest form of tele-health when Alexander Graham Bell called Mr. Watson after spilling sulfuric acid on his clothing.[14] Within the United States during the public health emergency, phone visits were a billable and reimbursable service, but the future of phone visits as a continued covered service remains uncertain.[15]

Online Patient Portal Communication is an asynchronous ocular telehealth modality where an established patient securely messages an eye provider through a patient portal. The conversation may involve medical decision-making or an exchange of information where the eye provider is fielding the patient's questions. The communication can take place over a 7-day period with documentation through the message exchange. The total time spent during the entire exchange (provided it is within a 7-day period) is used as the billing reference.[14]

SELECTING THE APPROPRIATE TYPE OF TELEMEDICINE VISIT
When to Consider a Video Visit
Video visits are optimal for those who desire a more personal connection to their provider and for external exams. While suboptimal compared to an in-person exam, especially for patients who require a fundus-copic exam, patients express high satisfaction from interacting with and having their concerns addressed via a video telehealth encounter.[16] As noted earlier, this synchronous telehealth to the home is best utilized if an in-person eye exam has already been performed elsewhere and the neuro-ophthalmic virtual video visit is more of an informative review to discuss diagnostic findings, educate, and plan next steps in care with the patient. Previously performed visual field testing, ocular imaging, and neuroimaging can still be presented visually to the patient in a virtual visit through screen sharing. The eye provider can instruct the patient to demonstrate neuro-ophthalmic signs over video platforms (e.g., ocular motility exam or even ice pack testing for myasthenia gravis).[17]

When to Consider Phone Visits
Phone visits may be used for the follow-up of a patient who has a known pathology with subjective outcome measures, such as ischemic cranial nerve palsy with accompanying diplopia, which is expected to recover over 6–12 weeks. If the diplopia is not recovered, the patient can then be brought into clinic or undergo further remote video visits to assess clinical progress. Phone visits enable physicians to adjust medications for patients with migraines or myasthenia gravis. Additionally, a physician can use phone visits to triage visual symptoms with a normal dilated eye exam by another provider or discuss medication compliance and tolerance, neuroimaging findings, and lab results.

When to Consider Online Portal Communication
Established patients may decide to reach out via online (EMR) portal regarding their condition. This asynchronous modality is best suited for communications that are not time-sensitive (e.g., medication refills, test results, treatment plans, overall condition, or scheduling). Online portal communication can also aid in sharing photographs or videos (e.g., external examination findings, OCT, visual fields) to aid in clinical evaluation. If there is a question or concern raised by the patient that may be better addressed with synchronous telehealth, one can convert to a video or phone visit.

When to Consider an Interprofessional Consultation (E-Consult)
Neuro-ophthalmologists are often asked by other providers to provide consultations regarding the diagnosis or management of a patient, but without the expectation of a clinic appointment (the so-called "curbside" consultation). This may be preferable for patients who are geographically distant and already have an engaged local physician. This option is ideal if the neuro-ophthalmologist determines that the patient requires related testing or medical care prior to an appointment or does not need their in-person examination.

IMPLEMENTATION STRATEGIES FOR TELE-NEURO-OPHTHALMOLOGY
Depending on the model used for telemedicine, there may be minimal technological requirements necessary for a successful neuro-ophthalmology telehealth encounter. As with most neuro-ophthalmology in-person care, much of the preparation comes before the provider and patient interaction.

Previsit
Patient selection
Neuro-ophthalmic conditions appropriate or not appropriate for telemedicine. Not every neuro-ophthalmology patient is a good candidate for telemedicine. A recent survey of 208 practicing neuro-ophthalmologists reported that diseases that have normal eye exams and/or prior ancillary testing were more amenable to telemedicine, while optic neuropathies may be better examined in person[2] (Tables 8.1–8.3).

TABLE 8.1
Neuro-Ophthalmologists' Perception of Telemedicine Utility for Select Neuro-Ophthalmic Conditions

>50% of Respondents Considered Telemedicine Helpful
- Migraine with aura
- Pituitary tumor with prior visual fields and MRI

>50% of Respondents Considered Telemedicine Not Helpful
- Nonarteritic anterior ischemic optic neuropathy (NAION)
- Possible arteritic anterior ischemic optic neuropathy (AAION)
- Optic atrophy

Credit: Adapted from HE Moss, KE Lai, MW Ko. Survey of telehealth adoption by neuro-ophthalmologists during the COVID-19 pandemic: benefits, barriers, and utility. *J Neuroophthalmol.* 2020;40:346–355.

TABLE 8.2
Examples of Diagnoses Amenable to Telemedicine

Diagnosis	Suggested Prior Testing
Afferent disease	
• Retrobulbar optic neuritis	VF, MRI brain/orbits with and without contrast
• Pituitary adenoma	VF, OCT ON, MRI sella with contrast
• Homonymous hemianopia	VF, MRI brain with and without contrast
• Transient visual loss (normal eye exam)	VF, echocardiogram, MRA or CTA head and neck
Efferent disease	
• Superior oblique myokymia	
• Blepharospasm	
• Follow-up of microvascular ischemic cranial nerve palsy	
• Bell's palsy	
• Myasthenia gravis[17]	Acetylcholine receptor antibodies
• Follow-up of Horner syndrome[17]	MRI brain with and without contrast, MRA or CTA head and neck (down to level of lung apex)
Other	
• Migraine with aura	
• Trigeminal neuralgia	
• Visual snow syndrome	MRI brain with and without contrast
• Giant cell arteritis (recommendations for initial management)	VF, fundus photos, FA, ESR, CRP, CBC

CT, computed tomography; *CTA*, CT angiography; *FA*, fluorescein angiography; *MRA*, magnetic resonance angiography; *MRI*, magnetic resonance imaging; *OCT*, optical coherence tomography; *ON*, optic nerve; *VF*, visual field.

TABLE 8.3
Examples of Neuro-Ophthalmic Diagnoses Incompatible With Telemedicine

Diagnosis

Afferent disease
- Papilledema/idiopathic intracranial hypertension
- Ischemic optic neuropathy
- Optic atrophy
- Sudden visual loss
- Unexplained visual loss
- Unexplained visual field defect

Efferent disease
- Unspecified diplopia
- Cranial nerve palsies (new)
- Nystagmus

Other
- Nonorganic (functional) visual loss
- "Rule out" diagnoses (e.g., rule out giant cell arteritis, rule out optic neuritis, etc.)

Further study is warranted to more precisely elucidate neuro-ophthalmic problems that are suitable for telehealth. Some criteria to consider when determining if a patient's problem is appropriate for telehealth evaluation include:

- **New vs established patients**
  New consultations for neuro-ophthalmology may not be easily assessed by telemedicine given the neuro-ophthalmologist may need to perform elements of the exam in person, such as the fundus exam. Misdiagnosis rates are reported of up to 60%–70% of referrals prior to neuro-ophthalmology evaluation, therefore, it can be difficult for the neuro-ophthalmologist to accurately predict if a patient's condition is amenable to telemedicine.[18,19] Established patients may be better suited for telemedicine, especially conditions for which there may be no need for a funduscopic examination.

- **Examination requirements**
  While telemedicine may be helpful for a myriad of neuro-ophthalmic conditions, afferent diseases requiring detailed slit lamp or funduscopic examination or efferent diseases requiring detailed assessment of ocular alignment/extraocular movements may be better examined in person. In contrast, referrals for subjective visual symptoms or conditions in which the eye exam is normal may be excellent candidates for telemedicine.

- **Prior examinations and testing**
  Unlike many other ophthalmology subspecialties, neuro-ophthalmology evaluation is often enhanced

by a detailed medical history including review of prior records and previous testing. If a patient has previously been evaluated by multiple eye care providers and neurologists and undergone testing such as laboratory studies, neuroimaging, visual fields, OCTs, or fundus imaging, the neuro-ophthalmologist may be able to avoid redundant testing and determine the appropriate diagnosis and management through careful abstraction of the medical records followed by telemedicine evaluation. In contrast, the patient with minimal or no prior records to review may need a comprehensive in-person eye exam as well as additional testing because common ocular diseases may not yet have been ruled out.

- **Urgency of problem**

  Many of the urgent or semiurgent problems encountered in neuro-ophthalmology (papilledema, transient visual loss, anisocoria, possible giant cell arteritis, etc.) may benefit from urgent workup or treatment prior to the neuro-ophthalmology evaluation. Certain forms of telemedicine (e.g., teleconsultation) may expedite coordination of care in urgent cases where the neuro-ophthalmologist's value is in determining the appropriate next steps in management rather than in the neuro-ophthalmologist's examination of the patient. For example, if the referring provider has strong clinical evidence to suspect giant cell arteritis, telemedicine may allow the neuro-ophthalmologist to recommend emergent laboratory workup, initiation of steroid therapy, and referral for temporal artery biopsy without having to physically examine the patient. This is especially helpful for situations in which access to neuro-ophthalmic care is limited, which is a common problem due to the significant shortage of providers.[3-5,20]

Special considerations. As with any telemedicine candidate, the patient must have suitable equipment (phone, tablet, or computer with webcam), access to the necessary applications, and sufficient broadband speed in order to have a high-quality examination.

Per the Federal Communications Commission (FCC), internet upload and download speeds of 2 megabits per second (Mbps) are sufficient for "standard-definition" telemedicine. However, for "high-definition" images that may be more useful for neuro-ophthalmic evaluation, 10 Mbps speeds are necessary.[21] In an analysis of broadband provider availability in neuro-ophthalmology patients, the authors found that while the vast majority of patients had access to at least 1 broadband carrier with speeds ≥ 2 Mbps (96.8%), slightly

fewer had access to at least 1 broadband carrier with speeds ≥ 10 Mbps (91.5%).[22]

Patients with speech barriers (e.g., aphasia, nonverbal, etc.) may have additional difficulty with telehealth examination in some situations, especially if there is reduced image quality. Telemedicine may either be a benefit or a barrier for patients requiring assistance from family. Patients who have difficulties with the examination (noncompliance, physical restrictions that prevent the examiner from obtaining any useful exam information) may benefit from telemedicine since in-person care would not provide any additional information.

Obtaining records and collateral information
Prior to the evaluation, all pertinent medical records should be accessible to the neuro-ophthalmologist in an organized fashion for review. These records may include:
- the referring provider's clinical exam
- pertinent previous eye or neurology exams
- ancillary testing (e.g., visual fields, optical coherence tomography, etc.)
- neuroimaging
- lab tests
- any other records pertinent to the patient's condition
Ideally, the neuro-ophthalmologist will have had sufficient time prior to the appointment to review those records and document any pertinent findings.

Important ancillary service considerations
Ophthalmic technicians may have a helpful role in synchronous or asynchronous telehealth, including obtaining medical history and assisting patients with many of the app-assisted tests of afferent and efferent visual pathways. Interpreters, social workers, or other ancillary service providers required for the encounter should receive instructions on how to utilize the telemedicine service. If necessary, additional time should be allotted to test the connection and ensure that all parties can communicate effectively.

Perivisit
Medical history
The medical history is obtained in a similar fashion to in-person care. It can be gathered by support staff before the neuro-ophthalmologist joins the synchronous telehealth encounter, or potentially filled out by the patient a few days prior to their telehealth encounter.

Examination
The key components of the neuro-ophthalmic examination include testing of afferent and efferent visual systems, and visualization of the fundus. The

neuro-ophthalmology group at Stanford University has created videos demonstrating how to perform various parts of the pediatric and adult eye exam via synchronous telehealth.[23]

Evaluation of the afferent visual system. Certain elements of the visual system can be evaluated via telemedicine using a combination of digital applications or printed aids. While some tests have been validated, many require assistance or may not provide the same type of information as in-person examinations (Table 8.4).

Accurate pupil examination by synchronous telehealth can be challenging. Because ambient lighting conditions can affect both visualization and pupil size, certain tests for assessing the pupil may not be as accurate. The video examination library at Stanford provides a helpful demonstration of remote pupil evaluation.[25] Here are some suggestions for pupil evaluation:

Evaluating anisocoria via telemedicine.
1. Using a diffuse fixed light set in front of the patient (e.g., flashlight on smartphone), take a screenshot of the patient with the diffuse fixed light shining directly toward the patient's nose.
2. Angling the diffuse light toward the patient's forehead, take another screenshot of the patient (simulates dimmer light relative to the direct light while maintaining enough ambient light to view pupils).
3. View the screenshots side-by-side to observe relative differences of anisocoria.

Evaluating a relative afferent pupillary defect via telemedicine. Sun and Odel described an adaptation of Hirschberg's method for evaluating a relative afferent pupillary defect (RAPD) using telemedicine[26] (validation studies have not yet been published):

1. Use a diffuse fixed light set in front of the patient (e.g., flashlight on smartphone) and orient the camera so that both eyes are closely framed in the screen.
2. Have the patient fixate on a distant target.
3. Using a large kitchen spoon, ask the patient to alternatively cover each eye.
4. Observe the revealed pupil: if it dilates rather than constricts, this is evidence of an RAPD.
5. For dark irides: patients can perform a swinging flashlight test on their own eyes. This method is subject to lighting variability and image quality but can still be used to detect RAPDs.

Evaluation of the efferent visual system. The video produced by Stanford is an excellent demonstration of gross assessments of ocular motility and alignment.[27]

Evaluation of the fundus. Although there are some techniques proposed for patient-site self-visualization of the fundus, the methodology still requires the use of some equipment not always readily available at home (self-illuminating magnifier) and can be technically challenging.[28] Previsit fundus photography may be helpful but does not always provide sufficient information for neuro-ophthalmic disease.

Ordering additional testing and arranging patient follow-up

Telemedicine patients who need additional serological testing, neuroimaging, lumbar punctures, or other diagnostic testing will need coordination of care with the provider's administrative staff. Instead of physically giving the patient an order, the provider's

TABLE 8.4
Validated Tests of the Afferent Visual System[24]

Test	Software	Viewing Distance	Assistance Needed
Visual acuity			
• PEEK Acuity	Android	Distance—2 m	Yes
• Visual Acuity XL	iOS	Distance—6 m	Yes
• Vision@home	Android and iOS	Distance—2 m	Yes—distance only
• Eye Chart Pro	iOS	Near—40 cm	Yes
		Distance—2.5 m	
Color vision			
• Eye Handbook (Ishihara)	Android and iOS		No
Visual fields			
• MRF Glaucoma	iOS (iPad)		No
• Visual Fields Easy	iOS (iPad)		No

Credit: Adapted from KE Lai, MW Ko, JC Rucker, et al. Tele-Neuro-Ophthalmology during the age of COVID-19. *J Neuroophthalmol.* 2020;40:292–304.

administrative staff will have to either electronically submit or fax the order to the patient's facility or hospital of choice.

Likewise, the patient should be counseled to expect additional contact from the provider's office to schedule follow-up and any other tests or referrals.

Postvisit
Billing and coding
Table 8.5 details the pertinent tele-neuro-ophthalmology CPT/HCPCS codes for billing. Also refer to Chapter 14, Billing and Coding, for more specific information.

Coordination of care and prolonged services
Neuro-ophthalmology patients often require additional coordination of care, such as discussing the case with referring providers, discussion of neuroimaging findings with a neuro-radiologist, or separately interpreting neuroimaging or lab tests. If this coordination takes place during the same day as the visit, the time spent in coordination of care should be added to the total time spent and can be used in determining the appropriate level of service billed. If the time spent in coordination is on a separate day and exceeds the thresholds for prolonged services, non-face-to-face prolonged services codes (CPT codes 99358, 99359) may be billable.

CASE EXAMPLES OF TELEHEALTH IN NEURO-OPHTHALMOLOGY
The following case examples are purely hypothetical and an amalgam of multiple neuro-ophthalmology patients. These examples illustrate how ocular telehealth might be utilized in neuro-ophthalmology. In some respects, many elements of the evaluation are identical to previous in-person models; for example, neuro-ophthalmologists often review more previous examinations and tests than other ophthalmology subspecialists even with in-person exams.[29] Most ocular telehealth visits in neuro-ophthalmology will therefore follow a hybrid model, in which the referring ophthalmologist acts as a telehealth facilitator gathering all of the data in person and asynchronously forwarding the information to the neuro-ophthalmologist for review. The neuro-ophthalmologist then performs the telehealth service (synchronous or asynchronous) directly with the patient following the review of the previously acquired data.

Synchronous Telehealth
In the following cases, the neuro-ophthalmologist performs a synchronous home-based visit directly with the patient.

Case 1: Optic neuritis
A 27-year-old Caucasian female is referred for neuro-ophthalmic evaluation of suspected optic neuritis. She was evaluated by an ophthalmologist who obtained the following information: documented history of a sudden onset of right eye pain with eye movements followed by decreased vision in the right eye 1–2 days later. The eye exam was normal aside from decreased visual acuity of 20/50 in the right eye (20/15 in the left eye) with decreased color vision and right RAPD. Visual fields, OCT of the optic nerve, fundus photos, and MRI of the brain and orbits with and without contrast were completed prior to the referral. The MRI revealed focal enhancement of the right optic nerve and there were several T2/FLAIR periventricular hyperintense lesions (Table 8.6).

TABLE 8.5
CPT/HCPCS Codes Pertinent to Neuro-Ophthalmology Evaluation[12]

Code	Description	Comments
Synchronous telehealth		
99202-99205 99212-99215	Office Evaluation and Management (E/M), New or Established	Similar documentation requirements as in-person visits
G2212 or 99417	Direct Prolonged Services, every 15 min	Time-based
99358-99359	Non-Face-To-Face Prolonged Services	Time-based
G2012	Virtual Check-In (video or phone)	≤10 min "Triage"
G2252	Virtual Check-In (video or phone)	11–20 min "Triage"
99441-99443	Telephone E/M	Time-based
Asynchronous telehealth		
G2010	Remote Evaluation of Pre-Recorded Patient Information	Patient must initiate submission
99421-99423	Online Digital E/M Communications	Time-based
99446-99449, 99451	Interprofessional Consult	Time-based

Credit: Adapted from MW Ko, KE Lai, A Gilbert, et al. Tele-Neuro-Ophthalmology: Updates and Future Implications. North American Neuro-Ophthalmology Society 47th Annual Meeting, Virtual; 2021.

TABLE 8.6
Considerations for Synchronous Telehealth Evaluation of Optic Neuritis

Previsit	Perivisit	Postvisit
• Ensure patient has appropriate equipment and broadband speeds • Copies of previous eye exams, visual fields, OCTs, fundus photos, and MRIs reviewed prior to evaluation	• Obtain medical history (ophthalmic technician-capable) • Check visual acuity, color vision, ±visual fields, pupils (ophthalmic technician-capable) • Refer to neurology for workup and management of multiple sclerosis	• Discussed case with referring doctor • Administrative staff arranges for neurology referral and follow-up appointment

Case 2: Myasthenia gravis

A 73-year-old Caucasian male is referred for neuro-ophthalmic evaluation of suspected myasthenia gravis. He was evaluated by an ophthalmologist who documented a 6-month history of progressive left upper eyelid ptosis and recent onset of painless binocular oblique diplopia that seemed to worsen throughout the day. The eye exam was normal aside from the aforementioned left upper eyelid ptosis and a right hypertropia and esotropia that changed to left hypertropia and exotropia in left gaze with bilateral abduction deficits, right adduction deficit, and left supraduction deficit. Fundoscopic examination was normal. Acetylcholine receptor antibody blood tests and MRI of the brain and orbits with and without contrast were completed prior to the referral. The MRI was normal and the acetylcholine receptor antibodies were strongly positive (Table 8.7).

Asynchronous Telehealth

The following example is where the neuro-ophthalmologist manages a clinical question from an established patient with a virtual check-in; in this case, via telephone.

Case 3: Virtual check-in

A 32-year-old female who has been seen previously for idiopathic intracranial hypertension leaves a message stating that she is having new-onset blurred vision and wants to know if she needs to be seen. At her last visit 2 months ago, she was symptom-free with no papilledema and normal visual function and had tapered her acetazolamide. The neuro-ophthalmologist calls the patient back and records that her blurred vision is transient, lasting up to a few minutes at a time, improves with blinking, and is associated with itching and burning. After reassuring her that this most likely represents dry eyes and a trial of artificial tears can be started, the neuro-ophthalmologist records that no urgent office visit is warranted (Table 8.8).

Case 4: Interprofessional consult (e-consult)

In this scenario, the neuro-ophthalmologist provides a professional opinion solely through record review.

A 72-year-old woman has sudden-onset painless vision loss in the right eye. She sees her ophthalmologist the same day, who notes that she has

TABLE 8.7
Considerations for Synchronous Telehealth Evaluation of Myasthenia Gravis

Previsit	Perivisit	Postvisit
• Ensure patient has appropriate equipment and broadband speeds • Copies of previous eye exams, labs, and MRIs reviewed prior to evaluation	• Obtain medical history (ophthalmic technician-capable) • Check visual acuity and pupils (ophthalmic technician-capable) • Check motility and alignment • Have patient perform an ice pack test at home 17 • Discuss starting pyridostigmine and/or steroids • Refer to neurology for workup and management of myasthenia gravis	• Discussed case with referring doctor • Administrative staff arranges for neurology referral and follow-up appointment

TABLE 8.8
Considerations for Virtual Check-In

Previsit	Perivisit	Postvisit
• Obtain patient consent for billing insurance for virtual check-in	• Obtain focused medical history • Determine if in-person visit is necessary	• CPT code G2012 or G2252 encapsulates this form of visit

hand motion vision in the right eye, pallid optic nerve edema in the right eye, and a normal optic nerve in the left eye. The patient reports having scalp tenderness, jaw claudication, and general malaise and myalgias. Concerned about giant cell arteritis, the ophthalmologist sent her to the ED for urgent ESR, CRP, and CBC, started her on steroids, and referred her to an oculoplastic surgeon for a temporal artery biopsy. The patient lives 6 hours away from the nearest neuro-ophthalmologist but both she and her ophthalmologist would like to get the neuro-ophthalmologist's input about her case but does not think she would be able to easily travel to see the neuro-ophthalmologist. She lives in a rural area where there is poor cell phone service and no broadband service providers (Table 8.9).

Case 5: Remote interpretation
In this example, the neuro-ophthalmologist interprets test results for another non-eye provider caring for a patient, but does not provide any care recommendations.

A 63-year-old male is being followed by neurosurgery department for a pituitary macroadenoma status post transsphenoidal resection. The department has an automated perimetry machine and OCT machine but contracts out to a neuro-ophthalmologist to interpret the test results (Table 8.10).

FUTURE DIRECTIONS

The future of telehealth for neuro-ophthalmology remains uncertain due to reimbursement issues. From the telehealth provider adoption perspective, there was a 17-fold increase in video visits by neuro-ophthalmologists during the early peri-COVID-19 period.[2] Positively, 74% of video visit users surveyed indicated that they plan to continue to use video visits following the public health emergency.[2]

Immediate questions for the future of telehealth include coverage and payment parity compared to in-person visits following the end of the global pandemic. Policymakers, regulators, providers, patients, and payers will play a critical role in whether or not adoption of ocular telehealth will be sustained. The necessary long-term needs for neuro-ophthalmic telehealth include

TABLE 8.9
Considerations for Interprofessional Consult (e-Consult)

Previsit	Perivisit	Postvisit
• Obtain patient consent for billing insurance for interprofessional consult • Obtain all pertinent clinical records, visual fields, OCTs, fundus photos, labs, biopsy reports	• Document total time spent in discussion with referring doctor, review of records, and in preparation of summary	• Use CPT code 99446-99449 for consults with verbal and written report to referring provider (time-based) • Use CPT code 99451 for written-only consults taking ≥ 5 min

TABLE 8.10
Considerations for Remote Interpretation

Preinterpretation		Postinterpretation
• Obtain patient consent for billing insurance for remote interpretation • Patient obtains test(s) from neurosurgeon's office • Obtain high-quality image of test(s) being interpreted	• Submit written summary of remote interpretation	• Use physician component modifier (− 26) for diagnostic test(s) being interpreted

research demonstrating tele-neuro-ophthalmology as non-inferior to an in-person evaluation, further validation of vision applications, and development of affordable, portable, easy-to-use quality digital ocular fundus imaging methods. These are all in progress.[30] Recently, artificial intelligence (AI) and deep learning are being studied in the detection of papilledema and other optic nerve disorders.[31]

Ultimately, the goal in the field of neuro-ophthalmology is to craft telehealth's integration into high-quality, individualized neuro-ophthalmologic patient care. Tele-neuro-ophthalmology adoption is necessary for expansion of patient access and extension of a limited workforce. It is also critical for the education of trainees and future neuro-ophthalmologists. Critical innovations in digital optical fundus photography, mobile vision testing applications, and artificial intelligence will facilitate further adoption of tele-neuro-ophthalmology and bring the specialty to the leading edge of healthcare delivery.

REFERENCES

1. Doximity. *2019 Telemedicine and Locum Tenens Opportunities Study Measuring Physician Interest in Emerging Employment Areas.* https://s3.amazonaws.com/s3.doximity.com/press/2019TelemedicineAndLocumTenensOpportunities-Study.pdf. Accessed 13.02.21.
2. Moss HE, Lai KE, Ko MW. Survey of telehealth adoption by neuro-ophthalmologists during the COVID-19 pandemic: benefits, barriers, and utility. *J Neuroophthalmol.* 2020;40(3):346–355.
3. Debusk A, Subramanian PS, Bryan MS, Moster ML, Calvert PC, Frohman LP. Mismatch in supply and demand for neuro-ophthalmic care. *J Neuroophthalmol.* 2021 Mar 23. https://doi.org/10.1097/WNO.0000000000001214. Epub ahead of print.
4. Frohman LP. Neuro-ophthalmology: transitioning from old to new models of health care delivery. *J Neuroophthalmol.* 2017;37(2):206–209.
5. Frohman LP. The human resource crisis in neuro-ophthalmology. *J Neuroophthalmol.* 2008;28(3):231–234.
6. Chauhan D, Ko MW, Moss HE, Mackay DD, Lai KE. A multicenter profile of tele-neuro-ophthalmology care in Indiana. In: *North American Neuro-ophthalmology Society 47th Annual Meeting; February 21*; 2021. Virtual.
7. Neurology. www.acgme.org. Accessed 13.02.21 https://www.acgme.org/Specialties/Program-Requirements-and-FAQs-and-Applications/pfcatid/37/Neurology.
8. Ophthalmology. www.acgme.org. Accessed 13.02.21 https://www.acgme.org/Specialties/Program-Requirements-and-FAQs-and-Applications/pfcatid/13/Ophthalmology.
9. *NANOS Illustrated Curriculum for Neuro-Ophthalmology. Novel.* Accessed 13.02.21 https://www.tetondata.com/resources/srOnline/Handouts/NANOS_Overview_Handout_STAT!Ref.pdf.
10. Ko MW. Tele neuro-ophthalmology: utility and adoption in a peri and post-COVID world. In: *Presented at the Mid-Winter Neuro-Ophthalmology Symposium; January 30; 2021.* Accessed 13.02.21 https://medicine.umich.edu/dept/ophthalmology/events/202101/mid-winter-symposium.
11. Krieger P, Conway J, Hasanaj L, et al. Telemedicine evaluations in neuro-ophthalmology during the COVID-19 pandemic: patient and physician surveys. In: *North American Neuro-Ophthalmology Society 47th Annual Meeting; February 21*; 2021. Virtual.
12. Ko MW, Lai KE, Gilbert A, Sun L, Moss HE. Tele-neuro-ophthalmology: updates and future implications. In: *North American Neuro-Ophthalmology Society 47th Annual Meeting; February 20*; 2021. Virtual.
13. *Virtual Check in Coverage.* www.medicare.gov. Accessed 13.02.21 https://www.medicare.gov/coverage/virtual-check-ins.
14. Aronson SH. The Lancet on the telephone 1876–1975. *Med Hist.* 1977;21(1):69–87.
15. *COVID-19 Frequently Asked Questions (FAQs) on Medicare Fee-For-Service (FFS) Billing-And-Medicaid- Programs-Basic-Health-Program-And-Exchanges-Additional-Policy-And-Regulatory.* Accessed 13.02.21 https://www.cms.gov/files/document/medicare-telehealth-frequently-asked-questions-faqs-31720.pdf.
16. *What Patients Like—and Dislike—About Telemedicine. Harvard Business Review;* 2020. Accessed 13.02.21 https://hbr.org/2020/12/what-patients-like-and-dislike-about-telemedicine.
17. *Teleneuro-ophthalmology. Practical Neurology.* Accessed 13.02.21 https://practicalneurology.com/articles/2020-june/teleneuro-ophthalmology.
18. Stunkel L, Newman NJ, Biousse V. Diagnostic error and neuro-ophthalmology. *Curr Opin Neurol.* 2019;32(1):62–67.
19. Stunkel L, Newman-Toker DE, Newman NJ, Biousse V. Diagnostic error of neuro-ophthalmogic conditions: state of the science. *J Neuroophthalmol.* 2021;41(1):98–113.
20. Williams RD. *Neuro-Ophthalmology's SOS: Save Our Subspecialty.* EyeNet; 2020.
21. Healthcare Broadband in America. *Early Analysis and a Path Forward.* Federal Communications Commission; 2010. Accessed 15.02.21 https://transition.fcc.gov/national-broadband-plan/health-care-broadband-in-america-paper.pdf.
22. Chauhan D, Ko MW, Moss HE, Mackay DD, Lai KE. Broadband access in tele-neuro-ophthalmology. In: *North American Neuro-Ophthalmology Society 47th Annual Meeting;* 2021. Virtual.
23. *Byers Eye Institute at Stanford—YouTube.* www.youtube.com. Accessed 15.02.21 https://www.youtube.com/channel/UCuyhdx6pjRmUD_mcuqWybJA.

24. Lai KE, Ko MW, Rucker JC, et al. Tele-neuro-ophthalmology during the age of COVID-19. *J Neuroophthalmol.* 2020;40(3):292–304.

25. Adult Patients: Pupil Exam. *Adult Patients: Pupil Exam. YouTube;* 2020. Accessed 15.02.21 https://youtu.be/Dzdw5Z-g8zc.

26. Sun LD, Odel JG. Going back one car in the train: evaluation of the relative afferent pupillary defect in the era of tele-neuro-ophthalmology. *J Neuroophthalmol.* 2020;40(3):442.

27. Adult Patients: Eye Movement Exam. *Adult Patients: Eye Movement Exam. YouTube;* 2020. Accessed 15.02.21 https://youtu.be/Yv9edG1ms2o.

28. Salzman IJ. *A Retina Telemedicine Technique.* EyeNet; 2020.

29. Hribar MR, Biermann D, Goldstein IH, Chiang MF. Clinical documentation in electronic health record systems: analysis of patient record review during outpatient ophthalmology visits. *AMIA Annu Symp Proc.* 2018;2018:584–591.

30. Grossman SN, Calix R, Tow S, et al. Neuro-ophthalmology in the era of COVID-19: future implications of a public health crisis. *Ophthalmology.* 2020;127(9):e72–e74.

31. Milea D, Najjar RP, Zhubo J, et al. Artificial intelligence to detect papilledema from ocular fundus photography. *New Engl J Med.* 2020;382(18):1687–1695.

Low Vision Ocular Rehabilitation Telehealth

CAROLYN IHRIG, OD, FAAO • THAO M. HARRIS, OD, FAAO

DESCRIPTION AND BACKGROUND

The terms "legal blindness" and "low vision" are often used interchangeably, but they have different meanings. The United States government determines eligibility for vocation training, rehabilitation, disability benefits, and tax exemptions based on the definition of legal blindness. According to the United States' definition of legal blindness, an individual is considered legally blind if their visual acuity, measured by the Snellen eye chart, is 20/200 or less in the better-seeing eye with best correction by conventional lenses, such as glasses and contacts. An individual is also considered legally blind if their visual field is 20 degrees or less in the better-seeing eye.[1] The vision must be stable or expected to last at least 12 months for eligibility under the category.

In 2007, Social Security updated the criteria of legal blindness regarding vision acuity using newer charts such as the ETDRS chart, which measures acuity in logMAR with the Snellen equivalent acuity between 20/100 and 20/200. Legal blindness when measured with the ETDRS chart is not being able to read *any* letters on the 20/100 line. If a patient reads 20/125⁺ or 20/100⁻, the individual is not considered legally blind, but if a patient reads 20/125, the individual is legally blind. The visual field requirement remains the same.

Low vision is the loss of vision through hereditary and congenital infections or trauma, which cannot be corrected by conventional glasses or surgical intervention.[2] Patients with low vision have partial vision, usually 20/70 or poorer in the better-seeing eye, not correctable by conventional lenses (Table 9.1). Functional low vision impairment refers to an individual with visual complications that interfere with their daily activities, whether it is visual acuity, peripheral vision loss, or contrast sensitivity reduction. Functional low vision is subjective, and this is where vision rehabilitation can help.[3]

Low vision rehabilitation (LVR) is a thorough assessment of a patient's functional vision and through therapy, utilizing optical or non-optical devices, helps an individual improve their activities of daily living (ADLs). The goals of LVR are individualized for specific tasks as simple as reading or for more advanced tasks such as driving. Ophthalmologists (MD), Optometrists (OD), and low vision therapists (LVTs) work together to help patients succeed in vision rehabilitation. MDs manage the disease component by medical or surgical intervention, while ODs help with co-management and assess/prescribe optical devices. Finally, LVTs help assist patients learn how to best use the devices, be it

Ocular Telehealth. https://doi.org/10.1016/B978-0-323-83204-5.00009-3

Credit: http://www.aoa.org.

TABLE 9.1
Visual Impairment Codes (Courtesy of the American Optometric Association)

	VISUAL IMPAIRMENT CODES						
	IMPAIRMENT LEVEL OF THE BETTER-SEEING EYE						
	Total Impairment NLP	Near-Total Impairment <20/1000=<5 Degrees	Profound Impairment 20/500–20/1000=<10 Degrees	Severe Impairment 20/200–20/400=<20 Degrees	Moderate Impairment 20/70–20/160	Near–Normal Impairment 20/30–20/60	Normal Impairment 20/10–20/25
Impairment level of lesser eye — Total impairment NLP	369.01	369.03	369.06	369.12	369.16	369.62	369.63
Near-total impairment <20/1000=<5 Degrees		369.04	369.07	369.13	369.17	369.65	369.66
Profound impairment 20/500–20/1000=<10 Degrees			369.08	369.14	369.18	369.68	369.69
Severe impairment 20/200–20/400=<20 Degrees				369.22	369.24	369.72	369.73
Moderate impairment 20/70–20/160					369.25	369.75	369.76

optical or non-optical. With recommendations from low vision ODs, a LVT provides consultation in low vision therapy and prepares the patient for home adaptive skills training.

CONSEQUENCES OF LOW VISION AND ACCESS FOR LOW VISION REHABILITATION SERVICES

Vision loss not only affects the individual but also their family, workplace, and society. Management of ocular disease with multiple doctor visits puts the burden on family and friends, as many of these low vision patients are not legally eligible to drive. Some may not be able to return to work if vision loss continues or is permanent. Loss of income may eventually result in these individuals requiring assistance via monetary savings, disability, or Medicare/Medicaid services. Financial constraints and loss of independence could result in depression, anxiety, and the feeling of isolation. For example, when compared to non-age-related macular degeneration (AMD) populations, patients with poor vision due to AMD are at a higher risk for depression with a higher prevalence observed with increasing severity. Specifically, female patients with AMD who live alone and have more comorbidities are at a particularly high risk of depressive symptoms. Moreover, AMD patients are more likely to be pessimistic about their future.[4,5] It is especially important that LVR is provided to prevent this downward spiral.

The Veterans Affairs Low Vision Intervention Trial (LOVIT) provided evidence of the effectiveness of in-person low vision rehabilitation services. This randomized clinical trial demonstrated that outpatient low vision rehabilitation services significantly improved the functional visual ability of Veterans with moderately and severely impaired vision compared to patients in a similarly impaired waitlist control group who received no low vision services and who lost their functional ability during the same interval of time. As a result of the trial, it was recommended that low vision rehabilitation services be offered as early as possible after visual impairment is diagnosed, due to the decline in functional ability over time observed in the waitlisted control group.[6,7,8] The study supports that low vision early intervention is important for those affected by vision loss, whether in the VA or in the private sector.

However, what happens to patients who cannot travel to an outpatient rehabilitation program? Often, they end up not receiving any low vision rehabilitation services, and the patient risks a decline in functional ability. Uncorrectable vision loss due to conditions such as macular degeneration and diabetic retinopathy often restricts the mobility and travel of older adults (especially by automobiles) and is one of the barriers to receiving low vision rehabilitation faced by partially sighted individuals who live in all regions. While public transportation is accessible in major cities, the ease and comfort of travel may not be suitable for everyone. This is where a telehealth modality is critical to bridging the gap in care and can mitigate access problems for patients. Both public and private sectors can use low vision telehealth to improve access for patients with visual impairment who may face difficulty in traveling to a clinic to have an in-person LVR visit.

Telehealth continues to advance and has been critical in improving health outcomes across all regions, especially rural regions.[9,10,11,12,13] Synchronous telehealth modalities to the home such as Doximity, Microsoft Teams, Zoom, FaceTime, and others use real-time interactive video conferencing to assess, treat, and provide care to patients remotely. As discussed in previous chapters, these modalities are limited for some aspects of eye telehealth because of the difficulty of obtaining important physical exam findings, such as funduscopy or slit lamp exam. However, these modalities have been used quite successfully for low vision rehabilitation because current ocular clinical reports can be provided to the low vision OD. In addition to synchronous telehealth to the home, clinic-based synchronous telehealth can also be used where a telehealth facilitator (e.g., technician) links the patient(s) at a health-care setting (e.g., a primary care clinic) to the low vision provider(s) at another location.

For proper low vision telehealth scheduling, it is important to note that urgent eye care is not a part of a low vision ocular rehabilitation telehealth evaluation. Any potential ocular emergency requires the patient to be referred to their primary optometrist or ophthalmologist. Effective delivery of low vision rehabilitation services utilizing synchronous telehealth requires significant planning. Steps for implementing low vision ocular rehabilitation telehealth services include: (1) building the team; (2) designating clinic space; (3) acquiring equipment; and (4) receiving current clinical reports.[14,15] See Chapter 12 for more details on implementation.

THE LOW VISION AND OCULAR REHABILITATION TELEHEALTH MODEL: INDEX CASE EXAMPLE
Goals of the Program

The main goal of low vision ocular rehabilitation is to prevent depression by addressing the psychological effects of low vision and empowering each patient with the knowledge of their clinical information and how to adjust and function with their low vision status. LVR uses tools and technologies that can help keep patients independent and be able to do their activities of daily living (ADL), work, and hobbies.

In general, a basic low vision ocular rehabilitation telehealth evaluation educates and counsels each patient based on their specific visual condition and its implications. The low vision OD introduces magnification and explains how magnification works and more importantly, how it does not work. The overall goal is to help the patient accept the use of magnification by learning why they are needed and how to properly use the recommended devices. A plan of care is recommended to improve each patient's visual functioning specific to each patient's special vision demands, needs, and adjustment to vision loss. Specifically, recommendations are given (with positive and negative points) of different devices (both optical and non-optical) specific to each patient.

In the future, additional low vision devices can be prescribed as per initial recommendations and training in their homes with a therapist or utilizing video home-based telehealth.

Planning and Set up of Clinic-Based Synchronous Telehealth

The U.S. Department of Veterans Affairs (VA) is recognized as a world leader in the development of telehealth.[16,17,18] In 2011, the VA began pursuing innovative care-delivery strategies, including low vision rehabilitation. In the VA, the hub-and-spoke model, applied to low vision ocular rehabilitation telehealth, maximizes efficiencies and effectiveness through strategic centralization of low vision rehabilitation providers at a single site (hub) and distributes basic low vision rehabilitation services via secondary sites (spokes), which are physically located remotely from the hub and much more convenient to the patient's home (e.g., primary care clinic).[19] This same model can potentially be duplicated in the private sector by having several low vision providers associated with a low vision rehabilitation center, or a low vision optometrist can reach out to local pre-existing medical clinics to provide care.

Spoke sites could include any location convenient to low vision patients who are unable to drive several miles to a specialty clinic. Examples include a local nonprofit agency, satellite clinic, rural hospital, community outpatient center, local optometrist's or ophthalmologist's private office, etc. Arrangements will be needed at the spoke site for space, internet connection capability, and a telehealth facilitator. The spoke site needs to have some basic low vision equipment and a video-capable telehealth cart or a computer with internet connection (e.g., webcam). Low vision equipment include a near visual acuity chart and low vision magnification devices, including electronic devices, if there is space available.

Referrals and Patient Recruitment

Patients may be referred to the program via a consultation from an ophthalmologist, an optometrist, or other health-care providers. If available, clinical reports are requested from the patient's local eye care provider in order to obtain current clinical information, which will not be re-evaluated during a low vision ocular rehabilitation evaluation.[20] It is important to note that urgent optometry or ophthalmology care is not a part of low vision ocular rehabilitation telehealth services. *Any potential ocular emergency requires the patient to be referred for in-person clinical care* (Fig. 9.1).

Pre-visit

The recommended team at the hub site includes a scheduler, a LV optometrist, and a LV therapist. Indirectly, the patient's local optometrist and/or ophthalmologist is also on the team as the most current eye exam report should be available for the LV optometrist prior to the low vision telehealth visit.

The telehealth facilitator at the patient site (spoke) and/or the scheduler at the provider site (hub) is responsible for making appointments after checking insurance information and coordinating any pre-visit materials, such as mailing visual acuity charts or necessary questionnaires to be completed in advance of the appointment. The scheduler's duty also includes making sure the patient has access to the desired video telehealth platform, which will be used to connect to the low vision provider. Video-capable equipment with access to the internet is required both at the provider site (hub) and at each patient site (spoke). Equipment may include readily available technology such as iPads with FaceTime or more complex technological alternatives such as a telehealth cart, desktop, or laptop webcam, or even a high-definition business-quality video device, which fosters a sense of "telepresence" – a "face-to-face" experience with remote participants over the network that simulates being in the same room.

Day of visit

On the day of the LV telehealth encounter, the patient will go to the spoke site location and be greeted by the telehealth facilitator. The telehealth facilitator will then sit the patient comfortably in a chair and set up the

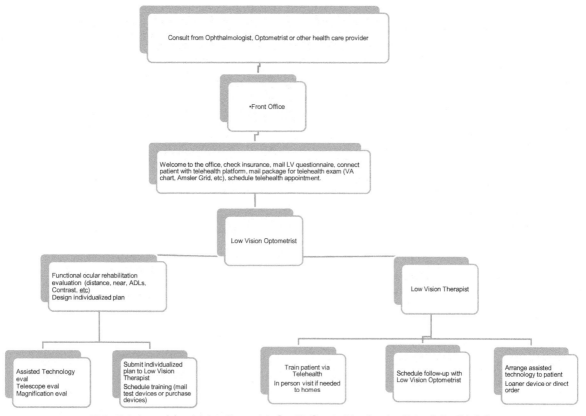

FIG. 9.1 Low vision telehealth model. Credit: Created by Carolyn Ihrig, O.D., F.A.A.O.

video equipment. The telehealth facilitator will have the demonstration low vision equipment kit ready. The low vision optometrist will then connect to the patient via video (Fig. 9.2).

A comprehensive history is gathered based on the patient's functional ability.[21,22] The LV doctor will go over current eye condition(s), vision, and functional loss the patient is experiencing. Throughout the low vision synchronous clinic-based telehealth consultation, the low vision optometrist asks specific questions, listens to the patient's answers, responds to the patient's questions, and introduces magnification and low vision rehabilitation. The patient is encouraged to set three goals, namely, distance, intermediate, and near. The telehealth facilitator will be instructed by the low vision optometrist to show the patient a particular magnifying tool, for example, and then the low vision optometrist will guide the patient on how to use the tool, observing the patient via the direct video connection and with the aid of the telehealth facilitator.

Modifications for Low Vision Synchronous Home-Based Telehealth

Home-based low vision ocular rehabilitation telehealth services can also be provided using two different methods. In the first method, the low vision optometrist makes a video call to the patient and a family member acts as the telehealth facilitator. In the second method, a low vision therapist travels to the patient's home and makes an in-home assessment of the patient, while acting as the telehealth facilitator for the low vision optometrist's synchronous telehealth encounter.

In the first strategy, home low vision ocular rehabilitation telehealth care can be provided to patients who have video access to a computer, laptop, tablet, or smartphone and use an agreed upon telehealth platform. If the patient does not have access to technology, they can ask family members or friends who do to assist the patient to connect to the telehealth provider during the session. Prior to the telehealth encounter, visual acuity charts are mailed or emailed to the patient

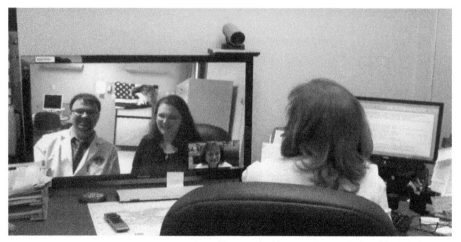

FIG. 9.2 Low vision evaluation via telehealth. Source: Carolyn Ihrig, O.D., F.A.A.O.

to print. If preferred, history materials, along with a sample "box" of common devices can be mailed to the patient's home.

After all necessary documents are sent and received, a telehealth appointment is set up for the patient with the LV optometrist. The patient's ocular health and refractive status is determined by a local optometrist/ophthalmologist before the LV telehealth services are scheduled.

Once the goals are established, the patient will use the acuity chart mailed prior to the exam to assess the acuity with the help of a family member. Based on the acuity, the LV optometrist will note the magnifiers, telescope, etc., that the patient may need. The low vision optometrist demonstrates and instructs the patient and the patient's family member on proper focusing techniques with specific low vision optical devices. The assistant or sighted family member guides the low vision patient as needed, and observes the provider through the monitor as needed to help the patient properly utilize optical and non-optical devices. The patient's family member or helper does not require specialized training on the proper utilization of low vision devices prior to the telehealth evaluation (Fig. 9.3).

In the second strategy, the low vision therapist travels to the patient's home with a laptop or tablet with a customized low vision rehabilitation travel kit, and once the therapist arrives, he/she connects to the low vision optometrist. In this option, the only home-based telehealth appointment is the low vision optometrist's ocular rehabilitation telehealth evaluation, followed by the therapist's in-person home assessment. Future home follow-up and training visits are scheduled by the therapist as needed.

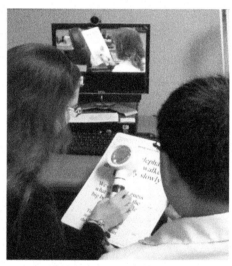

FIG. 9.3 Low vision evaluation via telehealth model. Source: Carolyn Ihrig, O.D., F.A.A.O.

After the initial telehealth exam is completed, the LV optometrist will submit a report of the patient's needs to the family members and discuss ordering devices. At the end of the exam, the patient will be seen by the low vision therapist or a future appointment will be scheduled with the LV therapist. It is also a good time to discuss a loan plan or loaner devices if the patient wishes to try before committing.

Low vision therapist follow-up
The final component of any low vision evaluation includes an assessment with the LV therapist. A synchronous telehealth consultation with a low vision

rehabilitation therapist (either home-based or clinic-based) typically follows the telehealth consultation by the low vision optometrist. With recommendations from the low vision optometrist, a low vision rehabilitation therapist provides consultation in low vision therapy and prepares the patient for home adaptive skills training.[23,24,25] An LVR therapist reviews and documents a comprehensive list of functional vision rehabilitation issues and assesses therapy recommendations. Proper training and education begin during the first session and continue in subsequent sessions. An in-person low vision therapy rehabilitation follow-up appointment is scheduled by the therapist at the patient's home to train and assess other areas of adaptive living skills as needed. The home visit may include a home safety[26] checklist, orientation and mobility training, computer access training, and other skills not readily and easily taught using clinic-based synchronous telehealth. The LV therapist will go over devices, whether purchased or loaned, which are recommended to the patient. Based on each individual practice protocol, the patient will have training with a LV therapist once the devices are attained and monitored on a monthly basis. Following the training, the LV therapist will set up an "exit" telehealth appointment for the patient with the LV optometrist.

Post-rehabilitation

Following several sessions, once the low vision team has completed addressing the patient's low vision rehabilitation goals, a survey or questionnaire is completed to obtain feedback about the overall low vision rehabilitation service experience, such as whether care was delivered in-person or via telehealth. The VA model has illustrated that a majority of the patients have provided positive feedback. Specifically related to telehealth, patients greatly appreciated the LV clinic-based synchronous telehealth services because it allowed them to receive services they would otherwise not have been able to receive.

LOW VISION AND OCULAR REHABILITATION TELEHEALTH BILLING

The detailed billing and coding guidelines for ocular telehealth are given in Chapter 14. One needs to assess the patient's insurance carrier and/or Medicare regarding payments to providers for telehealth vision rehabilitation services in satellite private offices and blind agencies. Medicare payment for telehealth services is established in 1834(m) of the Social Security Act and covered under the Medicare Fee-For-Service Program, and a limited number of services are reimbursed

with conditional requirements.[27,28,29,30] Medicare and Medicaid services do not cover low vision devices and low vision rehabilitation. Private practitioners may bill separately for an office visit or consultation, appropriate testing (i.e., visual fields), and follow-up care. There are also nonprofit organizations that can help these individuals cover low vision expenses.

Private insurance may cover certain expenses for the individuals when practitioners write letters declaring that the patient is legally blind. According to the American Optometric Association, a letter stating the patient "requires specialized services to maintain his independence/employment/educational access"; these services are to "restore the functioning of a malformed or damaged body part" may help patients get coverage for traditional noncovered services.

A complete encounter consultation includes 99242–99244 based on the number of elements met. These codes that are used in cases in which time is the key element for counseling and/or coordination of care with other physicians, other qualified health-care professionals, or agencies are provided consistent with the nature of the problem(s) and the patient's and/or family's needs. When using time as the key element, the time spent on counseling/coordination or care must be > 50% at the time of the examination. The best practice is to document or make medical notes on time spent, in 15-min increments, with the patient's care. The primary diagnosis is the ocular condition, and the secondary diagnosis will be the visual impairment code. Modifier code 95 (synchronous telemedicine service) is used for the telehealth clinic.

For visits without a consultation, 99201–99205 (new) or 99211–99215 (established) can be billed, based on the number of elements for history, exam, and medical decision making, or based on counseling and/or coordination of care with time as the key element. The primary diagnosis is the ocular condition, and secondary diagnosis will be the visual impairment code. Modifier code 95 (synchronous telemedicine service) is used for the telehealth clinic.

The American Medical Association made some changes, effective from January 1, 2021, regarding CPT evaluation and management of office, outpatient, and prolonged services. Time may be used to select a code level in office or other outpatient services (i.e., telehealth) and to determine whether counseling and/or coordination of care dominates the service. Time coding could be in-person or non-in-person care. These codes include 99202–99205 and 99212–99215. The primary diagnosis is the ocular condition, and the secondary diagnosis will be the visual impairment code.

TABLE 9.2
CMS-1734-F CY2021 List of Telehealth Eye Services

Code	Short Descriptor	Status *	Can Audio-only Interaction Meet the Requirements?
92002	Eye exam new patient	Temporary Addition—Added 4/30/20	
92004	Eye exam new patient	Temporary Addition—Added 4/30/20	
92012	Eye exam establish patient	Temporary Addition—Added 4/30/20	
92014	Eye exam&tx estab pt 1/>vst	Temporary Addition—Added 4/30/20	
97161	Pt eval low complex 20 min	Temporary Addition	
97162	Pt eval mod complex 30 min	Temporary Addition	
97163	Pt eval high complex 45 min	Temporary Addition	
97164	Pt re-eval est plan care	Temporary Addition	
97165	Ot eval low complex 30 min	Temporary Addition	
97166	Ot eval mod complex 45 min	Temporary Addition	
97167	Ot eval high complex 60 min	Temporary Addition	
97168	Ot re-eval est plan care	Temporary Addition	
97755	Assistive technology assess	Temporary Addition	
99441	Phone e/m phys/qhp 5-10 min	Temporary Addition—Added 4/30/20	YES
99442	Phone e/m phys/qhp 11-20 min	Temporary Addition—Added 4/30/20	YES
99443	Phone e/m phys/qhp 21-30 min	Temporary Addition—Added 4/30/20	YES

Credit: https://www.cms.gov/Medicare/Coding/ICD10.

For telehealth clinics, modifier code 95 (synchronous telemedicine service) is added. Effective from March 1, 2020, due to the COVID-19 public health emergency, telehealth services are covered by Medicare and insurance. See Table 9.2. The highlighted codes are relevant to low vision consultations.

CONCLUSIONS AND LESSONS LEARNED

Telehealth is helping to improve the overall healthcare system in many ways, especially for rural patients. The increased reach of low vision clinical care due to the addition of LV telehealth clinics demonstrates the power of telehealth modalities to improve the access for many ocular services, including low vision rehabilitation. More partially sighted and legally blind patients, who

could not travel in-person to a location that provided comprehensive low vision rehabilitation services, received care because of the use of telehealth. Clinic-based synchronous telehealth currently allows low vision rehabilitation with a low vision optometrist and a low vision rehabilitation therapist in a manner that is timely, without the need for the patient to travel long distances to receive services. Ocular telehealth, with a strong low vision team approach, involving highly qualified professionals dedicated to optimal vision rehabilitation, enables each patient to maximize his or her independent abilities by beginning low vision rehabilitation as early as possible.

While this chapter highlighted a VA program, low vision telehealth can become a reality outside the VA. For example, private low vision optometrists can use telehealth to provide services to older adults in the private sector. The ability to access a low vision optometrist remotely improves access to care for patients, particularly older people who already face travel barriers even without the challenges of visual impairment. Many older partially sighted patients, who are unable to drive safely, unfortunately forego low vision rehabilitation care because of the inconvenience and difficult travel distances when they have no other transportation resources or options. Utilizing low vision telehealth technologies can save money with reduced travel costs for the patient and reduce stress for patients when travel is reduced or eliminated.[31] Establishing[32] a 'virtual' network of low vision optometrists across the country can effectively eliminate the barriers associated with long distances and provider shortages. Most importantly, ready availability of low vision rehabilitation prevents depression, loss of function, and isolation that partially sighted individuals experience, ultimately leading to a more meaningful and higher quality of life for these patients.

REFERENCES

1. American Foundation for the Blind. *Low Vision and Legal Blindness Terms and Descriptions*; 2020. https://www.afb.org/blindness-and-low-vision/eye-conditions/low-vision-and-legal-blindness-terms-and-descriptions.
2. National Eye Institute. *Low Vision*; 2020. https://www.nei.nih.gov/learn-about-eye-health/eye-conditions-and-diseases/low-vision.
3. American Optometric Association. *Care of the Patient With Visual Impairment (Low Vision Rehabilitation)*; 2020. https://www.aoa.org.
4. Dawson SR, Mallen CD, Gouldstone MB, Yarham R, Mansell G. The prevalence of anxiety and depression in people with age-related macular degeneration: a systematic review of observational study data. *BMC Ophthalmol.* 2014;14:78.
5. Mylona I, Floros G, Dermenoudi M, Ziakas N, Tsinopoulos I. A comparative study of depressive symptomatology among cataract and age-related macular degeneration patients with impaired vision. *Psychol Health Med.* 2020;25(9):1130–1136. epub 2020 Feb 17.
6. Stelmack JA, Tang XC, Reda DJ, et al. Outcomes of the veterans affairs low vision intervention trial (LOVIT). *Arch Ophthalmol.* 2008;126(5):608–617.
7. Stelmack JA, Tang XC, Wei Y, Massof RW. Low-vision intervention study group: the effectiveness of low-vision rehabilitation in 2 cohorts derived from the veterans affairs low-vision intervention trial. *Arch Ophthalmol.* 2012;130(9):1162–1168.
8. Stelmack JA, Tang XC, Wei Y, et al. Outcomes of the veterans affairs low vision intervention trial II (LOVIT II). *JAMA Opthalmol.* 2017;135:96–104.
9. Ackerman MJ, Filart R, Burgess LP, Lee I, Poropatich RK. Developing next-generation telehealth tools and technologies: patients, systems, and data perspectives. *Telemed J E Health.* 2010;16(1):93–95.
10. Agha Z, Roter DL, Schapira RM. An evaluation of patient-physician communication style during telemedicine consultations. *J Med Internet Res.* 2009;11(3), e36.
11. Finkelstein SM, Speedie SM, Potthoff S. Home telehealth improves clinical outcomes at lower cost for home healthcare. *Telemed J E Health.* 2006;12(2):128–136.
12. Lawrence D. Let's meet onscreen. The use of video is expanding beyond rural areas. *Healthc Inform.* 2010; 27(4):26–28.
13. Yellowlees P, Odor A, Patrice K, et al. Disruptive innovation: the future of healthcare? *Telemed J E Health.* 2011;17(3):231–234.
14. Ihrig C. Steps to offering low vision rehabilitation services through clinical video telehealth. *J Vis Impair Blind.* 2016;110:441–447.
15. Ihrig C. Rural healthcare pilot clinic: low vision clinical video telehealth. *J Assoc Sch Coll Optometry Educ Podium.* 2014;40:14–16.
16. U.S. Department of Veterans Affairs. *VA Telehealth Services*; 2016. Retrieved from http://www.telehealth.va.gov. [Health Information Privacy, 2020].
17. National Advisory Committee on Rural Health and Human Services. *Telehealth in Rural America*; 2015. http://www.hrsa.gov/advisorycommittees/rural/publications/telehealthmarch2015.
18. U.S. Department of Health & Human Services. *Defining Rural Population*; 2015. Retrieved from http://www.hrsa.gov/ruralhealth/aboutus/definition.html.
19. Elrod JK, Fortenberry JL. The hub-and-spoke organization design: an avenue for serving patients well. *BMC Health Serv Res.* 2017;17(suppl. 1):457. DOI 10.1 186/s.
20. Sunness JS, El Annan J. Improvement of visual acuity by refraction in a low-vision population. *Ophthalmology.* 2010;117(7):1442–1446.
21. Boerner K, Wang SW. Goals with limited vision: a qualitative study of coping with vision-related goal interference in midlife. *Clin Rehabil.* 2012;26(1):81–93.
22. Colenbrander A. Assessment of functional vision and its rehabilitation. *Acta Ophthalmol.* 2010;88(2):163–173.
23. Bambara JK, Wadley V, Owsley C, Martin RC, Porter C, Dreer LE. Family functioning and low vision: a systematic review. *J Vis Impair Blind.* 2009;103(3):137–149.
24. McDonnall MC. Physical status as a moderator of depressive symptoms among older adults with dual sensory loss. *Rehabil Psychol.* 2011;56(1):67–76.
25. Wei H, Sawchyn AK, Myers JS, et al. A clinical method to assess the effect of visual loss on the ability to perform activities of daily living. *Br J Ophthalmol.* 2012;96(5):735–741.
26. Barstow BA, Bennett DK, Vogtle LK. Perspectives on home safety: do home safety assessments address the concerns of clients with vision loss? *Am J Occup Ther.* 2011;65(6):635–664.

27. Social Security Act, Title 18, Section 1834. n.d. Retrieved from https://www.ssa.gov/OP_Home/ssact/title18/1834.htm.

28. Health Information Privacy. *Summary of the HIPAA Security Rule*; 2020. https://www.hhs.gov/hipaa/for-professionals/security/laws-regulations/index.html.

29. Centers for Medicare and Medicaid Services. *Telehealth Services: Rural Health Series.* Baltimore, MD: Centers for Medicare and Medicaid Services, Department of Health and Human Services; 2015.

30. Centers for Medicare and Medicaid Services. *ICD-10*; 2020. https://www.cms.gov/Medicare/Coding/ICD10.

31. Ihrig C. Travel cost savings and practicality for low-vision telerehabilitation. *Telemed J E Health.* 2019;25(7):649–654.

32. Ihrig C. Home low vision ocular rehabilitation telehealth expansion due to COVID-19 pandemic. *Telemed J E Health* 2021. https://doi.org/10.1089/tmj.2021.0264. PMID: 34559013.

CHAPTER 10

Highlight on International Ocular Telehealth Programs in China and India

JIANJUN LI, MD, PHD • RENGARAJ VENKATESH, MD • BHARAT GURNANI, MD • RAVILLA D. THULASIRAJ, MBA

SECTION I: CHINA

JianJun Li, MD PhD

Introduction to the Current Situation of Ocular Telehealth in China

Ocular telehealth in China started in the early 21st century and its development is closely related to the development of a robust information technology network. China has a large population and a vast territory. There are large differences in the scope of ophthalmic medical services and the availability of ophthalmic subspecialty services among the different regions. Therefore, in order to improve access to eye care and improve eye care equity, China has carried out ocular telehealth research and related telemedicine services in recent years. The Beijing Institute of Ophthalmology is one of the earliest units to carry out tele-ophthalmic research and to operationalize pilot projects in China.

Compared with an in-person traditional visit, an eye telehealth encounter has the advantages of being time saving, labor saving, and money saving. Patients can receive an examination and treatment in their local hospitals and spend less time and money than if they were to travel a long distance seeking treatment

Ocular Telehealth. https://doi.org/10.1016/B978-0-323-83204-5.00010-X

in other places. The Chinese ocular telehealth program accepts consultation requests from remote ophthalmologists. Data gathered from the remote eye providers at each visit are stored in a cloud platform system, which can easily be queried and downloaded by the remote specialist through the internet, which is conducive to interprofessional consultations and referrals and provides an objective baseline for future follow-ups.

At present, the most common instrument used to obtain ophthalmic images is a digital fundus camera. It not only captures fundus images but also takes pictures of the external eye and the anterior segment. The images are small (hundreds of kilobytes (KB)), which is convenient for archiving, remote transmission, and fast download. In recent years, the trend is for digital fundus cameras to become more portable. Some studies have used smartphones for fundus photography, but image clarity and scope of photography are limited. Other commonly used methods to capture tele-ophthalmic images are slit-lamp anterior segment photography and optical coherence tomography (OCT); however, as the technical capabilities of grassroots medical units are limited, slit lamp and OCT testing are not widely carried out at present.

In recent years, telehealth units have provided image reading, asynchronous tele-ophthalmic consultation services, and even synchronous home-based video consultations in the form of WeChat and application programs (apps) through other mobile terminals, such as smartphones and tablet computers (e.g., an iPad). However, the scale using these newer technologies is not widespread because it is greatly affected by network transmission speed.

It should be emphasized that the current telehealth programs in China cannot replace traditional in-person diagnosis and treatment. Ocular telehealth in China is more suitable at present for the screening of common eye diseases, especially important blinding eye diseases (such as cataract, glaucoma, diabetic retinopathy, macular disease, etc.), and for screening eye complications in the prognosis of systemic chronic diseases. For the diagnosis of complex and severe eye diseases, telemedicine is not appropriate for patient care and is best used as an important consultation platform. In China, as in other places in the world, the purpose of carrying forward and developing eye telehealth is not to replace the traditional diagnosis and treatment service but to add a new entrance and a new way of patient management, complementing traditional diagnosis and treatment visits. It is a beneficial supplement to in-person care.

At present, tele-ophthalmology in China includes the following services: spoken and written consultation, image screening, and video consultation and archiving.

TYPES OF OCULAR TELEHEALTH SERVICES OFFERED IN CHINA
Part 1: Tele-Eye Spoken and Written Consultation
This telehealth service is designed to allow patients to directly consult remote doctors about the diagnosis and treatment of their eye disease(s) through text or telephone inquiries. In addition to internet websites, text consultation is mostly implemented through mobile apps. The disadvantage is the lack of image data or incomplete image data and poor image quality. At present, patients are the initiators of remote consultation, which are mostly mediated by third-party organizations in China, such as Haoda online or Chunyu Doctor.

Part 2: Tele-Ophthalmic Image Screening
Tele-ophthalmic image screening is of great importance for early detection of common blinding eye diseases and ocular complications of chronic diseases. This type of ocular telehealth service has been operational in some areas of China for several years and is therefore, a relatively mature program. Tele-ophthalmic image screening is an asynchronous telehealth program that includes both primary screening and advanced screening.

The initiators of primary screening are mostly primary medical units lacking a department of ophthalmology, such as community clinics, health examination centers, spectacle shops, townships, and rural clinics. The process is as follows: basic units collect a simple history of systemic chronic diseases, perform a simple visual acuity assessment (using a vision-screening card), and take non-mydriatic fundus images. If the fundus images are not clear as judged by the personnel taking the photographs, then they also take a 2D external eye image. Patient information is uploaded to the database; if possible, it is transmitted to the cloud platform. Eye doctors read the images remotely, and then the reading results are transmitted back to the community units.

The initiators of advanced screening are mainly primary medical units with better ophthalmic technology, such as county-level hospitals or non-ophthalmic specialized hospitals. The common process is to collect the history of chronic diseases, fill in the ocular chief complaint, conduct visual examination, and take fundus images with or without mydriasis. Patients are dilated if the hospital has access to ophthalmology and in patients with a resting pupil size of 4.0 mm or less. If the fundus image is not clear in a non-mydriatic patient, as judged by the telehealth facilitator, then there is an attempt to take fundus photos with mydriasis. Before dilation, the possibility of causing angle closure and intraocular pressure increase should be evaluated. Then, if the fundus image is not clear, external 2D eye images are taken with a fundus camera. The patient's data are uploaded to the database or cloud platform. Ophthalmologists can then read images remotely, and then the reading results will be transmitted back to the hospitals or to the patients themselves.

Readers at the image reading center evaluate the photo quality and determine whether it is necessary to transfer or consult for an in-person visit. If the readers think it is necessary to refer the patient for an in-person exam, they can directly click the referral and consultation link in the system software and make an appointment at the professional doctor's clinic of the ophthalmic center. If no referral is required, follow-up

and time to follow-up will be indicated on the image reading report. The image reading report of screening can be completed in real time or within an agreed time limit. When carrying out large-scale tele-ophthalmic services with a large number of patients, the image readers at the ophthalmic image reading center arrange shifts to read images. For emergency patients, through the coordination of operation management personnel, a "green channel" can be provided for emergency image reading and video consultation can also be applied if necessary (Figs. 10.1–10.4 show screen shots of the reading software and an example of the fundus image obtained during the telemedicine visit.).

Tele-ophthalmic image reading screening has developed rapidly in China in recent years. From 2013 to 2015, 7282 cases, 36276 cases, and 73571 cases respectively, were screened by the Research on Diagnostic Standard, Service Mode and Application Demonstration

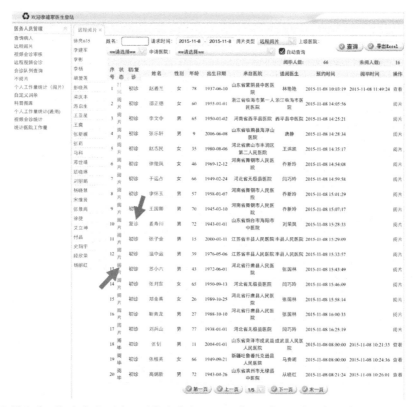

FIG. 10.1 List of patients in the tele-ophthalmic image reading software interface. Patient status includes: waiting to be read (*red arrow*), after reading, and reject (rejected by the image reader due to incomplete data or serious quality defects). The patients in the follow-up queue are marked in red (*blue arrow*). The source of the patient's primary hospital, the doctor transmitting the images, the time of image transmission, and the time of image reading completion are also shown in the software interface. In addition, the software can query and export patient data. (Credit: Li Jianjun MD PhD.)

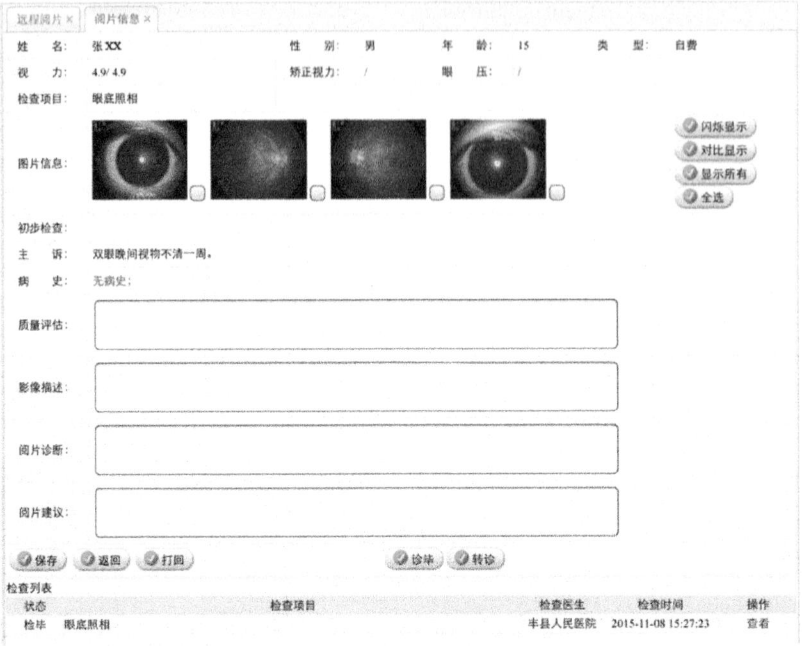

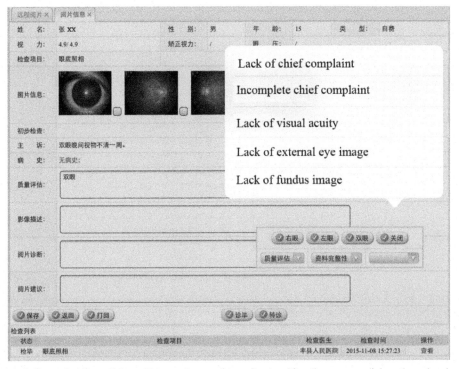

FIG. 10.2 Sample software interface for image interpretation. The eye provider is required to evaluate the quality of the transmitted data, describe the images, and make preliminary diagnosis and treatment suggestions. Free text entry boxes are available; provider customized entries can also be used. (Credit: Li Jianjun MD PhD.)

FIG. 10.3 Example of template options on the reading software. After the mouse click, a three-level entry menu appears, which can be customized. (Credit: Li Jianjun MD PhD.)

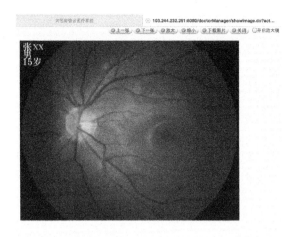

FIG. 10.4 Image viewing interface on the image reading software. Software tools for image reading include: page turning, zooming in, zooming out, image downloading, magnifying glass, and other functions. (Credit: Li Jianjun MD PhD.)

of Tele-ophthalmic Imaging, a project of the Beijing Institute of Ophthalmology. Fig. 10.5 shows the growth of cases over time, and Table 10.1 illustrates diagnoses made from the telemedicine program.

Studies have shown that hypertensive retinopathy and diabetic retinopathy are the most common ocular manifestations of systemic diseases in the tele-ophthalmic image reading screening of the

project. Cataract, macular epiretinal membrane, glaucoma, branch retinal vein occlusion, and other eye diseases are common in people over 50 years of age (Table 10.1). However, the satisfaction of patients with tele-ophthalmic screening needs further investigation.

The difficulties of image reading in tele-ophthalmic screening include: (1) identification of hard exudates, drusen, fundus reflection, and lens light path artifact; (2) identification of cotton wool spot and fundus reflection, lens artifact, and local retinal edema; (3) identification of severe NPDR or more on a single fundus image; (4) recognition of glaucomatous optic nerve change by non-glaucoma professional doctors; (5) identification of cataract requiring surgical treatment on a single fundus image; (6) in the absence of a chief complaint, central serous choroidoretinopathy is easily missed without careful comparison of both fundus images of the eyes; (7) identification of macular dystrophy (Stargardt disease, cone-rod cell dystrophy, etc.) on a single fundus image; and (8) in the absence of medical history, early hypertensive retinopathy with only vascular changes is easily overlooked.

Another tele-ophthalmic screening project is the "Diabetic Retinopathy Screening and Prevention Project in China" initiated by the Diabetes and Microcirculation Professional Committee of Chinese Microcirculation Society. In this project, doctors and nurses in the department of endocrinology take fundus photos without mydriasis, and the images are sent to a

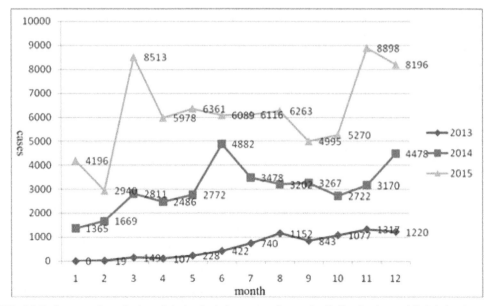

FIG. 10.5 Case number of tele-ophthalmologic image reading at the Beijing Institute of Ophthalmology from 2013 to 2015 (by month). (Credit: Li Jianjun MD PhD.)

TABLE 10.1
Diseases diagnosed by image reading in 2013–2015.

Disease	2013		2014		2015		TOTAL		Sort
	Cases	%	Cases	%	Cases	%	Cases	%	
Cataract	507	6.96	2587	7.13	12,642	17.18	15,736	13.43	1
Retinal arteriosclerosis	338	4.64	1540	4.25	5541	7.53	7419	6.33	2
DR	568	7.8	1472	4.06	5384	7.32	7324	6.25	3
Glaucoma and suspicious glaucoma	417	5.73	1032	2.84	3093	4.2	4542	3.88	4
Hypertensive retinopathy	12	0.16	617	1.7	3817	5.19	4446	3.8	5
Epiretinal membrane	221	3.03	657	1.81	1949	2.65	2827	2.41	6
Pathological myopia	207	2.84	407	1.12	1569	2.13	2183	1.86	7
BRVO	85	1.17	341	0.94	1140	1.55	1566	1.34	8
Subconjunctival hemorrhage	66	0.91	253	0.7	847	1.15	1166	1	9
Optic atrophy	50	0.69	292	0.8	800	1.09	1142	0.97	10
Pterygium	68	0.93	194	0.53	745	1.01	1007	0.86	11
AMD	56	0.77	175	0.48	662	0.9	893	0.76	12
Central serous choroidoretinopathy	47	0.65	165	0.45	477	0.65	689	0.59	13
CRVO	38	0.52	127	0.35	464	0.63	629	0.54	14
Posterior vitreous detachment	2	0.03	113	0.31	500	0.68	615	0.53	15
AION	13	0.18	83	0.23	335	0.46	431	0.37	16
Edema of optic disc	43	0.59	104	0.29	255	0.35	402	0.34	17
Macular hole	34	0.47	83	0.23	283	0.38	400	0.34	18
Retinitis pigmentosa	35	0.48	102	0.28	246	0.33	383	0.33	19
Vitreous hemorrhage	22	0.3	120	0.33	238	0.32	380	0.32	20
Retinal detachment	31	0.43	73	0.2	238	0.32	342	0.29	21
Myelinated fibers of retina	22	0.3	57	0.16	201	0.27	280	0.24	22
Corneal cloudiness and leukoplakia	21	0.29	58	0.16	195	0.27	274	0.23	23
Vitreous stellate degeneration	0	0	52	0.14	205	0.28	257	0.22	24
Ocular contusion	0	0	37	0.1	217	0.29	254	0.22	25
Uveitis	6	0.08	61	0.17	166	0.23	233	0.2	26
Concussion of retina	0	0	54	0.15	126	0.17	180	0.15	27

Cystoid macular edema	17	0.23	33	0.09	129	0.18	179	0.15	28
Ocular hypertension	0	0	25	0.07	141	0.19	166	0.14	29
CRAO	13	0.18	32	0.09	115	0.16	160	0.14	30
PCV	3	0.04	21	0.06	119	0.16	143	0.12	31
Optic neuritis	5	0.07	25	0.07	61	0.08	91	0.08	32
Congenital coloboma of iris and choroid	9	0.12	14	0.04	66	0.09	89	0.08	33
Keratitis	0	0	20	0.06	60	0.08	80	0.07	34
BRAO	3	0.04	18	0.05	52	0.07	73	0.06	35
Traumatic hyphema	3	0.04	15	0.04	47	0.06	65	0.06	36
Traumatic mydriasis	0	0	21	0.06	38	0.05	59	0.05	37
Idiopathic macular choroidal neovascularization	2	0.03	13	0.04	27	0.04	42	0.04	38
Optic disc vasculitis	0	0	12	0.03	17	0.02	29	0.02	39
Traumatic iridodialysis	2	0.03	5	0.01	18	0.02	25	0.02	40
Vogt–Koyanagi–Harada (VKH) syndrome	0	0	6	0.02	9	0.01	15	0.01	41
Stargardt disease	0	0	4	0.01	6	0.01	10	0.01	42

remote image reading platform. Artificial intelligence (AI) will automatically read the images first, which indicate the lesion points and objective quantitative reports, and then sends the results back to the endocrine clinic 3–5 min later. Unacceptable fundus images (blurry or abnormal images) are automatically transferred to ophthalmologists for reading. Patients obtain an electronic report through their official account of WeChat and receive follow-up reminders, patient education materials, and referral service information according to the severity of disease. From June 2016 to September 2020, the project has completed 1,016,400 cases of diabetic screening in more than 700 medical institutions in 30 provinces and cities; however, 464,000 cases were converted to manual reading due to poor image quality. Among 1,016,400 cases, 337,000 cases were diabetic retinopathy positive. A total of 148,000 cases were mild NPDR, 100,000 cases were moderate NPDR, and 89,000 cases were severe NPDR or more. A flowchart of the analysis of fundus images in this project is illustrated in Fig. 10.6.

Part 3: Tele-Ophthalmic Video Consultation

In the project of "Research on Diagnostic Standard, Service Mode and Application Demonstration of Tele-ophthalmic Imaging" of the Beijing Institute of Ophthalmology, both synchronous clinic-based video consultation, carried out between medical units and the reading center, and synchronous home-based video consultation are performed. China anticipates that the synchronous home-based video telehealth modality will likely have a greater demand in the future. The eye telehealth video encounter is made by appointment, and is generally completed within 1–7 days after the asynchronous telehealth visit (hybrid model). Ophthalmologists at the telemedicine center participate in video consultations according to their specialties. Video consultations are usually conducted

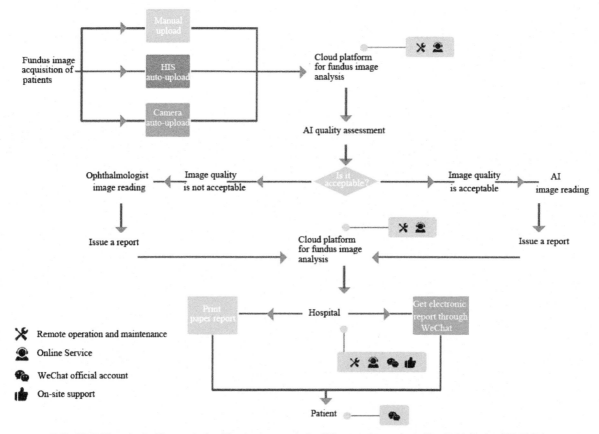

FIG. 10.6 Flowchart of the analysis of fundus images in the DR screening project. (Credit: Li Jianjun MD PhD.)

based on the diagnoses made from image reading. The technological process is as follows:

(1) After a discussion between the doctor and the patient at the primary hospital (spoke site), doctors in the primary hospital put forward video consultation requests in the software system. Fig. 10.7 shows a screen shot of the video platform.

(2) Patients are registered and provide informed consent at the primary hospitals.

(3) The coordinator of the remote image reading center makes an appointment with the relevant eye doctor and alerts the doctors in the primary hospital via the software system once the appointment has been made successfully. The doctors in the primary hospital inform the patient and prepare the relevant examination data.

(4) Video consultations are performed according to appointment time. Participants may include patients and their families, doctors and coordinators of the primary hospital, and doctors and coordinators of the remote consultation center (Fig. 10.8).

(5) At the end of the video consultation, the ophthalmologist at the remote center fills the consultation report via the software system and transmits it to the doctors in the primary hospital. Doctors in the primary hospitals are responsible for the treatment of patients according to the consultation results.

From 2014 to 2016, there were 540 cases of patients coming from 39 county-level hospitals within 16 provinces in the tele-ophthalmic project of the Beijing Institute of Ophthalmology. The average time interval between request for consultation and completion of consultation was 2.44 ± 2.66 days, and each video consultation time was 15–20 min. Data show that the most common reasons for tele-ophthalmic consultation were as follows: monocular optic disc edema, secondary glaucoma, glaucoma surgical complication management, retinal vein occlusion, and proliferative diabetic retinopathy (Table 10.2). While remote video consultation is a more time-intensive form of tele-ophthalmic service, it is a useful way to help treat more complex eye diseases. The referral mechanism after asynchronous image reading needs to be refined.

The factors to keep in mind with respect to a tele-ophthalmic video consultation are: (1) the remote identification of some types of secondary glaucoma is difficult; (2) the remote identification of monocular optic disc edema including AION is also difficult; (3) the anti-VEGF treatment of RVO combined with macular edema are common issues at the community hospital; and (4) public awareness of DM and diabetic retinopathy is still poor, and the treatment of PDR, especially at primary hospitals, is still difficult.

The accuracy of tele-ophthalmic video consultation needs to be compared with in-person diagnosis and treatment, but there should be no difference between video versus in-person patient counseling.

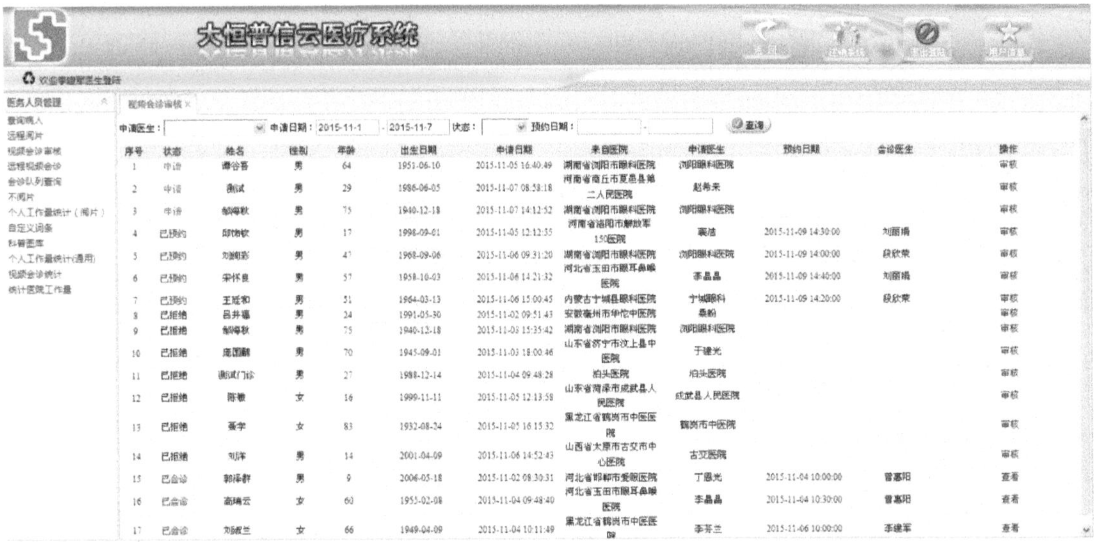

FIG. 10.7 Management interface of tele-ophthalmic video consultation program. The interface list shows the overall status of patients in the video consultation. (Credit: Li Jianjun MD PhD.)

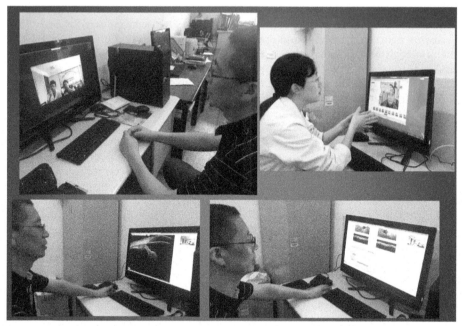

FIG. 10.8 Tele-ophthalmic video consultation for glaucoma and strabismus patients. (Credit: Li Jianjun MD PhD.)

Part 4: Tele-Ophthalmic Image Archiving

Tele-ophthalmic image archiving refers to an ocular telehealth system that allows different medical units to upload and store the patient's image and other medical records on the cloud platform. This will facilitate patients being able to have their cases reviewed by different doctors serving different medical units. Doctors in different units can access the medical record data with a password. This will lay the foundation for regional collaborative medical care. Even if the doctors in primary units read images by themselves, they can still upload images to the cloud platform database for archiving purposes alone. Another purpose of uploading images for archiving is to create and store a personal health file for each patient that he/she can view, which can reduce the chance of loss and damage of the patient's personal data as well as facilitate continuity of care for that individual patient.

FUTURE DIRECTIONS

In summary, there are many aspects of ocular telehealth that have been implemented and need to be further studied and improved upon in China. First of all, the tele-ophthalmic service has not been widely accepted and recognized. A considerable number of patients and doctors in primary hospitals are still skeptical about telemedicine, and ophthalmologists from larger hospitals are not enthusiastic enough about the program to be willing to participate. Second, it should be emphasized that ocular telehealth services are meant to supplement in-person eye care. Although the enthusiasm of third-party operators for tele-ophthalmology is high, it is necessary to recognize that not all patients are appropriate candidates for telehealth, depending on their eye care needs and medical condition. Third, there is a dispute on who takes the responsibility for patients in an ocular telehealth program, and it is urgent to formulate a detailed policy on this topic. Fourth, the access and referral standards of participating in tele-ophthalmic service units need to be established. It is also very important to further clarify what diagnoses and treatments are appropriate for telehealth and what needs to go directly to an in-person exam. Obviously, tele-ophthalmology cannot replace an in-person exam.

Using glaucoma as an example, tele-ophthalmic screening can only answer whether there is glaucomatous optic nerve damage and its degree. Due to the current limitations in diagnosis and treatment conditions at primary hospitals or clinics, most of them lack the data on angle examination, so it is difficult to distinguish open-angle glaucoma from closed-angle glaucoma, primary

TABLE 10.2
Disease composition of 540 video consultation cases at the tele-ophthalmic center of the Beijing Institute of Ophthalmology.

Diseases	Cases	%
Primary glaucoma and its surgical complications	55	10.19
AION and other optic disc edema diseases	43	7.96
RVO with cystoid macular edema	34	6.3
Secondary angle closure glaucoma	19	3.52
PDR and DME	18	3.33
Ocular hypertension	17	3.15
Unexplained visual loss	16	2.96
Wet AMD	16	2.96
Pathological myopia and macular damage	12	2.22
Recurrent central serous choroidoretinopathy	10	1.85
Blunt ocular trauma and its complications	10	1.85
Other macular diseases	9	1.67
Retinitis pigmentosa	9	1.67
Panuveitis	13	2.41
Chemical injury of cornea and conjunctiva	7	1.3
Unexplained optic atrophy	7	1.3
CRAO	6	1.11
VKH syndrome	6	1.11
Vitreous hemorrhage	6	1.11
Epiretinal membrane	6	1.11
PCV	5	0.93
Oculomotor paralysis	5	0.93
Hypertensive retinopathy	5	0.93
Lamellar macular hole	5	0.93
Suspicious glaucoma	5	0.93
Ametropia and amblyopia	5	0.93
Retinal detachment and related complications	5	0.93
Scleritis and superficial scleritis	5	0.93
Retrobulbar neuritis	4	0.74
Retinal vasculitis	4	0.74
Related problems of cataract surgery	4	0.74
Herpes simplex keratitis	4	0.74
Abducens paralysis	4	0.74
Vitreous degeneration and opacity	4	0.74
Leber hereditary optic neuropathy	3	0.56
Complicated cataract	3	0.56

Continued

TABLE 10.2
Disease composition of 540 video consultation cases at the tele-ophthalmic center of the Beijing Institute of Ophthalmology—cont'd

Diseases	Cases	%
Macular hole	3	0.56
Secondary optic nerve atrophy	3	0.56
Stromal keratitis	3	0.56
Corneal ulcer	3	0.56
Posner–Schlossman syndrome	3	0.56
Fungal keratitis	3	0.56
Normal tension glaucoma	2	0.37
Thyroid associated ophthalmopathy (TAO)	2	0.37
Punctate inner choroidal lesions (PIC)	2	0.37
Developmental glaucoma	2	0.37
Recurrent pterygium	2	0.37
Dry eye	2	0.37
Infectious keratitis	2	0.37
Iridocyclitis	2	0.37
Corneal laceration	2	0.37
Corneal thermal burn	2	0.37
Recurrent corneal erosion	2	0.37
Choroidal hemangioma	2	0.37
Syphilitic uveal inflammation	2	0.37
Morning glory syndrome	2	0.37
Papillitis	2	0.37
Unexplained optic neuropathy	2	0.37
Retinal phlebitis	2	0.37
Traumatic detachment of ciliary body	2	0.37
Congenital retinoschisis	2	0.37
Explosive injury of eye	2	0.37
Orbital wall fracture	2	0.37
Keratoconus	2	0.37
Toxic optic neuropathy	2	0.37
Syphilitic retinitis	2	0.37
Others	85	15.74

glaucoma, and secondary glaucoma. The correlation of tele-ophthalmic screening, and video consultation, with in-person diagnosis and treatment needs more detailed research studies. Fifth, the business model for tele-eye services needs to be further explored. Tele-ophthalmic service expenses have not been included in the reimbursement scope of basic medical insurance (including the reimbursement scope of the new rural cooperative medical system) in China. Commercial insurance for tele-ophthalmic services should be actively explored.

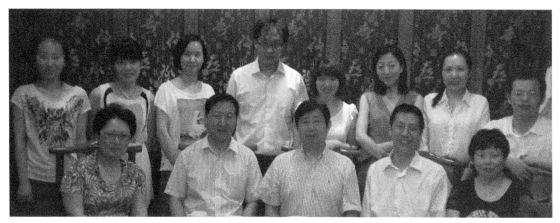

FIG. 10.9 The photo of the tele-ophthalmology research group at the Beijing Institute of Ophthalmology. (Credit: Li Jianjun MD PhD.)

Sixth, in addition to fundus photography, the standards of remote image acquisition and image reading of optical coherence tomography (OCT) and fundus fluorescein angiography (FFA) should be further established.

Other directions include expanding the method of video consultation based on a mobile terminal. It is also necessary to explore the methods of artificial intelligence, computer-based image processing, and automatic grading of ophthalmic images. For example, automatic assessment of fundus clarity, recognition of retinal arteriovenous nicking, identification and grading of fundus microangioma, hemorrhage, exudation and other lesions, classification of leopard pattern fundus, image enhancement of blurred fundus image, etc., Computer-based image processing will then create ideal conditions for "big data" analysis and disease-specific decision making. In China, at present, some companies are engaged in image analysis technology, cooperating with medical units to develop an improved automatic recognition system for diabetic retinopathy, which would then provide a better means for large-scale tele-screening of diabetic retinopathy.

The photograph depicted in Fig. 10.9 is of the tele-ophthalmology research group of the Beijing Institute of Ophthalmology.

REFERENCES FOR SECTION I

1. Zhang Q, Li JJ, Su BN, Xu L, Ren XL, Liu LJ, Wang S, Xu J, Peng XY. A preliminary study of screening disease spectrum in image reading center of teleophthalmology. Ophthalmology in China, 2015, 24(4): 220-225.

2. Liu LJ, Li JJ, Wu Q, Lu CL, Wang S, Duan XR, Deng SJ, Zeng HY, Zhang L, Shi XY, Ai LK, Wang LB, Xu L. Analysis of disease types in videoconferencing-based teleconsultation of Beijing Tongren Eye Center. Ophthalmology in China, 2016, 25(1): 9-12.

3. Kozak I, Payne J, Schatz P, et al. Telemedicine image-based navigated retinal laser therapy. Invest Ophthalmol Vis Sci, 2016, 57(12): 5853.

4. Li JJ, Xu L, Peng XY, Liu LJ, Wang S, Zhou D, Yang H, Ma YN, Wang NL. Quality standard for single fundus image of remote ophthalmology (Draft for comments). Ophthalmology in China, 2015, 24(1): 11-12.

5. Li JJ, Xu L, Peng XY, Liu LJ,Wang S, Liang QF, Yang H, Wang NL Quality standard of external eye and anterior segment image of remote ophthalmic fundus camera (Draft for comments). Ophthalmology in China, 2015, 24(2): 136-137.

6. Li JJ, Xu L, Wang YX, Liu LJ, Wang S, Yang H, ZhangL, Wang NL. Remote screening criteria for optic nerve damage in glaucoma(Draft for comments). Ophthalmology in China, 2015, 24(3): 152.

7. Su BN, Li JJ, Xu L, Liu LJ, Wang S, Lu CL, Wu Q, Wang LB. The quality evaluation of ocular images from primary hospitals in teleophthalmology. Ophthalmology in China, 2015, 24(4): 230-233.

8. Li JJ, Peng XY, Xu J, You QS, Liu LJ, Wang S, Zhang L, Xu L, Wang NL. Remote screening and diagnostic criteria for diabetic retinopathy (Draft for comments). Ophthalmology in China, 2015, 24(5): 292-293.

9. Li JJ, Wang S, Liu X, Liu LJ, Zhang L, Peng XY, Xu L, Wang NL. Remote screening and diagnostic classification criteria for hypertensive retinopathy (Draft for comments). Ophthalmology in China, 2015, 24(5): 294-295.

10. Li JJ, Xu L, Yang H, Zhang L, Wan XH, Liu LJ, Wang S, Wang NL. Evaluation criteria of fundus images for remote screening of cataract requiring surgical treatment (Draft for comments). Ophthalmology in China, 2015, 24(6): 367-368.

11. Li JJ, Peng XY, Liu NP, Chen WW, Hu AL, Wang S, Liu LJ, Xu L, Wang NL. Remote screening and diagnostic classification criteria for age-related macular degeneration (Draft for comments). Ophthalmology in China, 2015, 24(6): 363-364.

12. Rathi S, Tsui E, Mehta N, et al. The current state of teleophthalmology in the United States. Ophthalmology. 2017 Jun 21. pii: S0161-6420(17)30496-7. [Epub ahead of print]

13. Vaziri K, Moshfeghi DM, Moshfeghi AA. Feasibility of telemedicine in detecting diabetic retinopathy and age-related macular degeneration. Semin Ophthalmol, 2015, 30(2): 81-95.

14. Sreelatha OK, Ramesh SV. Teleophthalmology: improving patient outcomes?. Clin Ophthalmol, 2016, 10: 285-295.

15. Sim DA, Mitry D, Alexander P, et al. The evolution of teleophthalmology programs in the United Kingdom: beyond diabetic retinopathy screening. J Diabetes Sci Technol, 2016, 10(2): 308-317.

16. Li HK, Horton M, Bursell SE, et al. Telehealth practice recommendations for diabetic retinopathy, second edition. Telemed J E Health, 2011, 17(10): 814-837.

17. Li JJ, Zhang L, Peng XY. Some issues of diagnosis based on ocular fundus image reading in teleophthalmology. Ophthalmology in China, 2104, 23(4): 217-220.

18. Li JJ, Xu L, Yang H, Ma YN, Wang YX, Zhang L, Wang NL. The value of single fundus image in remote glaucoma screening. International Review of Ophthalmology, 2015, 39(3): 216.

SECTION II: INDIA: THE VISION CENTER MODEL OF TELEMEDICINE AT ARAVIND EYE CARE SYSTEM

Rengaraj Venkatesh MD, Bharat Gurnani MD, Ravilla D. Thulasiraj MBA

Introduction and Background

What Is Telemedicine and the Scope of Tele-Ophthalmic Care?

With increasing population sizes, increased life expectancy, better health facilities, and improved understanding of diseases and their management, the challenge is to make such advancements affordable and accessible in all areas of the world as well as meet the growing need for access to care. Telehealth offers an innovative approach to narrow the divide between rural and urban healthcare. Telehealth technologies have the potential to overcome existing disparities like uneven distribution of resources, infrastructure and provider shortage, and costs associated with the provision of and accessing healthcare. Telemedicine, with the right design, can also be an affordable, practical, and scalable supplement to the conventional in-person clinic visit. It also has the potential to democratize health care by bridging the urban–rural and associated competency divide.

Telemedicine has already made significant strides in non-ocular fields such as radiology and pathology. These were consult/support services and by design the radiology or pathology reports are expected with some time delay after the actual investigation. This asynchronous nature of requirement made it easier to adopt technology for remote reporting. However, when providing direct patient care, such as eye care, sometimes real-time input from a specialist is very helpful, especially when the patient is physically in the clinic. Eye telehealth technology, therefore, requires this ability and to achieve this goal requires appropriate workflows and supportive technology infrastructure to enable both synchronous and asynchronous care. This is evolving in the field of ocular telehealth, and some progress has been made. In India, eye providers now have a working telehealth model that provides real-time consultation by ophthalmologists to patients presenting at primary eye care centers. This tele-eye experience demonstrates an immense opportunity to manage the steadily increasing demand for eye care, especially in remote and underserved areas.

Why the Focus on Tele-Health in Primary Eye Care?

The 2019 Global Monitoring Report by the World Health Organization,[1] "identifies primary health care as the route to universal health coverage (UHC)" and establishes UHC's linkage to achieving the Sustainable Development Goals (SDG). UHC is defined by three

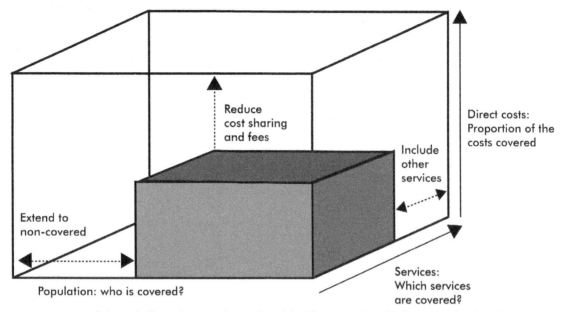

FIG. 10.10 Schematic illustrating care that ocular telehealth can provide. (Credit: Aravind Eye Care Center.)

components: health care access for all individuals and communities, comprehensive care, and financial protection (Fig. 10.10).

Since access is fundamental to timely, comprehensive, and affordable health care, primary health care (PHC) was recognized as a key strategy to achieve UHC. The same tenet is applied to eye care, where everyone in need of eye care can obtain care. In order to achieve this goal, a structured delivery of primary eye care through vision centers, was developed in India. Furthermore, studies show that established "eye camps," the only, decades-long strategy adopted to provide eye care to the masses, reached less than 7% of patients who wanted eye care services.[2] This study underscored the need for establishing a permanent facility closer to communities to provide eye care, so as to ensure easy access and make care affordable.

Primary eye care (PEC) is the delivery of appropriate, accessible, affordable, and high-quality eye care with good community participation.[2] PEC also includes promotion of eye health, prevention and treatment of conditions that may lead to visual loss, as well as low vision services. To make this a reality, the first step was to define the scope of the Indian vision centers. To better define the activities, it is useful to adopt a healthcare framework that spans the full spectrum—prevention, diagnosis, treatment, follow-up, and rehabilitation. This ensured a comprehensive design, an important component of UHC. Applying this framework to the

major eye conditions, the following scope of service or activity matrix at vision centers, emerged (Table 10.3):

Primary eye care services include:
1. Patient education about maintaining healthy vision
2. Comprehensive ocular examination including screening for asymptomatic eye diseases
3. Performing refractions and prescribing glasses
4. Triaging patients for more specialized care and referring to base hospital for further care
5. Counseling about management plan
6. Active participation in blindness prevention program.

Why Is PEC Necessary for India and Elsewhere?

Blindness and disability are major public health problems in India. Availability and easy access to basic eye care services are essential for universal coverage and eliminating preventable or treatable blindness. In developed countries in North America, Western Europe or the Pacific Rim, where there is relatively less scarcity in terms of providers and allied health personnel resulting in easier access to care and better financial enablement, there is still a need for eye care in remote regions. However, in developing countries, with a paucity of ophthalmologists and allied ophthalmic personnel, and these individuals being located mostly in large urban conglomerations, most of the community doesn't have any easy access to eye care and therefore

TABLE 10.3
Scope of services offered at vision centers.

| | Case Finding | INTERVENTION | | | | Compliance to Follow-up |
		Curative	Prev.	Referral	Rehab	
Cataract	√			√		√
Ret. Error	√	√				√
Child. Blindness	√		√	√		√
D. Retinopathy	√[a]			√		√
Glaucoma	√[a]			√		√
Cornea	√	√	√	√		√
Low Vision	√			√	√	√

[a]Supported by low-cost imaging and Artificial Intelligence technologies.

do not receive it. In this context, the telemedicine enabled PEC model, when integrated with secondary and tertiary levels of eye care, offers a viable solution which can eventually lead to universal eye health.[3]

PEC in developing countries like India is provided by Allied Ophthalmic Personnel who work through local centers located in the rural areas. These centers have been termed as vision centers (VCs). In India, these VCs have been established both by the Government and by several other hospitals to ensure eye care for rural population. Larger hospitals running VCs include Aravind Eye Care System (AECS), LV Prasad Eye Institute (LVPEI), Dr. Shroff's Charity Eye Hospital (SCEH), Sadguru Netra Chikitsalaya, HV Desai Eye Hospital, and Vivekananda Mission Asram Netra Niramay Niketan. There are close to 340 VCs presently run by these hospital systems, annually handling more than 1.3 million outpatient visits. The Government of India has also prioritized the development of vision centers under the "National Vision Management Program".

Need for Linking Tele-ophthalmology and Primary Eye Care

In developing countries like India, a nation with an aging population, increasing prevalence of systemic pathologies, better neonatal and geriatric services, and emerging treatments ensuring longer survival, there is a growing need for providing basic and timely eye health services. Effective management of ocular complications associated with chronic diseases is dependent on timely diagnosis and intervention.

Having thus defined the scope and goals of eye care, the next step was to ensure matching resources to make this happen. The key amongst them being human resources and equipment. This had to be thought through in the context of scale and location. The locations would typically be quite remote rural areas and the scale would be relatively small given that each of these VCs would have a service area population of about 50,000. Some challenges stem out of this. On the staffing front, given the paucity of both optometrists and ophthalmologists, their preference to work in larger cities for better social life and professional career growth opportunities, ability to recruit and retain eye providers at the VCs was an unrealistic expectation. The most realistic option was to use ophthalmic technicians. In India, opportunities exist to become a mid-level ophthalmic assistant, where the individual trains for 2 years in basic eye care, creating a workforce that can help bridge the competency gap between the technician and an eye provider, in order to ensure comprehensiveness and high quality care is provided.

A VC, though small in size with just one or two staff members, still needed to be managed carefully, to ensure adequate supplies, staffing at all times, and financial solvency. For adequate population coverage, a large number of VCs would be required and this resulted in logistical challenges involved in managing them, for the most part, remotely.

Both these challenges—bridging the clinical competency gap and managing the VCs remotely—could best be addressed by leveraging technologies like telehealth, electronic medical record, and vision center management systems.

With tele-ophthalmology, ophthalmologists can diagnose and suggest treatment and remotely follow patients, without extensive travel or physical contact. This has been important, especially during the COVID-19 pandemic. Patients benefit, as they receive the same level of care at a local center without travelling long distances, saving them significant cost and travel time, and increasing their likelihood of follow-up.

THE AECS MODEL OF PRIMARY EYE CARE THROUGH VISION CENTERS—A HYBRID TELEHEALTH MODEL
How Do VCs Work to Provide PEC?

(1) **Population coverage, accessibility, other eye care services in the vicinity**

A vision center is a permanent facility to provide primary eye care in the community and serves as the first point of contact for patients. Eye care services are provided at these centers by skilled eye care technicians.[4] An important step while planning a VC is estimating the demand for services based on local population density, service area characteristics, and local economy. At Aravind, each VC is designed to serve a population of 50,000—60,000. Most VCs are set-up in small rural towns with a reasonably sized population, since they tend to be a hub for surrounding smaller villages and many people access it for trade and other reasons. Thus, patients have familiarity with the larger rural 'hub' town. Aravind also ensures, to prevent duplication, that there is no eye care in the vicinity before establishing a permanent VC. At the same, Aravind ensures that the VCs are located within a reasonable distance (30–50 miles) from the base hospital for the referred patients to easily access follow up eye care.

(2) **Human Resources and Equipment**

Non-physician workers staff the VCs and serve as an extension of the main medical organization, thereby representing the hospitals at the community level. Aravind employs two staff members in each VC. One staff member is trained to do eye examinations (vision technician) and the other does administrative duties, such as patient registration, sales of medicines/glasses and counseling. These individuals tend to be people who already have a few years of work experience at the base hospital. They are additionally trained for 3–6 months to use technology deployed in the VC such as EMR and fundus imaging. Married female employees from the local community are preferred as this helps in staff retention—they receive a long-term employment opportunity in their hometown. The VC requires an area of approximately 700 square feet with two or three rooms and a washroom facility. One room is dedicated for examination with a slit lamp, loose lenses, and a retinoscope for refraction, and equipment for tele-ophthalmology. A second room is used for optical sales, medication sales, counseling, and a combined or separate patient waiting room.

(3) **Details of clinical service**

The VCs perform three basic functions—*Recognizing* or detecting eye conditions, *Refracting* and provision of spectacles, and *Referring* a patient to the base hospital.[5] Apart from these, staff at VCs are also involved in opportunistic screening of eye diseases and create awareness about common eye problems.

Once the patient registers, the technicians ask about the presenting complaints, refract the patient, perform the ocular examination in the form of comprehensive adnexal and anterior segment examination using a slit lamp, undilated fundoscopy in all, and dilated fundoscopy in needed cases, applanation tonometry, gonioscopy and anterior and posterior segment imaging as needed. All these findings are entered in the Electronic Medical Records (EMR) in the cloud, which can be reviewed simultaneously by the tele-eye doctor at the base hospital. VC staff then present the complaints and examination findings via video conferencing using Google Hangouts or similar software. Based on the chart review, presentation by the technician, and talking to the patient, the remote ophthalmologist at the base hospital arrives at a diagnosis and a care plan. The doctor at the base hospital through synchronous video interacts with the patient and explains the treatment plan.

This allows patients to clarify any questions they may have and promotes trust on the whole process, thus leading to better adherence to prescribed treatment. The final prescription is virtually signed by the eye provider (Fig.10.11).

Regardless of the ocular complaints, patients above 40 years are also routinely evaluated for common systemic medical disease by obtaining blood pressure, blood sugar levels, and are referred to local primary care or internal medicine physician if needed. This opportunistic screening, to some extent enables timely detection of systemic conditions, which otherwise might be missed till advanced stages of the disease. Typical daily patient volumes varies across VCs, largely depending on the age of the Vision Center. Most centers start with 10–15 patients daily and gradually increase to 30 + patients a day within two years. The patients are charged a nominal amount of (Rs. 20) 30 US cents, which is good for 2 additional visits within 3 months. Most patients receive a prescription for glasses or medication, both of which can be purchased at the VC. Local pharmacies seldom have any of the ophthalmic drugs, so providing them at the VCs, ensure better compliance. Typical spend on medicines would $1 to 2 and under $ 10 for glasses. Ten to 15 % of patients are referred to the base hospital either for cataract surgery or specialty consultation (Fig. 10.12)

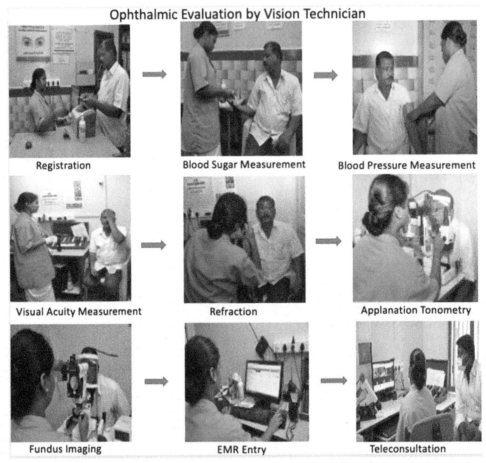

FIG. 10.11 Image depicting ophthalmic evaluation by vision technician and workflow of patients presenting to vision center. (Credit: Aravind Eye Center.)

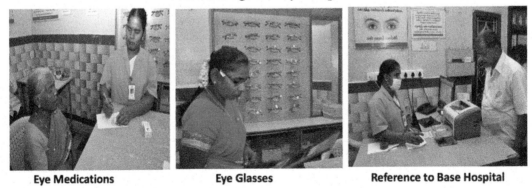

FIG. 10.12 Image depicting counseling and dispensing of medication, glasses and referral to base hospital. (Credit: Aravind Eye Center.)

What Type of Technology Is Used at a VC?

Technology is important for maintaining, recording the patient data, and connecting to the base hospital. All VCs have the same EMR software and this is connected to the base hospital system. The EMR in the cloud facilitates seamless collaboration during the real-time video interaction between the VC technician and the remote eye provider. In addition, the common EMR facilitates easy referral as well as referral attendance. The EMR allows the remote eye provider to enter his/her management plan and send out a signed prescription for medicines/glasses that gets printed out at the Vision Centre.

USE OF LOW-COST IMAGING DEVICES IN PEC

Smartphone assisted anterior and posterior segment photography is a low-cost technology. At our VCs, ophthalmic technicians are trained for either smartphone assisted slit lamp anterior segment imaging and fundus imaging or portable fundus camera imaging.[6]

This has made documentation and detection of subtle ophthalmic pathologies easier. These images can be uploaded in the EMR, which are then accessed by the eye provider at the base hospital. This good yet low-cost imaging promotes early detection of vision threatening conditions and avoids unnecessary referrals to the base hospital.

DEPLOYMENT OF ARTIFICIAL INTELLIGENCE

Artificial intelligence (AI)[7] is useful in healthcare—computer-algorithms analyze medical data to provide instant diagnosis or suggest referrals. AI and deep learning (DL) can be applied in fields such as ophthalmology where large amounts of image-based data need to be analyzed. AI and DL have already been proven to help in early diagnosis of conditions such as diabetic retinopathy (DR),[8] age-related macular degeneration (ARMD),[9] retinopathy of prematurity (ROP),[10] glaucoma,[11] and other eye disorders with high diagnostic accuracy, consistency, and durability. Currently AI for detection of DR is being piloted in some of the Vision Centers. Such deployment of AI based technology is expected to be the future of VCs, which will enable the technician to get an instant diagnosis, make more appropriate referrals, and improve efficiency.

TECHNOLOGY AND PATIENT CARE

Technology, especially the EMR, has helped in maintaining patient medical records, patient tracking with

an unique ID number, easy referrals, post-operative check-ups at VC, prescribing medications at the VC, and regular follow up.

PATIENT SATISFACTION AND QUALITY ASSURANCE—CLINICAL AND NON-CLINICAL AUDITS

Quality monitoring at VCs take into account both clinical and non-clinical aspects. Key performance indicators (KPIs) are a critical way to track VC success. The number of patients seen, glasses prescribed and ordered, volume and compliance of cataract surgeries and specialty cases are closely monitored. The KPIs include non-clinical metrics such as revenues, costs, equipment downtime, punctuality, and extensive assessment of patient satisfaction.

PERFORMANCE MANAGEMENT

The VC technicians have regular meetings at the base hospital with the VC manager and remote eye provider at frequent intervals to check on performance management—including reviewing new and established patient charts. Since the goal of Vision Centers is to achieve universal eye health, the performance monitoring is driven by the denominator or the estimated eye care need in the community. The following (Table 10.4) gives a rough estimate of the need in a population of 50,000.

TABLE 10.4 Eye care need for a vision center population.	
Eye Care need for a population of 50,000	**Estimate**
Those in need of any form of eye care (25% of population):	12,500
Annual need:	
• Cataract Surgeries (based on CSR of 10,000)	500
• Spectacles (20% would need & change in 5 years)	2000
Ongoing care:	
• Glaucoma (1%)	500
• Diabetics (3%)	1500
• Incurably Blind and Low Vision (0.1% of each)	50+50

GENERAL BENEFITS OF VCs AND TELE-OPHTHALMOLOGY IN EYE CARE SERVICE DELIVERY

There are many benefits that VCs provide to the local patient population including:

- Instant service—VCs serve as the first level of response and care for patient eye needs. By responding to basic eye care requirements in the VCs through ocular telehealth modalities, almost 85% of patients with ocular problems requiring simple interventions can be managed at the VC. This also reduces the burden on secondary and tertiary centers.

- Reducing barriers and costs—Many studies have examined barriers in the utilization of eye care services.[12] These include economic barriers,[12] travel logistics, lack of felt need, lack of accompaniment, fear of surgery,[13] and lack of awareness. VC's, by design, addresses most of these barriers and makes the services more accessible.

- Improve health-seeking behavior—Prior to VCs, people in need of eye care used to wait weeks or months for eye camps to come to their community. With VCs, they can now access eye care at any time, which allows for timely diagnosis of asymptomatic eye disease and earlier intervention. In addition, patients can successfully complete their follow-up visits without traveling for long distances—patients with slowly progressive ocular pathologies like DR, glaucoma, and ARMD can be safely followed at VC. Tele-ophthalmology and the EMR help with monitoring progression and referrals.

- Reduction of healthcare disparities due to gender—We find that VCs serve a higher number of women compared to eye hospitals. Women are less dependent on others when trying to visit a Vision Centre in their local area compared to traveling long distance to a base hospital. In addition, VC's help to overcome the cultural barriers to accessing care, especially because many VCs have a female vision technicians.

- Benefits to the whole community—Establishing VCs in remote areas expands employment opportunities for community members, especially women, and strengthens the local economy.

CONCLUSION

Vision Centers are positioned at the primary level and thus serve a fairly well-defined population. Their establishment in the community allows, for the first time, monitoring coverage—that is, provision of eye care services targeted to the needs in the community. The capability to monitor and therefore know which communities are or are not adequately served is what will ultimately help achieve universal eye health. Vision Centers enabled with appropriate technologies like EMR, imaging, compliance tracking systems and AI, ensure comprehensive eye care to the Vision Center's catchment. Vision Centers, by being located in close proximity to the community, by developing registries for patients with chronic conditions, are uniquely capable of ensuring convenient follow up care for patients. In fact, secondary and tertiary level eye care services are less effective than Vision Centers for the management of chronic conditions like glaucoma or diabetic retinopathy. The effectiveness of treatments for these conditions is largely dependent on patient's compliance to regular follow-up and medication use, which may not occur at base hospitals due to distance and appointment wait times. Vision Centers not only promote the ocular health of the community, they reduce eye care disparities, and also enhance the effectiveness of secondary and tertiary level eye care services.

REFERENCES FOR SECTION II

1. Sood S, Mbarika V, Jugoo S, et al. What is telemedicine? A collection of 104 peer-reviewed perspectives and theoretical underpinnings. *Telemed J E Health*. 2007;13(5):573–590.
2. https://www.aao.org/clinical-statement/definition-of-primary-eye-care- -policy-statement.
3. Misra V, Vashist P, Malhotra S, Gupta SK. Models for primary eye care services in India. *Indian J Community Med*. 2015;40(2):79–84. https://doi.org/10.4103/0970-0218.153868.
4. Khanna RC, Sabherwal S, Sil A, et al. Primary eye care in India—the vision center model. *Indian J Ophthalmol*. 2020;68(2):333–339.
5. Sharma M, Jain N, Ranganathan S, et al. Tele-ophthalmology: need of the hour. *Indian J Ophthalmol*. 2020;68(7):1328–1338.
6. Quellec G, Bazin L, Cazuguel G, Delafoy I, Cochener B, Lamard M. Suitability of a low-cost, handheld, nonmydriatic retinograph for diabetic retinopathy diagnosis. *Transl Vis Sci Technol*. 2016;5(2):16. Published 2016 Apr 20.
7. Ting DSW, Pasquale LR, Peng L, et al. Artificial intelligence and deep learning in ophthalmology. *Br J Ophthalmol*. 2019;103(2):167–175.
8. Gunasekeran DV, Ting DSW, Tan GSW, Wong TY. Artificial intelligence for diabetic retinopathy screening, prediction and management. *Curr Opin Ophthalmol*. 2020;31(5):357–365.

9. Dutt S, Sivaraman A, Savoy F, Rajalakshmi R. Insights into the growing popularity of artificial intelligence in ophthalmology. *Indian J Ophthalmol.* 2020;68(7):1339–1346.

10. Gensure RH, Chiang MF, Campbell JP. Artificial intelligence for retinopathy of prematurity. *Curr Opin Ophthalmol.* 2020;31(5):312–317.

11. Mayro EL, Wang M, Elze T, Pasquale LR. The impact of artificial intelligence in the diagnosis and management of glaucoma. *Eye (Lond).* 2020;34(1):1–11.

12. Brilliant GE, Lepkowski JM, Zurita B, Thulasiraj RD. Social determinants of cataract surgery utilization in South India. The Operations Research Group. *Arch Ophthalmol.* 1991;109(4):584–589.

13. Snellingen T, Shrestha BR, Gharti MP, Shrestha JK, Upadhyay MP, Pokhrel RP. Socioeconomic barriers to cataract surgery in Nepal: the South Asian cataract management study. *Br J Ophthalmol.* 1998;82(12):1424–1428.

CHAPTER 11

Ocular In-Home Monitoring Devices

AKSHAR ABBOTT, MD • STEPHANIE J. WEISS, DO

INTRODUCTION

Home telehealth modalities have been a staple of disciplines outside of eye care for decades. Prominent examples include home glucose measurement, home blood pressure checks, and home diabetic foot checks. Additionally, the ability for patients to interact with providers via telehealth, whether audio or video, has been broadly applied across many disciplines outside of eye care for years. Bringing the ease, accessibility, and comfort of home telehealth from these specialties into eye care presents patients and providers with a new landscape of challenges and opportunities that will likely redefine the relationship between patients and their eye providers for decades to come.

Many factors are responsible for the recent rapid rise in home-based ocular telehealth paradigms of care. Most obviously, the wrenching changes brought on by the COVID-19 pandemic are responsible for a rapid adoption of home ocular telehealth as well as an increased willingness to imagine what types of care must still be provided in a healthcare setting and what types are safe and effective to provide at home. In parallel to these dramatic societal changes, technological advances in internet access, miniaturization, and patient familiarity with small-scale personal technology platforms such as the smartphone, have created ripe conditions for these changes. Beyond sociological and technological considerations, it is no coincidence that, in a time of renewed focus on health equity in medicine, healthcare systems and providers are being pushed to think about how better to expand access to quality eye care.

Home tele-eye devices hold enormous promise not only in navigating a changing landscape of care but in empowering patients to reimagine how these tools will reduce the burden of time and financial expenditure required to acquire quality healthcare. By allowing patients to interact with the healthcare system from the comfort of their own homes, these devices allow patients to better balance the demands of their lives without sacrificing their eye health. Long visits to eye care specialists, in many cases requiring the aid of family members or the personal expense of transportation, may someday be replaced with iterative home monitoring interspersed with regular follow-ups in-person.

For those patients whose sense of well-being is negatively impacted by the emotional burden of having a chronic blinding disease that requires ongoing follow-up, home ocular telehealth may also offer some level of comfort as they may be liberated from the worry of declining ocular health between visits. Instead of only getting annual or semiannual updates as to the status of their disease, the ability to perform self-checks between visits may allow them to spend less of their time wondering how their eyes are doing or worrying that their condition is worsening in some avoidable way between appointments.

While most readers of this text will be well acquainted with the workflow and clinical scheduling demands of patients with chronic eye diseases, it is important to at least review the extent of care required by these patients to better frame how shifting some of their healthcare time expenditure into the home setting may be substantially beneficial to their overall quality of life.

One prominent example arises from patients who have irreversible blinding diseases of age-related macular degeneration (AMD). In the setting of AMD, patients with non-neovascular (colloquially known as "dry") macular degeneration primarily require semiannual-to-yearly visits with an office exam and optical coherence tomography (OCT) imaging. In addition, they are required to monitor their own vision at home using an Amsler grid, essentially a small graph with regularly intersecting lines and a central dot for fixation. If the patient notices an increase in distortion in the lines of the Amsler grid, they are to notify their provider so that they may come into the office for an additional visit. If the subsequent exam and OCT show evidence of conversion to neovascular (known as "wet") macular degeneration, the patient needs to begin a series of regular visits for the purpose of treatment with intravitreal injections. If the patient experiences a change in their Amsler grid but their exam and OCT findings remain stable, then they may simply need continued observation despite having experienced the feeling of a medical emergency and having often gone to great lengths on short notice to arrange transportation and potentially ask family members to accompany them. In aggregate, whether a patient has "dry" or "wet" macular degeneration, their burden of care is very high and requires frequent follow-up visits, constant observation, and continuous doubt as they weigh whether their perception of the Amsler grid merits a short notice trip to a healthcare setting or signals further irreversible vision loss.

Another valuable example can be found in patients with glaucoma, which represents a family of diseases with the often painless, insidious loss of the peripheral visual field over time, in many cases related to elevated intraocular pressure (IOP). Working against this often asymptomatic disease process, these patients require frequent office visits to measure their intraocular pressure in addition to OCT and visual field testing to evaluate for progression of optic nerve damage and visual field loss. However, pressures detected at routine eye exams represent only single moments in time and may insufficiently map the extent of fluctuations and numeric range of intraocular pressure that a patient may experience within a given 24-hour time frame. Home monitoring of intraocular pressure can provide the physician treating the patient with a much clearer picture of the patient's intraocular pressure over time, and give the physician a better understanding of what combination of topical eye drops, laser, and surgery may be required to maintain safe intraocular pressures. Patients benefit as well, as home monitoring can alleviate some of the ongoing concern that their IOP may be elevated between office visits or that their in-office IOP measurements may not be reflective of their actual underlying disease, leaving them vulnerable to silent vision loss.

These simple, rough sketches of patient care paradigms in macular degeneration and glaucoma easily lead the reader to understand the potential benefits of ocular in-home monitoring devices. For concerned patients, these devices may provide a higher quality of life by reassuring them on an ongoing basis that they are stable and likely to catch important findings quickly so that they may maximally act to rapidly address them. For those patients who have difficulty navigating the healthcare system, live far from their providers, or do not have a large social or family network upon which to rely for transportation and support, these devices may be a lifeline for them by moving their care into the home without sacrificing the quality of care. For providers, the ability to have more robust data for each patient may enable them to provide better care and achieve better outcomes by rapidly detecting and acting upon new findings. In addition, this increased density, high-quality data may facilitate training and developing the next-generation artificial intelligence models in eye care that require significant amounts of data for development. The rest of this chapter discusses examples of existing in-home monitoring devices for common ocular conditions. Some are commercially available at the time of writing, others are still under development. Discussion of these technologies is meant to be informative, may not be comprehensive of all in-home monitoring devices, and inclusion here does not signal endorsement by any of the authors. None of the authors have any financial interest in the technologies discussed below.

SPECIFIC HOME MONITORING DEVICES
Amsler Grid
The Amsler grid, a ubiquitous feature of ophthalmic offices and in the homes of macular degeneration patients, dates back to 1947 and is named after the Swiss ophthalmologist Marc Amsler. A square grid with regularly spaced lines at right angles with a fixation dot located centrally (Fig. 11.1), the Amsler grid is used by patients to track changes in the apparent distortion of the grid that may come from corresponding distortions in the topography of the retina and the retinal pigment epithelium. This lightweight, easy-to-use, low technological footprint tool is the mainstay of first-generation home eye monitoring devices. The most notable limitation of this device is the minimum visual acuity required to resolve the grid in a sufficiently clear manner to detect subtle changes, a task that may prove

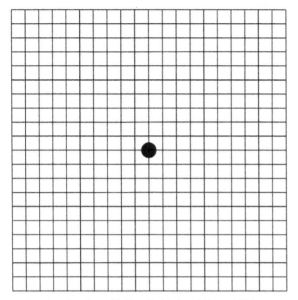

FIG. 11.1 Amsler grid. (Credit: Akshar Abbott, MD.)

increasingly difficult as a patient's vision declines or their central scotoma deepens, making fixating on the target dot progressively more difficult.

Additionally, some authors have highlighted concerns over the efficacy of patient-directed home monitoring with the Amsler grid, with one study finding only an estimated 30% ability to detect changes.[1] While alternate testing systems such as Macular Computerized Psychophysical Test have been put forth, the Amsler grid remains a mainstay of age-related macular degeneration management. It is from this device and its limitations that most home ophthalmic devices take some inspiration, especially preferential hyperacuity perimetry devices such as the ForeseeHome.

ForeseeHome Device

The ForeseeHome device (Notal Vision, USA) is a small table-mounted electronic vision testing device that allows patients to lean forward and place both eyes into the viewer, where they are confronted with an image of dots arranged in a straight line across their field of view. The patient uses a mouse to indicate where they feel that the device image may be distorted, and the onboard software compares the patients' test responses both to their own previous tests and to a normative database. Each test covers 500 dots shown three to five times and is estimated to take 3 min per eye (Figs. 11.2 and 11.3).

The results are communicated over cellular networks to a central monitoring service,[2] and physicians may review these results remotely to alert patients who need to be seen in clinic as a result of their testing.[3]

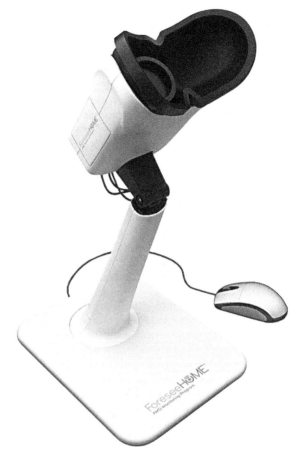

FIG. 11.2 ForeseeHome Device. (Credit: Used with permission from Notal Vision.)

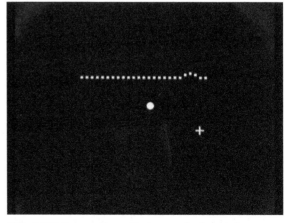

FIG. 11.3 ForeseeHome Device—patient view of screen. (Credit: Used with permission from Notal Vision.)

The device is rented from the company, eliminating the need for a large upfront payment by patients that may discourage use.

The HOME study was an unmasked, controlled, randomized clinical trial evaluating whether home-monitoring with the ForeseeHome device allowed for early detection of choroidal neovascularization (CNV) in age-related macular degeneration patients and better visual acuity outcomes over the study period as compared to control patients receiving standard care.[4] The study included 1520 patients with non-neovascular age-related macular degeneration and a mean age of 72.5 years who were deemed to be at high risk for developing choroidal neovascularization. Patients in the standard care group were provided instructions by their ophthalmologists covering standard parameters for notifying the clinic of vision changes. In the ForeseeHome group, patients were provided the device at home and instructed to test daily, with results generated by those tests remotely communicated to clinical centers that would in turn notify patients and instruct them to present to the clinic for an examination in the case of a possible change. Overall, the patient group being monitored with ForeseeHome device exhibited a statistically significantly smaller decline in visual acuity from baseline visual acuity to time of CNV detection.[4] Additionally, the study demonstrated that lesions in the ForeseeHome group tended to be smaller (as measured on OCT and fluorescein angiography) at the time of detection, potentially suggesting benefit in ForeseeHome monitoring, allowing for the detection of smaller lesions at an earlier stage.[5] A secondary analysis of the data demonstrated that triggered visits brought on by alerts from the device were found to be associated with a lesser degree of vision loss than those triggered by conventional standard care home self-monitoring, defined as Amsler grid and self-monitoring for vision changes.[6]

Though the results of the HOME study have been encouraging, other investigators detected trends worth noting. One study highlighted the difficulties in ensuring that patients use the device frequently enough to generate meaningful measurements, with more than a quarter of patients failing to use the device more than two times per week and more than half of patients failing to use it more than three times per week.[7] Almost a quarter of patients stopped using the device within a year.[7] Additionally, there seem to be some age-related differences in patients who were able to successfully establish a baseline measurement against which further testing could be meaningfully compared. As the younger people were more successful, this may be an indication that older patients may experience more difficulty with navigating the user experience as compared to their younger peers.[7] These challenges in establishing appropriate baselines may provide insight as to why > 90% of the alerts registered by the device over the course of the study were later deemed to represent false positives. Alternatively, given that age-related macular degeneration is known to progress over time, these findings raise the question of whether or not the device becomes more difficult to use appropriately as a patient's vision declines.

Taken together, the literature surrounding the ForeseeHome device demonstrates intriguing promise for the potential to monitor patients at home in a standardized way, leveraging technology to facilitate early warnings regarding potential progression from non-neovascular macular degeneration to the onset of choroidal neovascularization. Ultimately, like any home health intervention requiring patient buy-in and self-motivated behavioral change such as regularly taking glaucoma drops or checking one's blood sugars, it appears that the promise of this device will not be fully realized without adequate strategies to encourage persistent adherence and appropriate use. The next-generation Notal home monitoring device is the Notal Home OCT, which is an artificial intelligence-based, patient-operated, home SD-OCT platform, for which trials remain ongoing (Fig. 11.4).

Smartphone-Based Apps

Smartphone-based vision-tracking apps hold promise for the future of ocular home monitoring. As smartphones have become more ubiquitous and more powerful, the potential horizons of home monitoring applications have expanded dramatically.

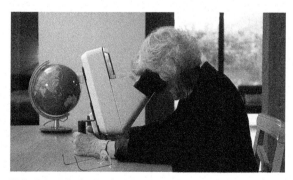

FIG. 11.4 Patient using the Notal Vision Home OCT Device (not commercially available). Credit: Used with permission from Notal Vision.

One such application, MyVisionTrack (Genentech, USA), features a smartphone-based shape discrimination hyperacuity test (adapted from a previous desktop version of the program),[8] designed to combine ease of use and portability by evaluating radial shape discrimination that may occur in age-related macular degeneration.[9] Patients are initially presented with two circles and one distorted shape and asked to tap on the distorted shape. Next, they are shown a series of similar prompts with declining distortion of the key shape in each successive series of images, with the goal of determining the smallest amount of detectable distortion as a proxy signal for visual function. A recent single-arm, prospective, open-label, 16-week, multicenter pilot study sought to assess the utility of this app in 160 patients with active CNV in at least 1 eye, with best-corrected visual acuity (BCVA) letter score of 24 or higher by Early Treatment Diabetic Retinopathy Study scoring.[10] Patients were given direct instruction in how to use the app prior to the study, as well as up to 7 days to become comfortable with its use prior to the initiation of the study period. Possibly owing to the ability to send push notifications reminding patients to use the device, compliance with daily testing was 84.7% and weekly testing was 98.7%.

Ultimately, further head-to-head data will be needed to compare this type of intervention to the comparatively lower tech and easier to use Amsler grid. Additionally, comparisons will need to be made relative to other platforms such as the home OCT and the ForeseeHome device. Smartphone applications may still retain limitations owing to the lower order program complexity necessitated by the host platform; it may be difficult to scale down the benefits of more complex and powerful in-office imaging and exam equipment without losing their ability to meaningfully assess visual function in the home setting.

Though these apps are likely to have a place in eye care as smartphones advance and are capable of hosting more complex content, at this point the marginal utility of smartphone-based vision testing does not seem to favor wide-scale adaptation over and above other platforms.

iCare HOME Tonometer

The iCare HOME (Revenio, Finland) is a rebound tonometer. Held in the patient's hand and aligned with the eye with the aid of markers on the device, the iCare HOME projects a disposable probe via electromagnetic propulsion such that the probe impacts on the corneal surface (Fig. 11.5A, B). By detecting the recoil time, with quicker recoils correlating with higher intraocular pressures, the device measures the intraocular pressure.

The accessibility and simplicity of this device allow for high satisfaction and compliance rates among in-home users. In one study, patients trained to use the iCare HOME were asked questions regarding the ease of use and acceptability of the device. This study reported 78.5% of patients found the technology easy to use, and 80.6% of patients would be willing to use the device at home.[11] Other studies have supported the idea that, in general, patients find this device easy to understand and use comfortably.[12] However, the mechanism by which the iCare HOME establishes intraocular pressure limits the utility of the device when measuring eyes with significant astigmatism or with above or below average corneal thickness.[13]

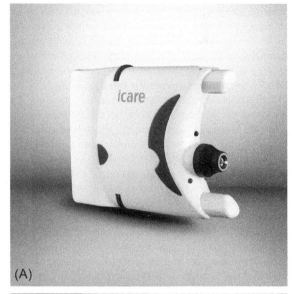

(A)

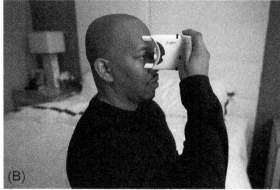

(B)

FIG. 11.5   A and B The iCare HOME tonometer (A) and a patient using an iCare HOME Device (B). (Credit: Used with permission from iCare.)

Differing results have been reported regarding the reliability of iCare HOME measurements when compared with the gold standard of intraocular pressure measurement, Goldmann applanation tonometry. In one study of 128 patients, the mean difference between measurements by patients using the iCare HOME device and Goldmann applanation measurements performed by an ophthalmologist was 0.7 mm Hg and was statistically significant.[14] This difference was significantly widened as a function of increasing corneal thickness, highlighting central corneal thickness as an important confounding factor of the iCare HOME's core technology. Every 10% increase in corneal thickness predicted a 1.2% increase in the difference between iCare HOME measurement and Goldmann measurement.[14] Another French study found that the iCare HOME device measurement performed by patients overestimated intraocular pressures relative to those measured by Goldmann applanation tonometry by 1.31 mm Hg—a result the authors found to be statistically significant.[15] However, they did not find a correlation between central corneal thickness and widened error measurement between the two modalities.[15]

The variations in intraocular pressures recorded by the iCare HOME device also raise the obvious point that the timing of measurement affects the collected data and with it, a provider's understanding of a given patient's range of intraocular pressure.[16,17] In an effort to address some of the data gaps created by intermittent self-directed interactive pressure measurement, excepting the hours of sleep or measurements made during activities in which handling measurement devices would be impossible, a new generation of implantable intraocular pressure measurement devices has arisen. Most prominent are the Sensimed Triggerfish Contact Lens and the Eyemate implantable intraocular pressure measurement device.

Sensimed Triggerfish Contact Lens

The Sensimed Triggerfish Contact Lens (Sensimed AG, Switzerland) is a wireless ocular telemetry sensor (OTS) composed of a silicone contact lens with embedded platinum-titanium strain gauge circuitry that tracks changes in corneal curvature caused by intraocular pressure changes and relays these changes wirelessly to a recording hub. Given the understanding that central corneal thickness can fluctuate over the course of the day, some observers indicate a note of caution in interpreting intraocular pressure data gleaned from corneal curvature changes, as there is potential that the contact lens being used to measure corneal curvature could itself be inducing corneal edema, warping, or other changes.[18,19,20] In general, studies have shown this contact lens to be well-tolerated by patients over a 24-hour period of time, though the exclusion of patients with significantly above or below average corneal curvature may be important to enhance maximum tolerability and safety.[21] This profile appears to be similar for wear in patients with and without glaucoma.[22]

As important as device tolerability is to the potential clinical utility of this device, reproducibility of measurement remains a critical piece as well. In one 2012 study comparing measurements taken during two 24-hour monitoring sessions in one cohort of patients who were glaucoma suspects and another cohort with a known diagnosis of glaucoma, the reproducibility of the measurements was found to be similar, despite a lack of control activities and movements throughout the two sessions.[23]

Despite limitations to interpreting the data gleaned from this device, alongside other limitations to real-world use, this technology still represents an intriguing opportunity. The experience of clinical practice demonstrates that traditional ocular measurement is limited to observation in the clinic, and that the metrics that eye care providers use to make medical decisions may vary outside the range documented during a given patient's history within the clinical setting.[24]

This technology may also provide an opportunity to generate a wealth of data regarding the intersection of sleep and intraocular pressure, including the prevalence of nocturnal IOP spikes that would otherwise not have been detected previously. Beyond the timing of sleep, investigators have focused on sleep position, with a recent Canadian group utilizing the Triggerfish contact lens in a study of patients with both primary open-angle glaucoma and normotensive glaucoma.[25] While the results did not reach statistical significance, this study did find more pressure elevation in patients in the flat position than those in the head-up position, highlighting the need for future research as to whether sleeping position recommendations could be made for glaucoma patients.[25]

The prospect of monitoring patients not just in their homes, but in the multiple physiologic states they might find themselves in over the course of their lives, may give us greater insight into how patients' pressures fluctuate on a daily basis[26] and may open opportunities to better understand the disease processes underlying glaucoma itself.[27,28,29,30,31] Several recent studies have found a lack of significant fluctuations in intraocular pressure for patients with this device onboard during activities one may expect to cause an elevation in intraocular pressure such as exercise[32] or playing woodwind instruments.[33]

Beyond the clinic, potential exists in the realm of surgery as well. The 24-hour monitoring will allow a deeper understanding of changes to intraocular pressure dynamics induced by different procedures in glaucoma, such a canaloplasty,[34] trabectome,[35] selective laser trabeculoplasty,[36,37] cataract surgery,[38] and other filtration procedures.[39] Unfortunately, the data so far has not supported a role for intraocular pressure measurement, even in surgeries in which intraocular pressure measurement might be a concern.[40] The Triggerfish device is both CE Marked in Europe and FDA approved in the United States.

Eyemate

The Eyemate (Implandata GmbH, Germany) is an implantable, wireless intraocular pressure transducer, sheathed in biocompatible silicone that is placed into the ciliary sulcus during intraocular surgery. Drawing power from a paired external device as well as relaying measurement data to said device, the Eyemate lacks an internal power source and does not require direct manipulation by the patient.[41] It does not appear that routine electromagnetic signals interfere with the function of this technology.[42] In general, surgical implantation is well-tolerated when performed in conjunction with cataract surgery, without unexpected adverse events,[43] and with a favorable safety profile in the first 12 months after implantation.[44]

A recent study examining variability in intraocular pressure in 22 patients with implanted Eyemate devices had the patients measure their pressures at predetermined time frames during the day, collecting 92,860 measurements over 15,811 measurement days.[45] Though interpretation of the data may be confounded by the significant range of measurements (ranging from 1 to 277 daily), interesting trends nevertheless emerged in the measurements. In general, intraocular pressure appeared to vary least in the nighttime and most in the early morning.[45] By highlighting the time-based differential variability of intraocular pressure in glaucoma patients, the Eyemate has the potential to allow for additional subdivision of patients not simply by maximum intraocular pressure but also in terms of the short- and long-term variability of their intraocular pressure readings. This quantitative basis of determining multiple intraocular pressure data points outside of office visits may both allow for the plotting of more accurate intraocular pressure curves for each patient and additionally may prove a fruitful avenue for future research into whether disease processes we currently understand to be similar are actually distinct pathological phenomena.

Novel applications of this technology include monitoring intraocular pressure longitudinally in patients who have had ocular keratoprosthesis surgery, a subset of patients in whom accurate tonometry is challenging due to the absence of traditional corneal distension mechanics for the measurement of intraocular pressure. A 2019 study evaluating postoperative IOP changes in patients receiving a Boston Keratoprosthesis demonstrated that Eyemate measurements corresponded with finger palpation performed by glaucoma specialists in the study, accurately stratifying intraocular pressure results between normal, soft/hypotonic, borderline, and hypertonic categories.[46] Additionally, the Eyemate device captured peaks on postoperative day one, as well as a longitudinal increase in intraocular pressure after surgery, expanding providers' understanding of the natural history of intraocular pressure changes following keratoprosthesis surgery while at the same time providing a quantitative basis for disease management and further research investigation.[46] The Eyemate is not currently FDA approved in the United States, but is commercially available in Europe.

SUMMARY

Ocular home monitoring devices are on the verge of revolutionizing both paradigms of clinical care and eye providers' understanding of ophthalmic pathology itself. Though there are some hurdles to clear, including patient buy-in and willingness to incorporate behavior changes to their routines, significant absence of head-to-head randomized controlled studies comparing these new technologies to existing monitoring techniques, these technologies show immense promise and are likely to change how eye providers and patients conceptualize and manage care for chronic eye diseases.

REFERENCES

1. Zaidi FH, et al. The Amsler chart is of doubtful value in retinal screening for early laser therapy of subretinal membranes. The west London survey. *Eye (London, England)*. 2004;18(5):503–508. PubMed https://doi.org/10.1038/sj.eye.6700708.
2. Han DP. The ForeSeeHome device and the home study: a milestone in the self-detection of neovascular age-related macular degeneration. *JAMA Ophthalmol*. 2014;132(10):1167–1168. Silverchair https://doi.org/10.1001/jamaophthalmol.2014.1405.
3. Chaikitmongkol V, et al. Early detection of choroidal neovascularization facilitated with a home monitoring program in age-related macular degeneration. *Retin Cases Br*

Rep. 2015;9(1):33–37. PubMed https://doi.org/10.1097/ICB.0000000000000085.

4. AREDS2-HOME Study Research Group, et al. Randomized trial of a home monitoring system for early detection of choroidal neovascularization home monitoring of the eye (HOME) study. *Ophthalmology.* 2014;121(2):535–544. PubMed https://doi.org/10.1016/j.ophtha.2013.10.027.

5. Domalpally A, et al. Imaging characteristics of choroidal neovascular lesions in the AREDS2-HOME study: report number 4. *Ophthalmol Retina.* 2019;3(4):326–335. PubMed https://doi.org/10.1016/j.oret.2019.01.004.

6. Chew EY, et al. Effectiveness of different monitoring modalities in the detection of neovascular age-related macular degeneration: THE home study, report number 3. *Retina.* 2016;36(8):1542–1547. PubMed https://doi.org/10.1097/IAE.0000000000000940.

7. Yu HJ, Kiernan DF, Eichenbaum D, Sheth VS, Wykoff CC. Home monitoring of age-related macular degeneration: utility of the ForeseeHome device for detection of neovascularization. *Ophthalmol Retina.* 2021;5(4):348–356. https://doi.org/10.1016/j.oret.2020.08.003.

8. Wang Y-Z, et al. Handheld shape discrimination hyperacuity test on a mobile device for remote monitoring of visual function in maculopathy. *Invest Ophthalmol Vis Sci.* 2013;54(8):5497. DOI.org (Crossref) https://doi.org/10.1167/iovs.13-1.

9. Vazquez NP, et al. Radial shape discrimination testing for new-onset neovascular age-related macular degeneration in at-risk eyes. *PLoS One.* 2018;13(11), e0207342. PLoS Journals https://doi.org/10.1371/journal.pone.0207342.

10. Kaiser PK, et al. Feasibility of a novel remote daily monitoring system for age-related macular degeneration using mobile handheld devices: results of a pilot study. *Retina.* 2013;33(9):1863–1870. DOI.org (Crossref) https://doi.org/10.1097/IAE.0b013e3182899258.

11. Cvenkel B, et al. Self-measurement with Icare home tonometer, patients' feasibility and acceptability. *Eur J Ophthalmol.* 2020;30(2):258–263. PubMed https://doi.org/10.1177/1120672118823124.

12. Dabasia PL, et al. Evaluation of a new rebound tonometer for self-measurement of intraocular pressure. *Br J Ophthalmol.* 2016;100(8):1139–1143. PubMed https://doi.org/10.1136/bjophthalmol-2015-307674.

13. Liu J, et al. Icare home tonometer: a review of characteristics and clinical utility. *Clin Ophthalmol.* 2020;14:4031–4045. PubMed https://doi.org/10.2147/OPTH.S284844.

14. Takagi D, et al. Evaluation of a new rebound self-tonometer, Icare home: comparison with Goldmann applanation tonometer. *J Glaucoma.* 2017;26(7):613–618. PubMed https://doi.org/10.1097/IJG.0000000000000674.

15. Valero B, et al. Reliability and reproducibility of introcular pressure (IOP) measurement with the Icare® home rebound tonometer (model TA022) and comparison with Goldmann applanation tonometer in glaucoma patients. *J Fr Ophthalmol.* 2017;40(10):865–875. PubMed https://doi.org/10.1016/j.jfo.2017.06.008.

16. Qassim A, Mullany S, Awadalla MS, et al. A polygenic risk score predicts intraocular pressure readings outside office hours and early morning spikes as measured by home tonometry. *Ophthalmol Glaucoma.* 2021;4(4):411–420. https://doi.org/10.1016/j.ogla.2020.12.002.

17. Huang J, et al. Diurnal intraocular pressure fluctuations with self-tonometry in glaucoma patients and suspects: a clinical trial. *Optom Vis Sci.* 2018;95(2):88–95. PubMed https://doi.org/10.1097/OPX.0000000000001172.

18. Hubanova R, et al. Effect of overnight wear of the Triggerfish® sensor on corneal thickness measured by Visante® anterior segment optical coherence tomography. *Acta Ophthalmol.* 2014;92(2):e119–e123. Wiley Online Library https://doi.org/10.1111/aos.12241.

19. Mansouri K, Shaarawy T. Continuous intraocular pressure monitoring with a wireless ocular telemetry sensor: initial clinical experience in patients with open angle glaucoma. *Br J Ophthalmol.* 2011;95(5):627–629. https://doi.org/10.1136/bjo.2010.192922. Epub 2011 Jan 7 21216796.

20. Hubanova R, et al. Effect of overnight wear of the Triggerfish® sensor on corneal thickness measured by Visante® anterior segment optical coherence tomography. *Acta Ophthalmol.* 2014;92(2):e119–e123. Wiley Online Library https://doi.org/10.1111/aos.12241.

21. Dunbar GE, et al. The sensimed triggerfish contact lens sensor: efficacy, safety, and patient perspectives. *Clin Ophthalmol.* 2017;11:875–882. PubMed https://doi.org/10.2147/OPTH.S109708.

22. Lorenz K, et al. Tolerability of 24-hour intraocular pressure monitoring of a pressure-sensitive contact lens. *J Glaucoma.* 2013;22(4):311–316. PubMed https://doi.org/10.1097/IJG.0b013e318241b874.

23. Mansouri K, Medeiros FA, et al. Continuous 24-hour monitoring of intraocular pressure patterns with a contact lens sensor: safety, tolerability, and reproducibility in patients with glaucoma. *Arch Ophthalmol.* 2012;130(12):1534–1539. PubMed https://doi.org/10.1001/archophthalmol.2012.2280.

24. Shioya S, et al. Using 24-hr ocular dimensional profile recorded with a sensing contact lens to identify primary open-angle glaucoma patients with intraocular pressure constantly below the diagnostic threshold. *Acta Ophthalmol.* 2020;98(8), e1017–23. PubMed https://doi.org/10.1111/aos.14453.

25. Beltran-Agulló L, et al. Twenty-four hour intraocular pressure monitoring with the SENSIMED triggerfish contact lens: effect of body posture during sleep. *Br J Ophthalmol.* 2017;101(10):1323–1328. PubMed https://doi.org/10.1136/bjophthalmol-2016-308710.

26. Mansouri K, Weinreb RN. Meeting an unmet need in glaucoma: continuous 24-h monitoring of intraocular pressure. *Expert Rev Med Devices.* 2012;9(3):225–231. PubMed https://doi.org/10.1586/erd.12.14.

27. Mansouri K, Gillmann K. Intereye symmetry of 24-hour intraocular pressure-related patterns in untreated glaucoma patients using a contact Lens sensor. *J Glaucoma.*

2020;29(8):666–670. PubMed https://doi.org/10.1097/IJG.0000000000001563.

28. Pajic B, et al. Continuous IOP fluctuation recording in normal tension glaucoma patients. *Curr Eye Res.* 2011;36(12):1129–1138. PubMed https://doi.org/10.3109/02713683.2011.608240.

29. Kim YW, et al. Twenty-four-hour intraocular pressure-related patterns from contact lens sensors in normal-tension glaucoma and healthy eyes: the exploring nyctohemeral intraocular pressure related pattern for glaucoma management (ENIGMA) study. *Ophthalmology.* 2020;127(11):1487–1497. PubMed https://doi.org/10.1016/j.ophtha.2020.05.010.

30. Moraes D, Gustavo C, et al. Association between 24-hour intraocular pressure monitored with contact Lens sensor and visual field progression in older adults with glaucoma. *JAMA Ophthalmol.* 2018;136(7):779–785. PubMed https://doi.org/10.1001/jamaophthalmol.2018.1746.

31. Esen F, et al. Diurnal spikes of intraocular pressure in uveitic glaucoma: a 24-hour intraocular pressure monitoring study. *Semin Ophthalmol.* 2020;35(4):246–251. PubMed https://doi.org/10.1080/08820538.2020.1809683.

32. Bozkurt B, et al. The evaluation of intraocular pressure fluctuation in glaucoma subjects during submaximal exercise using an ocular telemetry sensor. *Indian J Ophthalmol.* 2019;67(1):89–94. PubMed https://doi.org/10.4103/ijo.IJO_585_18.

33. de Crom RMPC, et al. Intraocular pressure fluctuations and 24-hour continuous monitoring for glaucoma risk in wind instrument players. *J Glaucoma.* 2017;26(10):923–928. PubMed https://doi.org/10.1097/IJG.0000000000000747.

34. Rekas M, et al. Assessing efficacy of canaloplasty using continuous 24-hour monitoring of ocular dimensional changes. *Invest Ophthalmol Vis Sci.* 2016;57(6):2533–2542. PubMed https://doi.org/10.1167/iovs.16-19185.

35. Tojo N, Hayashi A. Can a contact lens sensor predict the success of trabectome surgery? *Graefes Arch Clin Exp Ophthalmol.* 2020;258(4):843–850. PubMed https://doi.org/10.1007/s00417-019-04576-9.

36. Tojo N, Oka M, et al. Comparison of fluctuations of intraocular pressure before and after selective laser trabeculoplasty in normal-tension glaucoma patients. *J Glaucoma.* 2014;23(8):e138–e143. PubMed https://doi.org/10.1097/IJG.0000000000000026.

37. Lee JWY, et al. Twenty-four-hour intraocular pressure related changes following adjuvant selective laser trabeculoplasty for normal tension glaucoma. *Medicine.* 2014;93(27):e238. PubMed https://doi.org/10.1097/MD.0000000000000238.

38. Tojo N, Otsuka M, et al. Comparison of intraocular pressure fluctuation before and after cataract surgeries in normal-tension glaucoma patients. *Eur J Ophthalmol.* 2019;29(5):516–523. PubMed https://doi.org/10.1177/1120672.

39. Osorio-Alayo V, et al. Efficacy of the SENSIMED triggerfish® in the postoperative follow-up of PHACO-ExPRESS combined surgery. *Arch Soc Esp Oftalmol.* 2017;92(8):372–378. PubMed https://doi.org/10.1016/j.oftal.2017.04.003.

40. Vitish-Sharma P, et al. Can the SENSIMED Triggerfish® lens data be used as an accurate measure of intraocular pressure? *Acta Ophthalmol.* 2018;96(2):e242–e246. PubMed https://doi.org/10.1111/aos.13456.

41. Dick HB, Schultz T, Gerste RD. Miniaturization in glaucoma monitoring and treatment: a review of new technologies that require a minimal surgical approach. *Ophthalmol Therapy.* 2019;8(1):19–30. https://doi.org/10.1007/s40123-019-0161-2. Epub 2019 Feb 6 30725339.

42. Invernizzi A, et al. Influence of electromagnetic radiation emitted by daily-use electronic devices on the Eyemate® system in-vitro: a feasibility study. *BMC Ophthalmol.* 2020;20(1):357. PubMed https://doi.org/10.1186/s12886-020-01623-6.

43. Choritz L, Mansouri K, van den Bosch J, et al. Telemetric measurement of intraocular pressure via an implantable pressure sensor-12-month results from the ARGOS-02 trial. *Am J Ophthalmol.* 2020;209:187–196. https://doi.org/10.1016/j.ajo.2019.09.011. Epub 2019 Sep 20 31545953.

44. Enders P, Cursiefen C. Device profile of the EYEMATE-IO™ system for intraocular pressure monitoring: overview of its safety and efficacy. *Expert Rev Med Devices.* 2020;17(6):491–497. https://doi.org/10.1080/17434440.2020.1761788. nEpub 2020 May 12. 32339024.

45. Mansouri K, Rao HL, Weinreb RN, ARGOS-02 Study Group. Short-term and long-term variability of intraocular pressure measured with an intraocular telemetry sensor in patients with glaucoma. *Ophthalmology.* 2021;128(2):227–233. https://doi.org/10.1016/j.ophtha.2020.07.016.

46. Enders P, Hall J, Bornhauser M, et al. Telemetric intraocular pressure monitoring after Boston keratoprosthesis surgery using the Eyemate-IO sensor: dynamics in the first year. *Am J Ophthalmol.* 2019;206:256–263. https://doi.org/10.1016/j.ajo.2019.02.025. Epub 2019 Mar 5 30849343.

CHAPTER 12

Principles of Ocular Telehealth Implementation

LOREN J. LOCK, MS • ALEJANDRA TORRES DIAZ, BS •
ANNETTE L. GIANGIACOMO, MD • YAO LIU, MD, MS

OVERVIEW

This chapter presents general principles guiding the establishment and maintenance of ocular telehealth programs, with a focus on implementation for long-term sustainability. While many successful ocular telehealth initiatives have been established globally (see Chapter 10), this chapter focuses the discussion on the implementation of primary care–based teleretinal diabetic retinopathy screening within multi-payer health systems in the United States.[1-3] Using this as the index case example, the authors illustrate general principles of ocular telehealth implementation that are applicable to a variety of settings. First, the importance of engaging key stakeholders in the development and design of the ocular telehealth program is discussed. Then, aspects of training personnel participating in the program are highlighted.

STAKEHOLDER ENGAGEMENT
Definition and Purpose

Stakeholder engagement is an often overlooked, yet essential, component of establishing and maintaining a successful ocular telehealth program.[3,4] This process involves engaging individuals needed to allocate organizational resources and obtain buy-in to support the planning and implementation process, such as senior health system leadership or administrators. Stakeholder engagement should also involve individuals who may be affected by and/or directly participate in implementing the ocular telehealth program. These often include providers (both those referring patients and those providing the telehealth interpretation), clinic administrators, staff, patients, and external organizations. Comprehensively considering the needs of a broad range of stakeholders and including their diverse perspectives can be invaluable for informing the development and ongoing evaluation of a robust ocular telehealth program to maximize its impact and sustainability.

Identifying Key Stakeholders

To identify key stakeholders, one often starts by asking "Who are the relevant stakeholders that will be affected by or participate in this program?" Also consider,

Ocular Telehealth. https://doi.org/10.1016/B978-0-323-83204-5.00012-3

"From whom will one need official approval to move forward?" and "What knowledge, resources, or commitments will one need from those individuals or groups?" It can be helpful to create a list or diagram to help identify all relevant stakeholders. Some useful tools could include reviewing an organizational chart for the clinic or health system, as well as creating an end-to-end workflow diagram (see "Setting the Stage and Mapping the Workflow" section).

Once an initial list of stakeholders is obtained, plan to meet with them either one-on-one or in a group setting as appropriate to discuss the telehealth program. Consider asking the stakeholders if they believe anyone is missing from the current list of key stakeholders who would be valuable to include. It is not always obvious which individuals or roles within an organization are highly influential, and it can be highly beneficial to identify stakeholders with considerable influence who may be willing to publicly champion the ocular telehealth program.

Meeting With Stakeholders

When meeting with stakeholders in a group setting, it can be useful to divide different types of stakeholders into separate groups or to create mixed stakeholder groups. For example, in the authors' work in primary care clinics, the team chose to hold meetings among patient stakeholders separately from clinical stakeholders (e.g., clinicians, medical assistants, clinic managers, schedulers, and electronic health record (EHR) staff) due to differences in power dynamics and terminology use.[3] In addition, by dividing stakeholders into smaller groups, more participants can be included to provide meaningful input and perspectives.

For clinical stakeholders' meetings, inviting a mix of people with varying roles within the organization can be particularly helpful to fill in critical information gaps that may only be known to certain members of the organization. For example, EHR staff can provide information on existing EHR functionalities to leverage for the ocular telehealth program, and schedulers may have unique knowledge on the existing workflows used for scheduling patients' next primary care clinic visit. Thus, when a clinical stakeholder group has members that encompass a wide variety of roles and responsibilities, the meetings and project can often move forward more efficiently.

Since clinical teams can be quite hierarchical depending on the organizational culture, using tools such as the Nominal Group Technique (NGT)[5] can help ensure that less vocal members of a group share their insights and have an equal voice in decision-making.

Using NGT, each participant in the group sequentially offers one idea until no new ideas are generated. Each participant then votes for 2–3 ideas, after which the top 2–3 ideas endorsed by the group are identified through tallying the votes. The top ideas selected are then advanced. This technique can be used, for example, to choose which implementation strategies to try first when implementing an ocular telehealth program. It can also be helpful to engage an experienced meeting facilitator, such as a professional practice facilitator.[6,7] This facilitator can promote a culture of respectful inquiry and ensure that all ideas are given adequate consideration, with all group members encouraged to contribute to the discussion.

Finally, it is important to be mindful of stakeholders' time and to reduce barriers to participation. Clinical staff attendance and active participation in meetings can be greatly enhanced by leveraging time already designated for staff meetings during regular work hours whenever possible and blocking clinic schedules with permission from clinic supervisors or administrators. Meeting participants generally appreciate receiving information on how specific elements of their feedback have contributed to moving the project forward as well as having refreshments provided at meetings.

Applying Implementation Science

This section provides a brief overview of implementation science, which is the field from which much of the work in this chapter is derived. The National Institutes of Health (NIH) defines implementation science as "the study of methods to promote the adoption and integration of evidence-based practices, interventions and policies into routine health care and public health settings."[8] This field directly addresses the slow adoption of evidence-based practices into clinical settings.[9] Major principles from implementation science include: involving stakeholders early in the implementation planning process to assess organizational readiness; continuing to elicit and incorporate stakeholder input throughout the implementation process to tailor the program to the unique needs and resources of the organization; and providing stakeholders with ongoing feedback and data obtained from evaluating program outcomes.[10]

Implementation science frameworks can help guide the development, execution, and evaluation of ocular telehealth programs. Most of the frameworks can be categorized as providing guidance with assessing the factors or *determinants* of successful implementation, the *process* of implementation or the *evaluation* of implementation outcomes (Table 12.1). They can also be used in research

TABLE 12.1
Frequently Used Implementation Science Frameworks for Clinical Practice and Research[10]

Name	Description
Reach, Effectiveness, Adoption, Implementation, and Maintenance (RE-AIM)[11]	RE-AIM evaluates program outcomes by assessing factors including reach, effectiveness, adoption, implementation, and maintenance
Consolidated framework for implementation research (CFIR)[12]	CFIR investigates factors associated with implementation outcomes across five domains: intervention characteristics, outer setting, inner setting, characteristics of individuals, and process of implementation
Integrated promoting action on research implementation in health services (i-PARIHS)[13]	PARIHS posits that successful implementation is a function of the *evidence* that supports the intervention, the *context* into which it is being introduced, and how the intervention is *facilitated*; Used in the VA Implementation Facilitation Guide[11]
Expert recommendations for implementing change (ERIC)[14]	ERIC provides a standardized nomenclature for describing a wide variety of implementation strategies
Stages of implementation completion (SIC)[15]	SIC is an eight-stage tool describing an implementation process and milestones across three phases: pre-implementation, implementation, and sustainability

to identify generalizable principles for improving adoption and uptake of ocular telehealth programs. Using principles of implementation science, the authors have developed a practical, free, online toolkit for implementing teleretinal diabetic eye screening in primary care called I-SITE (Implementation for Sustained Impact in Teleophthalmology, www.hipxchange.org/I-SITE). This tool provides useful pearls that can apply to other ocular telehealth programs, even if those programs do not focus strictly on diabetic teleretinal screening.

Key Stakeholder Perspectives
Overview of clinical stakeholder perspectives
Prior to engaging with clinical stakeholders to establish or make changes to an ocular telehealth program, it is important to consider how stakeholders perceive their roles in the organization and telehealth program as well as their perceived barriers and facilitators to using the program. Often this centers upon barriers and facilitators around adopting or using the program. For example, asking the stakeholders in a teleretinal diabetic eye screening program: "What makes it hard to ensure that every patient with diabetes obtains eye screening?" "What has helped in the process of referring patients for screening?" and "What has not helped in the process of referring patients for screening?" can provide useful insights into what is working well and what challenges exist. Some results from the authors' individual interviews and stakeholder meeting discussions in a primary care–based teleretinal diabetic eye screening program are summarized in Table 12.2.[2,16]

Barriers and facilitators for health system administrators
Health system administrators are typically senior members and key decision-makers in the organization, often holding "C-level" executive titles such as Chief Medical Officer or Chief Executive Officer. Approval and allocation of resources are needed from these organizational leaders to move forward with an ocular telehealth program. In large organizations, there may also be a specific leadership committee (or multiple committees) that must first evaluate a project before it can be approved, a process that can require multiple rounds of presentations, written proposals, and discussions. Thus, understanding the perspectives of key decision-makers in an organization is a vital first step. Since these individuals and committees are typically very busy, it can be beneficial to first engage with either another member within the organization who could help champion the effort (e.g., an influential clinician or a clinical administrator, such as a Director of Population Health or Quality Improvement) or any person who is trusted and well-known to the organization. Identifying internal champions creates an opportunity for the champions to introduce the ocular telehealth program to organizational leaders and increases the odds that the proposal will receive a comprehensive review.

Key barriers for ocular telehealth adoption by health system administrators may include the cost of equipment, physical space needed for the equipment, information technology (IT) infrastructure (e.g., for image storage and transfer), time needed for provider and staff training, lack of consensus around billing codes, and limited insurance coverage for telehealth services.[17] A central concern for health system administrators is an analysis of the expected return on investment for the ocular telehealth program. Administrators may also be

TABLE 12.2
Barriers and Facilitators to Adoption and Use of a Primary Care–based Teleretinal Diabetic Eye Screening Program Among Key Clinical Stakeholders[2,16]

Role	Barriers	Facilitators
Health system administrators	• Cost of cameras and image storage system • Physical space for camera equipment • Lack of information technology (IT) infrastructure • Time required to train providers and staff • Variability in insurance coverage • Limited reimbursement • Uncertain return on investment	• Education regarding the program's alignment with organizational mission and existing initiatives (e.g., for diabetes care) • Participation in insurer-based quality improvement incentive program • Calculation of expected clinical and financial outcomes • Leverage existing IT infrastructure when possible (e.g., X-rays or mammograms)
Referring Providers and clinical staff	• Difficulty in identifying eligible patients for screening • Lack of time to explain the program to patients • Lack of knowledge about insurance coverage and patient out-of-pocket costs • Lack of knowledge about and confidence in teleretinal imaging • Limited knowledge of diabetic eye disease	• Education about diabetic eye disease, data on program's clinical effectiveness along with patient success stories, insurance coverage, and patient out-of-pocket costs • Streamlined ordering/referral processes • Suggested scripts for discussing the program with patients • Patient education materials
Imaging Staff	• Camera equipment difficult to use • Camera location far from patient care area and/or in a shared room where it is frequently unavailable • Lack of knowledge about and confidence in teleretinal imaging • Infrequent imaging leading to poor retention of imaging skills • Limited knowledge of diabetic eye disease	• User-friendly, touch-screen cameras with autofocus/autocapture • Standardized protocols for image capture with step-by-step screenshots in printed guides located near the camera • Use of a selective pupil dilation protocol with 0.5% tropicamide to reduce ungradable images • Camera location near patient care area • Training smaller number of staff to increase the frequency of imaging to enhance skills retention • Education about diabetic eye disease, data on program's clinical effectiveness along with patient success stories
Interpreting eye care providers	• Lack of familiarity with image grading and referral recommendations • Limited reimbursement for image grading • Concerns about clinical liability	• Education about diabetic eye disease, data on program's clinical effectiveness along with patient success stories • Calculation of expected reimbursement from grading multiple images per hour • Standardized protocols for image grading, reporting, and recommendations to follow up eye care • Artificial intelligence to provide clinical decision support, streamline interpretation/reporting process, and risk stratification

concerned about the burden of the program on providers and staff who are already stretched thin with their existing duties. For example, teleretinal diabetic eye screening performed in primary care clinics can add a variety of additional tasks for already overburdened primary care teams focused on the management of multiple acute and chronic systemic medical conditions.

Key facilitators for ocular telehealth adoption by health system administrators include provision of information on the ocular telehealth program and its expected benefits and outcomes. This includes detailed information regarding how the program aligns with the organization's mission and existing initiatives, the size of the population served by the ocular telehealth program, the extent of the unmet need that would be filled by the program (e.g., projected increase in diabetic eye screening rates), and the expected clinical and financial outcomes (e.g., projected number of patients identified and treated for vision-threatening eye disease, as well as projected financial incentives from health insurers earned through meeting certain healthcare quality measures). Much of this baseline data may be obtained with the assistance of the organization's quality improvement and billing/compliance staff. Projected patient volumes, costs, and program revenue can help provide reassurance regarding the expected burdens on staff and clinicians, as well as a compelling value proposition. Prior studies of return on investment of teleretinal diabetic eye screening have found that they can result in savings to the patients and health system as well as increased revenue to the health system through quality incentives.[18–20] Finally, an illustrative patient vignette or story can complement the data presented and provide a valuable and persuasive case illustrating the problem solved and the benefits to be gained from the ocular telehealth program.

With regard to future trends, there has been a major increase in telehealth adoption by health systems and broadening of telehealth insurance coverage resulting from the COVID-19 pandemic. On the health system administration and societal level, there is now a greater acknowledgment and acceptance of the central role that telehealth can play in increasing healthcare access. Long-term plans for expanding insurance coverage for telehealth are encouraging. Additionally, rapidly evolving imaging technology will continue to advance the field by providing higher quality imaging at lower cost using devices with greater portability. Advances in artificial intelligence will continue to provide important opportunities to support image interpretation, clinical decision support, and risk stratification. The use of cutting-edge telehealth technology not only benefits patients but also can be a market differentiator for health systems that can apply patient-centered telehealth technology to attract and expand their patient population.

In summary, resource allocation for an ocular telehealth program requires approval from health system leadership. Given this, those planning to create or change an ocular telehealth program must analyze and understand the key decision-makers, as well as determine the program's alignment with the organizational mission and financial considerations, particularly around return on investment. Understanding these factors is critical for successfully moving the project forward with the strong support of organizational leaders.

Barriers and facilitators for Referring Providers and clinical staff

Referring Providers are those who are referring patients or entering orders for patients to receive ocular telehealth. These providers can come from a variety of different training backgrounds, and they may be non-eye care providers depending on the type of ocular telehealth program. Therefore, these stakeholders may have limited familiarity not only with ocular telehealth in general but also may have limited knowledge of the ocular condition that the program is designed to address. Likewise, clinical staff who are supporting the Referring Provider and/or who may be involved in acquiring imaging and tests for ocular telehealth may not understand the rationale for the ocular telehealth program and its potential to improve patient care. This can lead to difficulty in identifying patients who are eligible for the program, a lack of confidence in discussing and recommending the program to eligible patients, discomfort about patient costs and insurance coverage, concerns about the quality and reliability of the service, and even fears about potential clinical liability.[2,21] Furthermore, there has been an increasing focus on burnout in healthcare due to the high burden of tasks placed on providers and staff. Thus, adding an ocular telehealth program to clinical practice could be negatively perceived as yet another task put upon the shoulders of already overextended personnel.

In anticipation of these potential barriers, providing the essential clinical knowledge and evidence for the ocular telehealth program while emphasizing the benefits to patients can greatly ease concerns and engender positive attitudes toward the ocular telehealth program. The goal of providing information to providers and staff is to simultaneously convey the knowledge they need and to get them excited about offering this innovative program to increase patient access to vision-saving eye care.

A presentation at a regularly scheduled staff meeting can address common questions regarding the ocular condition, the problem solved using ocular telehealth, direct patient benefits (i.e., improved access and better clinical outcomes), evidence that the program is effective, and a detailed discussion of costs and insurance coverage. Again, a compelling patient story can provide an important introduction to engage the attention of providers and staff who are often highly motivated by the prospect of improving patient care and enhancing their patients' quality of life through saving sight. Of note, a strong recommendation from a patient's primary care provider has been found to have the greatest impact on a patient's decision to obtain teleretinal diabetic eye screening in primary care.[2,22] In particular, such presentations can be important opportunities to identify clinical champions among Referring Providers and staff who will provide strong, public support for the program. As Referring Providers can leverage patient trust and have a major impact on both patient acceptance and use of ocular telehealth, it is crucial to obtain their buy-in.

Once Referring Providers and clinical staff are aware of the clinical importance and usefulness of the ocular telehealth program, tools should be provided to make their role in the program as easy as possible. This might include streamlining identification and referral of eligible patients as well as providing suggested scripts for how to discuss the program with patients.[2,23] In addition, an easy way to convey information to patients while requiring less personnel time is offering patient education materials for patients to read while they are waiting to be seen by their provider. Regularly sharing data on program outcomes and eliciting feedback from providers and staff about opportunities to further improve the program can help to sustain the program's momentum past the initial wave of enthusiasm and maintain its effectiveness.[3] Specific implementation strategies targeting Referring Providers, clinical staff, and patients are discussed in "Strategies to Increase Clinical Stakeholder Engagement" section.

Since ocular telehealth programs have traditionally focused on technical and validation aspects of image acquisition, transfer, and interpretation, there has been less attention paid to engaging upstream Referring Providers and clinical staff who are mainly responsible for identifying and persuading patients to obtain ocular telehealth. Without their support, buy-in, and active contributions, ocular telehealth programs are at high risk for underutilization. Thus, addressing the barriers and facilitators to engaging Referring Providers and clinical staff can greatly strengthen the long-term effectiveness of an ocular telehealth program.

Barriers and facilitators for Imaging Staff (telehealth facilitators)

Imaging Staff play a crucial role in obtaining high-quality images and/or data from patients in an ocular telehealth program. These imagers may be drawn from a variety of different roles, including medical assistants, technicians, nurses, diabetes educators, or clinic managers. An eye care background may not be needed for Imaging Staff who receive on-the-job training for the ocular telehealth program. However, there can be significant barriers in engaging with imagers who, in the case of teleretinal diabetic eye screening in primary care, may lack familiarity and knowledge of diabetic eye disease. Their initial reaction may be to perceive imaging negatively, as another burden (i.e., "yet one more thing") they must do with no increase in their compensation. In addition, a lack of familiarity with or difficulty in using the camera equipment can also contribute to imager frustration and lack of confidence in obtaining high-quality images. Furthermore, the location of the camera is very important as well. It can be time-consuming and inconvenient for imagers to have camera equipment located far from patient care areas. This can be exacerbated if the room where the camera is located is shared with other equipment (e.g., EKG machines, X-ray, etc.) or shared with a staff office that causes it to be frequently unavailable due to being in use by others. Finally, there can be limited retention of skills among Imaging Staff if patient volumes are low or if there is high staff turnover. Thus, careful consideration of the imager experience is needed when designing the ocular telehealth workflow, and obtaining feedback from imagers early on can be invaluable for addressing their needs to enhance the success of the ocular telehealth program.

Facilitators for Imaging Staff include making the imaging experience as easy and convenient as possible with regard to camera selection and location, as well as educating them about the importance of the ocular telehealth program in improving patient outcomes. Camera selection is a critical component contributing to whether Imaging Staff will successfully adopt the ocular telehealth program. Many eye cameras have traditionally been designed for use by professional ophthalmic photographers that allow for a multitude of operator-controlled adjustments to maximize image quality. However, in ocular telehealth programs the Imaging Staff may have little or no prior eye care background, and the complexity of a traditional camera user interface can be quite daunting for these individuals. For example, the use of a traditional joystick, while used routinely in slit lamps and other eye care equipment, can be highly non-intuitive and cumbersome for use by Imaging Staff. A major advance for ocular telehealth programs has been the development of user-friendly, touch-screen cameras with autofocus/autocapture imaging. Thus, the simple touch-screen interface overcomes a major barrier for Imaging Staff. Trying various cameras is essential to ensure that Imaging Staff are comfortable with the technology and can obtain high-quality images with minimal training. While many organizations will be naturally drawn to purchasing the lowest cost camera equipment, purchasing a slightly more expensive unit that provides substantially higher quality images with lower ungradable rates can often be well-worth the investment to ensure that Imaging Staff do not lose confidence in their ability to obtain images. Furthermore, the camera should be located in a convenient and easily accessible area that minimizes patient travel in the clinic.

Low rates of ungradable images contribute not only to the quality of the ocular telehealth program but are also critical to ensuring the sustained engagement of Imaging Staff. Detailed training materials with standardized protocols for image capture with step-by-step screenshots should be available in printed guides located near the camera. These reference materials can be very helpful for Imaging Staff who may have experienced a long gap since their training or the last time they performed imaging. Having a lead imager among the Imaging Staff who can help troubleshoot and answer questions, provide refresher training, and/or onboard new imagers, particularly in organizations with high staff turnover, can also be highly valuable. Some organizations may choose to use a selective pupil dilation protocol wherein a nurse or staff member with medication administration privileges can instill 0.5% tropicamide eye drops when needed to reduce ungradable retinal images for patients with small pupils.

Finally, as with all clinical stakeholders, education of Imaging Staff about diabetic eye disease, data on the ocular telehealth program's clinical effectiveness, and patient success stories can help motivate participation in the program and overcome initial misgivings about having additional duties. By providing easy-to-use camera equipment and aligning the work of the ocular telehealth program with improved patient outcomes, Imaging Staff can gain a sense of accomplishment with learning a new skill to help patients. This can also reduce burnout by augmenting the meaningfulness of their work.

Barriers and facilitators for Interpreting Providers

Barriers and facilitators among Interpreting Providers in ocular telehealth programs have been less well-studied[24]

in part because such programs are often initiated by eye care providers who are highly motivated to perform the image interpretation. However, as an ocular telehealth program expands, recruiting additional eye care providers to perform image interpretation can be challenging due to a variety of financial, licensure, and liability concerns. Since many ocular telehealth programs provide relatively small reimbursement amounts per patient compared to in-person office visits and procedures, some eye care providers may consider it "not worth their time" to provide the interpretation service. In addition, interstate clinical licensure requirements limit the ability of Interpreting Providers to provide services to patients in states in which they have not yet obtained licensure. Finally, eye care providers may feel uncomfortable regarding the possible liability associated with providing interpretations.

Similar to discussions about the ocular telehealth program with Referring Providers, conversations about the program with potential Interpreting Providers should emphasize the clinical benefits of the program for improving patient care. However, greater attention should be focused on the logistical and financial aspects for Interpreting Providers. Interpreting Providers should be reassured that with proper training and experience, they can perform a high volume of interpretations within a relatively short time period that results in a reasonable hourly compensation rate. Furthermore, interpretations can be performed at their convenience, such as at home or to fill in unused time in an in-person eye clinic or operating room (i.e., while waiting for patients to be roomed or for operating room cleaning and turnover). Streamlined interpretation and reporting forms as well as standardized interpretation and follow-up protocols can further increase ease of use and reduce time burdens on Interpreting Providers.[25] Additionally, the program can augment the complexity of patients seen by the Interpreting providers in their in-person clinical practice. The ocular telehealth program can provide care to patients with normal findings who are satisfied with their vision and do not require in-person evaluation. The in-person eye clinic will then have more appointments available for more complex patients who may require procedures, such as refraction, laser, or surgery, which provide greater reimbursement.

With regard to regulatory issues and liability, Interpreting Providers currently need to be licensed in each state in which the patient's imaging originates. This can be achieved in large ocular telehealth programs by pursuing licensure in multiple states, but the process can be time-consuming and costly to maintain. Instead, ocular telehealth programs may choose to partner with existing reading centers that have eye care providers already credentialed in multiple states. Concerns regarding liability should be discussed with each organizations' legal counsel. When discussing concerns with Interpreting Providers, it is helpful to note that ocular telehealth programs using protocols that have been well-validated and/or endorsed by respected national organizations (e.g., American Diabetes Association) are considered to be providing standard of care or best care practices. Patient information regarding the ocular telehealth program may emphasize that the program is designed to answer specific diagnostic questions (e.g., diabetic eye screening) and include its limitations, if applicable, such as that it may not be a substitute for a comprehensive in-person evaluation. Reporting language may include phrases often seen in the radiology literature that list possible pathologic conditions noted in the imaging for which "clinical correlation" is needed to confirm the diagnosis when appropriate.

The growth and expansion of ocular telehealth programs can be limited by the availability of Interpreting Providers if insufficient attention is paid to common barriers and facilitators to engagement that are experienced by these stakeholders. Recent advances in artificial intelligence interpretation will augment the pool of available Interpreting Providers and provide clinical decision support and risk stratification that could further increase the efficiency and productivity of ocular telehealth programs. In addition, eye care providers have become increasingly familiar and comfortable with providing telehealth-based care in the setting of the COVID-19 pandemic and thus many of their concerns resulting from being unfamiliar with ocular telehealth may be reduced.

Strategies to Increase Clinical Stakeholder Engagement

In this section, the authors present suggested processes and strategies to increase clinical stakeholder engagement within an ocular telehealth program. Much of this information is derived from the team's implementation program, I-SITE (Implementation for Sustained Impact in Tele-ophthalmology).[26] The authors' program allows clinical stakeholders who are participating in the ocular telehealth program to tailor implementation of the program to the unique resources and needs of their organization. The process for creating a successful ocular telehealth program includes convening key clinical stakeholders in an implementation team, mapping the existing workflow, identifying stakeholders' barriers and facilitators to the program's success, and systematically

TABLE 12.3

Systematic Approach to Optimizing an Ocular Telehealth Program Using Stakeholder Input[26,27]

Strategy	How Strategy Might be Applied in Practice
Organize implementation teams and team meetings	Create a local implementation team of Referring providers, administrators, clinical staff, IT/EHR staff, and other stakeholders involved in implementation; Convene the team regularly to share barriers and facilitators to implementation, share best practices, and refine the program
Assess for readiness and identify barriers and facilitators	Identify barriers and facilitators for key stakeholders
Assess and redesign workflow	Observe and map the existing workflow, then identify and implement specific changes to improve processes
Plan–do–study–act (PDSA) cycles	Implement small changes in a cyclical fashion: select a small change to improve the workflow, decide how the outcome of the change will be measured, implement the change for a short period of time, analyze the data, and decide whether to keep the change, further refine it, or abandon it

testing refinements to the workflow (Table 12.3). Note that the examples provided in the following sections are based on a teleretinal diabetic eye screening program in primary care, but the general principles can be applied more broadly to ocular telehealth programs for optimizing utilization and sustainability.

Creating a local implementation team

The odds of an ocular telehealth program's success are greatly increased by having a group of clinical stakeholders within the organization to inform and shape its implementation from the outset. Such a group can also be brought together once the program has already been established to improve its outcomes. This group, which we will refer to as the local implementation team, ideally has representatives from all roles involved in ocular telehealth implementation. This team should include providers, staff members, information technology staff, as well as individuals who have the ability to communicate and persuade members at all levels of the organization. This person may be a quality improvement coordinator or clinic administrator who, in conjunction with a health system administrator such as the Chief Medical Officer, can help coordinate authorization of space and personnel time as well as coordinate staff delegation of roles within the ocular telehealth program. When the implementation team meets, they should discuss the current state of the ocular telehealth program, reflect on what is working well and what barriers are being encountered, share best practices, and decide on the next steps to refine the program.[3,26]

Implementation facilitation

It can be challenging to guide an interdisciplinary local implementation team to make collaborative decisions for developing and refining an ocular telehealth program. Teams can benefit from having the expert guidance of a skilled practice facilitator whenever possible to lead the discussion and increase the effectiveness of meetings. In addition to offering professional expertise, the practice facilitator is a neutral third party who can reduce both perceived or real hidden agendas by individuals within the organization, as well as overcome any organizational and interpersonal politics that could result in "team" decisions that mainly represent the viewpoints of only the most vocal or powerful members of the group. Experienced practice facilitators are often trained in well-validated quality improvement methods such as the Institute for Healthcare Improvement (IHI) Model and Lean Six Sigma.[6] The following processes we describe here apply principles from the NIATx Model for healthcare quality improvement.[28] Sources of trained practice facilitators include the nearly 200 practice-based research networks (PBRNs) in the United States and organizations or an External Quality Review Organization (EQRO).[6,29] One alternative to hiring a practice facilitator is having an individual (either internal or external to the organization) experienced in quality improvement methods serve as the facilitator.

Setting the stage and mapping the workflow

Prior to discussing barriers and strategies to improve ocular telehealth implementation, members of the local implementation team first need to have a clear idea of the existing or proposed workflow. A possible starting point would be creating a step-by-step flowchart that maps the ocular telehealth process from beginning to end. To begin gathering some of this information, some members of the implementation team might consider performing a "walk-through" in which they physically complete the clinical process from the perspective of a patient, provider or clinical staff member involved in the ocular telehealth program.[30] The information gathered during the walk-through can be used to create an initial flowchart diagram for eliciting additional details and perspectives during local implementation team meetings.

Each local implementation team meeting should begin with a brief review of the goals and purpose of the team; a review of the minutes from the last meeting; a discussion of how feedback from the last meeting helped advance the project; and a timed agenda for the planned discussion items.

Doing so reinforces the importance of the project, uses meeting time efficiently, and provides participants with a clear understanding of the value of their contributions to motivate continued participation. It is very helpful to schedule these meetings at times that are most convenient for the local implementation team members. With the support of the health system administrators, implementation team members may even be authorized to block out time from clinical schedules to prevent them from being distracted by competing clinical duties.

Identifying strategies to overcome key barriers

Once the clinical workflow is mapped, the local implementation team should identify (1) which steps in the workflow create the most significant barriers to the desired change (e.g., low utilization of the ocular telehealth program) and (2) the highest impact and most feasible strategies to overcome those barriers. For example, in a teleretinal diabetic eye screening program with low utilization, primary care providers and staff might report that the most significant barrier to increasing use of the program is difficulty in identifying patients eligible for screening. Team members may describe several reasons for this difficulty, including lack of knowledge among providers and staff about patient eligibility requirements, poor EHR documentation regarding the date of the last diabetic eye screening exam, and lack of reminders to ask patients about diabetic eye screening.

In this example, to address the lack of knowledge about ocular telehealth, the team might invite an eye care provider experienced with teleretinal screening to explain the importance of diabetic eye screening, discuss the evidence regarding benefits and outcomes from teleretinal screening, and answer common patient questions regarding the program at a regularly scheduled provider and staff care meeting. Based on this information, the local implementation team may develop suggested scripts for discussing the program with patients and refine patient education materials on teleretinal screening. To address the lack of documentation in the EHR, the clinic may create a standardized workflow for obtaining diabetic eye screening exam notes from patients' eye doctors and standardize the documentation of that information, including specifying a location in the EHR to make it easy to find the date of the last diabetic eye screening. The team might also create a reminder in the EHR to flag patients who either lack documentation of diabetic eye screening or patients for whom more than a year has elapsed since the last screening date. A low-cost alternative for health systems with more limited EHR capabilities is for medical assistants to use a simple color paper–based flagging system to alert primary care providers when a patient has diabetes and to remind the medical assistant to complete information regarding a patient's diabetes-related health maintenance tests (e.g., date of last diabetic eye screening, last hemoglobin A1c testing, last urine microalbumin testing, etc.).[3]

The I-SITE online toolkit has a worksheet used to help streamline the implementation team's discussion of strategies to improve ocular telehealth implementation.[26] The process starts with team members brainstorming barriers individually, then sharing ideas with the group sequentially, and using the Nominal Group Technique to vote on the top 2–3 barriers. Team members then use the same process to identify strategies to overcome those barriers. At the end of the meeting in which the top 2–3 strategies based on their impact and feasibility, individual members of the local implementation team should be tasked with implementing those strategies measuring the outcomes, and reporting back on their progress at the next meeting.

Plan–do–study–act (PDSA) test cycles
Once teams have identified how they want to address specific barriers in their tele-eye care workflow, they can use Plan–Do–Study–Act, or PDSA, test cycles to systematically test and refine the strategies that they have chosen to implement. These cycles consist of the following four steps:[26]

Plan: After identifying one or two aspects of a workflow that a team might want to change, team members should decide how that change will be implemented. Teams should set a specific goal for the change they intend to make and identify how that change will be made.

Do: Teams should then implement the change and collect outcomes data.

Study: Teams evaluate and measure the impact of the change. Is the change having the intended effect? If not, where are the challenges being encountered? How might those be addressed?

Act: Teams decide whether to adopt, abandon, or adapt the strategy. If adaptations are not needed, it can be widely adopted in the organization.

To monitor outcomes from the changes implemented, clinical administrators and staff should create standardized reports and share this information at regularly scheduled staff meetings, for example, on a quarterly basis. Providing regular updates to all providers and clinical staff (i.e., audit and feedback) involved in the ocular telehealth program can be highly beneficial for maintaining their engagement. These presentations also provide an opportunity to foster friendly competition across clinics and staff by creating clinic- and individual-specific reports. For example, in a teleretinal diabetic eye screening program, recognition can be given to the clinic with the highest screening rate, the Referring Provider with the highest number of referrals to the program, and the Imager with the lowest rate of ungradable images.

Examples of implementation strategies
The local implementation team, which should consist of a variety of stakeholders within the organization, can design and test strategies to achieve the organization's goals for the ocular telehealth program using the process described in the preceding sections. In this section, we describe a few examples of specific strategies to increase Referring Provider and clinical staff engagement within a primary care–based teleretinal diabetic eye screening program (Table 12.4).

Conduct patient outreach. To reduce the burden on Referring Providers and clinical staff to identify patients due for screening, yearly automated reminders (e.g., by mail, phone, or text message) can be sent to patients who had teleretinal screening previously and are due again for diabetic eye screening. These reminders are best followed up with a phone call by an individual who can schedule the appointment for the patient to obtain screening.

Referring provider and clinical staff education. Educating Referring Providers and clinical staff about the use and benefits of ocular telehealth can increase support for implementation efforts and boost ocular telehealth utilization. Educational meetings

TABLE 12.4

Examples of Implementation Strategies to Increase and Sustain Utilization in a Teleretinal Program for Diabetic Eye Screening[26,27]

Strategy Name	How Strategy Might be Applied in Practice
Remind clinicians	Develop reminder systems to help Referring Providers and clinical staff remember to ask patients about diabetic eye screening
Intervene with patients to enhance uptake and adherence	Contact patients who are due for diabetic eye screening or who lack recent documentation of diabetic eye screening in the EHR
Conduct educational meetings	Hold regular meetings to educate multiple stakeholders—including Referring Providers, administrators, staff, community members, and patients—about the importance of the program, answer questions, and obtain feedback on implementation
Audit and provide feedback	Provide stakeholders with a summary of the program's clinical outcomes over time (e.g., compared to a baseline or prior outcomes) as well as provider- and clinic-level data to motivate increased or continued utilization of the program
Alter financial incentives	Offer performance-based financial incentives for Referring Providers that are aligned with those of the organization for achieving diabetic eye screening targets

provide an opportunity to explain what will be implemented, how it will be implemented, and its benefits for patients and clinical stakeholders.[27] All members of the organization involved in the ocular telehealth program should be offered education about the program. This includes Referring Providers and their clinical staff, Imaging Staff, information technology (IT) staff, clinic administrators, and clinic managers. In a busy clinical setting, it is helpful to request time during regularly scheduled provider and staff meetings to provide this critical education regarding the ocular telehealth program.

Audit and provide feedback. The team should choose the measures they will use to evaluate outcomes ideally prior to beginning the project. Assessing these measures at baseline, conducting consistent and ongoing audits of the data, and sharing and eliciting feedback are valuable means to keep stakeholders engaged in the project's goals. Sharing and eliciting feedback might occur during regularly scheduled provider and staff meetings, a quarterly newsletter distributed via e-mail, or a data dashboard within the EHR. Examples of outcome measures for teleretinal diabetic eye screening include the screening rate (i.e., proportion of patients with diabetes who have had screening within the past year), number of imaging orders placed and photos taken, rate of ungradable images, and follow-up rates for in-person eye care among patients who screened positive for vision-threatening eye conditions (Table 12.5).

Financial incentives. Although offering financial incentives to providers based on their performance on healthcare quality measures remains somewhat controversial,

TABLE 12.5

Examples of Outcomes Measures in a Teleretinal Diabetic Eye Screening Program

Outcome Measure	Description
Diabetic eye screening rate	Proportion of patients with diabetes who have met diabetic eye screening guidelines (either via a dilated eye exam or teleretinal imaging)
Teleretinal imaging order rate	Number of imaging orders entered per month or quarter
Teleretinal imaging use rate	Number of patients with teleretinal photos completed per month or quarter
Ungradable rate	Proportion of patients with ungradable photos on teleretinal imaging
Follow-up rate for in-person eye care among screen positives	Proportion of patients with abnormal results on teleretinal screening who attended a follow-up in-person eye exam within the recommended time frame

many health systems employ these performance-based bonuses to better align the incentives of individual providers with those of the organization. These performance-based bonuses compensate physicians for meeting certain healthcare quality metrics such as targets for diabetic eye screening, hemoglobin A1c testing, etc. Performance-based financial bonuses can be an effective method for increasing provider referrals for teleretinal diabetic eye screening in primary care.[31]

In summary, the previous sections have provided just a few examples of implementation strategies that can be tailored to an individual program and organization. These examples are by no means exhaustive. More information on implementation strategies can be found by reviewing the Expert Recommendations for Implementing Change (ERIC) strategies[14] and the I-SITE online toolkit.[26]

Patient Engagement
Barriers and facilitators for patients

Studies conducted in the United States about patient attitudes toward ocular telehealth have been overall positive, with evidence of high patient satisfaction and willingness to pay for these services. However, several important barriers to patient use of ocular telehealth remain. In a VA study, patients were very satisfied with their ocular telehealth experience when they had testing performed by ophthalmic technicians in primary care clinics and their results were evaluated remotely by eye care specialists.[32] Ramchandran et al. found that patients in a multi-payer health system were willing to pay at least as much for teleretinal diabetic eye screening as for screening performed in-person.[33] Most patients also reported feeling comfortable having teleretinal screening in their primary care clinic and would recommend the service to others.

Barriers to patient use of ocular telehealth include a lack of familiarity with this technology and logistical barriers—such as time, transportation, and out-of-pocket costs (Table 12.6).[2,33] Furthermore, with regard to teleretinal diabetic eye screening, many patients had misconceptions about the value of diabetic eye screening and did not understand the consequences of not following recommended eye screening guidelines. Significant facilitators to patient use of ocular telehealth include provider endorsement and convenience.[2] Among urban, low-income adults, facilitators of tele-ophthalmology exam receipt included the convenience of obtaining imaging at the primary care clinic, the peace of mind resulting from having the screening done, and a provider explanation of the reason for screening.[33]

TABLE 12.6
Barriers and Facilitators to Teleretinal Screening Among Patients With Diabetes

Barriers	Facilitators
• Lack of knowledge/ familiarity with teleretinal screening • Lack of knowledge about diabetic eye screening • Lack of knowledge about diabetic eye disease • Time required for appointment • Cost of screening • Transportation to appointment	• Provider endorsement/ leveraging provider trust • Convenience of screening (e.g., allow walk-in availability, camera located in primary care clinic) • Offering screening at low cost and insurance coverage of screening • Patient education about the importance of screening and availability of effective eye treatments to prevent vision loss

---

Engaging patients in ocular telehealth programs by soliciting their feedback and providing patient education materials can result in more effective and sustainable ocular telehealth programs. Patient advisory groups can provide practical feedback on an ocular telehealth program by offering valuable patient perspectives and insight into opportunities to improve the program. Patient advisory groups can be recruited via mailings to eligible patients, flyers placed in patient waiting areas, and by asking providers and clinical staff to discuss the opportunity with patients who may enjoy providing input into the program. Once created, patient advisory groups can contribute toward developing and refining patient education materials; providing feedback on the patient experience; and offering concrete recommendations regarding costs, scheduling, and patient-facing workflows for ocular telehealth.

While substantial research has increased the field's understanding regarding patient attitudes, knowledge, and beliefs toward ocular telehealth, additional work is needed to better understand similarities and differences around barriers and facilitators, as well as effective strategies to increase patient use of ocular telehealth, particularly for underserved minority populations. A better understanding of patient perspectives will allow teams to create ocular telehealth programs best-suited to effectively address the specific needs of their diverse communities.

Engagement With External Organizations

Engaging with external organizations can be useful for improving the community's understanding of the ocular telehealth program and facilitating the program's success. These include local eye care providers, governmental regulatory agencies and insurers, and community-based/nonprofit organizations.

Perhaps the most important group to consider are local eye care providers external to the organization who might initially feel somewhat threatened by an ocular telehealth program. Implementation teams should notify eye care providers in their communities that they are establishing such a program and communicate how the program's goals align with those of the local eye care providers. For example, in a teleretinal diabetic eye screening program, emphasis should be placed on screening patients who are not currently seen by an eye care provider. This will reinforce that the eye care provider and teleretinal program will not compete for the same patients. Local eye specialists can also be invited to partner in the ocular telehealth program by agreeing to see patients who screen positive and need follow-up in-person eye care. By focusing on the mutual goal of preventing blindness and on the benefits of the ocular telehealth program for the external partner, the perceived threat of the ocular telehealth program can be more appropriately framed as a "win–win" for both organizations.

In addition to external eye care providers, governmental regulatory agencies and insurers play a large role in ocular telehealth programs by determining how these services are covered and reimbursed. Ocular telehealth leaders at each organization should advocate for increased coverage of telemedicine services at the state and federal levels, as well as policies that facilitate interstate medical licensure for telehealth providers. Finally, notifying community organizations and nonprofits such as Lions Clubs can foster rewarding partnerships. Nonprofit organizations and patient advocacy groups can partner in advocacy as well as provide funds to support the development and sustainability of an ocular telehealth program. For example, organizations might pay for screening vouchers among low-income patients, contribute to purchasing equipment, and host community events to raise awareness about the ocular telehealth initiative.

Relevant stakeholders exist both inside and outside the organization implementing the ocular telehealth program. Reaching out to external organizations, including local eye care providers, engaging in governmental and insurer-targeted advocacy, and forming partnerships with community/nonprofit organizations can contribute greatly to successful implementation.

Summary of Stakeholder Engagement

Ensuring that adequate attention has been paid to address barriers and facilitators for the various stakeholders involved in an ocular telehealth program can be invaluable for successfully achieving and sustaining the effectiveness of the program. Allocation of necessary resources by health system administrators, obtaining buy-in and input from providers and clinical staff, consideration of the patient experience, and maintenance of relationships with external organizations all contribute to successful implementation. Although it is ideal to involve stakeholders from the initial design and development stages of the ocular telehealth program, groups of stakeholders can be engaged at any time to address issues that arise during implementation and enable the program to achieve its goals long term.

TRAINING PERSONNEL

This section provides an overview of the types of personnel training needed to establish and perform the daily operations for an ocular telehealth program. Telehealth practice guidelines[25] should be referenced when creating standardized training and recertification processes for ocular telehealth personnel.

Clinic Administrators and Information Technology (IT) Staff

Clinical administrators and IT staff are often responsible for developing and providing training for ocular telehealth personnel. They will need to create standardized protocols for image capture, transfer, and grading; the end-to-end ocular telehealth workflow (i.e., including order entry by Referring Providers, the results notification process, and management of follow-up in-person eye care when needed); and a program manual. The program manual should contain all training documents and protocols; specific technical information regarding network settings, Wi-Fi passwords, security details, etc.; and contact information for staff who can assist with troubleshooting issues that can be easily referenced by ocular telehealth personnel when needed. Ocular telehealth guidelines[25] should be referenced for creating these materials in conjunction with obtaining input from personnel involved in the program to ensure that the workflows, training, and documentation are as streamlined and user-friendly as possible. Ideally, clinical personnel not familiar with the ocular telehealth program's details should be able to quickly review key diagrams and components from the manual and have a solid understanding of the purpose of the program, their role, how to perform and troubleshoot tasks, and who to ask for additional information.

Referring Providers and Clinical Staff

Identifying which providers are best suited to identifying and referring eligible patients for the ocular telehealth program is the first step in training Referring Providers and clinical staff. For a teleretinal diabetic eye screening program, the Referring Providers are typically primary care providers. However, possible additional Referring Providers include diabetes educators, podiatrists, and pharmacists who routinely interact with a large number of patients with diabetes. When including varying groups of Referring Providers, consider designing an EHR workflow that maximizes ease of use and is flexible enough that all referrers can participate.

Education and training of Referring Providers should address both the rationale and benefits of the ocular telehealth program as well as provide a step-by-step walk-through of the Referring Provider and clinical staff roles (e.g., identification of eligible patients, educating patients about the ocular telehealth program, ordering the imaging in the EHR, results notification, etc.). Given the challenges of creating workflows for varied personnel, it is imperative to have clinical administrators and IT staff work together to develop a process that is adapted to the needs of all users.

During initial training, the most common questions from Referring Providers and clinical staff are regarding patient eligibility criteria. Thus, these criteria must be clearly outlined, documented, and shared with Referring Providers and clinical staff. Referring Providers can obtain assistance from their clinical support staff in reviewing medical records and talking with the patient to determine their eligibility to participate in the ocular telehealth program. For example, in a teleretinal diabetic eye screening program, patients who do not have a documented dilated eye exam or teleretinal diabetic eye screening within the past 10 months in the EHR may be eligible. If the patient endorses having had a dilated eye exam with an outside eye care provider from whom no documentation was received, then the clinical support staff are tasked with requesting those records from the outside eye care provider. If, however, no documentation is available and the patient cannot remember the timing of their last screening, then Referring Providers are encouraged to order teleretinal imaging if the patient is willing to participate in screening.

Referring Providers and clinical staff are also typically interested in determining how the imaging will be billed, reimbursed, and ordered. Patient insurance coverage and reimbursement for ocular telehealth varies by insurer and by region. For further information on billing, coding, and reimbursement refer to Chapter 14. Order entry is typically completed in the EHR. In some organizations, a delegation protocol may be developed that allows clinical staff to identify eligible patients and place orders on behalf of the Referring Provider. In addition, best practice alerts in the EHR or a patient rooming checklist that reminds Referring Providers and clinical staff to ask patients questions to determine their eligibility can be highly useful. The local implementation team (see "Creating a Local Implementation Team" Section) can aid in the design of implementation strategies that enhance Referring Provider and clinical staff workflows.

Finally, Referring Providers and clinical staff should be familiar with the results notification process by which they receive results from the Interpreting Provider and how patients will be notified of their results. Results reporting from Interpreting Providers should include not only the findings from the imaging tests but also specific recommendations for further follow-up when needed (i.e., time frame and what type of provider (optometrist, ophthalmologist, etc.) In addition, Referring Providers should be aware of processes by which they will refer patients who screen positive for vision-threatening eye conditions in the ocular telehealth program for further in-person eye care.

Imaging Staff/Telehealth Presenter or Facilitator

A wide variety of clinical staff can be trained to perform imaging in an ocular telehealth program. For example, clinic staff who may be trained to perform ocular imaging include medical assistants, nurses, radiology and laboratory technicians, clinic managers, and scheduling personnel. In general, it is best to have a limited number of Imaging Staff to ensure that there is always an imager available when needed, but also allow each imager to perform an adequate volume and frequency of imaging to maintain their skills. It is best to adapt or utilize existing imaging workflows whenever possible to make the imaging workflow easier for staff to learn, such as those used for chest X-rays or mammograms. To minimize staffing costs, it is also best to train existing personnel rather than hire new staff given uncertainty regarding imaging volumes during the initial stages of the program.

An imaging protocol should include all information documenting the entirety of the workflow from beginning to end. This workflow should include instructions on how to utilize and maintain any imaging equipment, instructions on documentation and order review to be performed in the EHR, and instructions on how to check that all images were transferred correctly. The imaging protocol should be documented in an imager training manual tailored to each imaging site and should also include troubleshooting instructions. Imagers may provide feedback on drafts of the imaging manual to ensure that they are comprehensive yet easy to use. Step-by-step photos and screenshots are recommended to help imagers recall the steps of the imaging process. This is especially helpful when they are new to the imaging process or may have experienced a lengthy period of time between imaging patients. The contact information for whom imagers should contact regarding urgent and nonurgent questions should also be made readily available in the manual, a copy of which should be located near the camera for easy reference. For further technological considerations please see Chapter 13.

On the day of training, all training-related materials should be prepared in advance and distributed, including the imager training manual, educational materials providing information regarding the importance and benefits of the ocular telehealth program, and a training checklist to document imagers' ability to perform the essential tasks. The training should not simply be focused on equipment operation. Time must be also dedicated to functions related to use of the EHR. For example, Imaging Staff may need to demonstrate proficiency with entering and releasing imaging orders. Imaging Staff should take turns participating in and observing others' move through the entire imaging process from end to end using a test patient's information. Imagers should be shown examples of good quality and poor quality images so that they can confirm whether the image quality is adequate and retake the images if needed. They should also be provided instruction on common problems and how to troubleshoot them. Among the imagers, having 1–2 "lead imagers" who are in charge of troubleshooting and training new imagers can be very helpful given that there can be significant staff turnover in some organizations. In addition to the basic steps of image acquisition, challenging scenarios should be discussed such as what to do if images have not been transferred correctly or if a patient has ungradable images due to small pupils, etc. Once all the checklist proficiencies have been demonstrated, Imaging Staff members should have documented certification of training stored in the organization's records.

In order to maintain image quality, Interpreting Providers should notify Imaging Staff regarding any suboptimal, incomplete, or ungradable images. Common issues range from having a missing image in a series, a poorly centered image, unexplained glare, lack of focus, or even dust buildup on the lens that requires cleaning. The Interpreting Provider can offer advice based on the issue and suggest modifications to obtain improved images. Ongoing evaluation and feedback to imagers with respect to image quality and ungradable rates can be helpful for identifying any issues and assess the need for refresher training. The frequency of refresher training for imagers should be tailored to the organization's needs, with more frequent refresher trainings in settings where there is high staff turnover.

Interpreting Providers

The role of the Interpreting Provider is to provide a timely assessment and report with recommendations for follow-up in-person eye care when indicated. Interpreting Providers in most ocular telehealth programs are eye care specialists. Interpreting Providers should be reminded that the audience for the report is the primary care provider and patient. Therefore, it is very helpful for the report and recommendations to be written without acronyms and in language easily understood by non-eye care specialists. A clear and realistic time frame regarding how quickly images must be reviewed and reported should be determined by each organization in partnership with the Interpreting Providers. In addition, there should be standardized information regarding thresholds for recommending patients to obtain follow-up eye care, including within what time frame and with what type of eye care provider (e.g., optometrist or general ophthalmologist for glaucoma suspects and retina specialist for vision-threatening diabetic eye disease). We recommend creating the report in the form of a letter addressed to the patient and providing contact information for local eye care providers if follow-up eye care is needed.

Similar to the training for Imaging Staff, all training-related materials should be prepared in advance and distributed on the day of training, including the Interpreting Provider manual, educational materials regarding the importance and benefits of the ocular telehealth program, and a training checklist to document Interpreting Providers' ability to perform their essential tasks. The training should not simply be focused on image evaluation. Time must be dedicated to functions related to use of the EHR. For example, providers may need to demonstrate proficiency with accessing and manipulating images to maximize their ability to make the interpretation and to send their interpretation reports back to the Referring Provider.

Interpreting Providers should be shown examples of good quality and poor quality images so that they can understand when the image quality is adequate and identify when images are ungradable. They should also be provided instruction on common imaging artifacts. Typically, an image assessment test is used to confirm that the Interpreting Provider has the knowledge needed to perform their role. Ideally, each of the Interpreting Providers should be observed walking through the entire process from end to end. Once all of the checklist proficiencies have been demonstrated, Interpreting Providers should have documented certification of training completion stored in the organization's records.

Quality assurance procedures for maintaining image interpretation quality involve having a second Interpreting Provider perform an "over-read," or reassess an image. Most research-based ocular imaging programs require 5% over-reads.[25] The Interpreting Provider should be providing ongoing feedback to Imaging Staff regarding the image quality and any problems identified should be addressed quickly. Refresher trainings may be necessary to reduce interpretation drift among individuals, which is a common phenomenon that occurs over time in which individual Interpreting Providers may change their evaluation standards in a manner that deviates from those set by the organization.

Summary of Training Personnel

Providing standardized training with clearly defined workflows documented in an easy-to-use program manual can greatly facilitate onboarding new staff and providing refresher training for existing staff. Given the potential for significant personnel turnover in many organizations, particularly among Imaging Staff, empowering trained staff with the knowledge, skills, and reference documents to provide high-quality training to new staff greatly enhances the resilience of the ocular telehealth program. Again, stakeholder engagement principles should be applied in the training process by providing personnel with the appropriate background knowledge regarding the purpose and benefits of the ocular telehealth program and inviting their input on making the workflows and manual as user-friendly as possible. Continued feedback on how to improve the training process, and how to further refine workflows and documentation should be elicited. By addressing the training needs of personnel, the ocular telehealth program is positioned to successfully achieve its goals of providing high-quality eye care access to patients in our communities.

CONCLUSION

The application of implementation science principles has informed the stakeholder engagement considerations and methods used in this chapter. Together with conducting personnel training, working closely with stakeholders to design and implement an ocular telehealth program is critical for launching and refining these programs in a manner that maximizes their impact. Continued research into strategies and methods to ensure the successful establishment and sustained effectiveness of these programs will further advance widespread adoption of ocular telehealth.

REFERENCES

1. Hussey P, Anderson GF. A comparison of single- and multi-payer health insurance systems and options for reform. *Health Policy.* 2003;66(3):215–228.
2. Liu Y, Zupan NJ, Swearingen R, et al. Identification of barriers, facilitators and system-based implementation strategies to increase teleophthalmology use for diabetic eye screening in a rural US primary care clinic: a qualitative study. *BMJ Open.* 2019;9(2), e022594.
3. Liu Y, Carlson JN, Torres Diaz A, Lock LJ, Zupan NJ, Molfenter TD, Mahoney JE, Palta M, Boss D, Bjelland TD, Smith MA. Sustaining gains in diabetic eye screening: outcomes from a stakeholder-based implementation program for teleophthalmology in primary care. *Telemed J E Health.* 2021;27(9):1021-1028. https://doi.org/10.1089/tmj.2020.0270. Epub 2020 Nov 19. PMID: 33216697; PMCID: PMC8558054.
4. Moullin JC, Dickson KS, Stadnick NA, et al. Ten recommendations for using implementation frameworks in research and practice. *Implement Sci Commun.* 2020;1:42.
5. Nominal Group Technique. *CHESS/NIATx;* 2020. https://chess.wisc.edu/niatx/content/contentpage.aspx?NID=147. Updated 2020. Accessed 09.09.20.
6. Agency for Healthcare Research and Quality. *Descriptive Information about AHRQ-Registered Practice-based Research Networks.* https://pbrn.ahrq.gov/sites/default/files/docs/page/2015AHRQPBRNDataSlides.pdf. Accessed 15.12.20.
7. AHRQ. *Module 1. Practice Facilitation as a Resource for Practice Improvement. Agency for Healthcare Research and Quality;* 2013. https://www.ahrq.gov/ncepcr/tools/pf-handbook/mod1.html. Updated May 2013. Accessed 01.04.21.
8. NIH Fogarty International Center. *Frequently Asked Questions About Implementation Science;* 2021. https://www.fic.nih.gov/ResearchTopics/Pages/ImplementationScience.aspx. Accessed 28.02.21.
9. Colditz GA, Emmons KM. Accelerating the pace of cancer prevention- right now. *Cancer Prev Res (Phila).* 2018;11(4):171–184.
10. National Institutes of Health Office of Disease Prevention. *Dissemination and Implementation (D&I) Research. U.S.*

Department of Health and Human Services; 2020. https://www.prevention.nih.gov/research-priorities/dissemination-implementation. Accessed 28.02.21.

11. RE-AIM. *RE-AIM;* 2021. https://www.re-aim.org/. Accessed 28.02.21.

12. CFIR Research Team-Center for Clinical Management Research. *Consolidated Framework for Implementation Research;* 2021. https://cfirguide.org/. Accessed 28.02.21.

13. Harvey G, Kitson A. PARIHS revisited: from heuristic to integrated framework for the successful implementation of knowledge into practice. *Implement Sci.* 2016;11:33.

14. Powell BJ, Waltz TJ, Chinman MJ, et al. A refined compilation of implementation strategies: results from the expert recommendations for implementing change (ERIC) project. *Implement Sci.* 2015;10:21.

15. Chamberlain P, Brown CH, Saldana L. Observational measure of implementation progress in community based settings: the stages of implementation completion (SIC). *Implement Sci.* 2011;6:116.

16. Liu Y, Torres Diaz A, Benkert R. Scaling up teleophthalmology for diabetic eye screening: opportunities for widespread implementation in the USA. *Curr Diabetes Rep.* 2019;19(9):74.

17. Rathi S, Tsui E, Mehta N, Zahid S, Schuman JS. The current state of teleophthalmology in the United States. *Ophthalmology.* 2017;124(12):1729–1734.

18. Brady CJ, Villanti AC, Gupta OP, Graham MG, Sergott RC. Tele-ophthalmology screening for proliferative diabetic retinopathy in urban primary care offices: an economic analysis. *Ophthalmic Surg Lasers Imaging Retina.* 2014;45(6):556–561.

19. Ellis MP, Bacorn C, Luu KY, et al. Cost analysis of teleophthalmology screening for diabetic retinopathy using teleophthalmology billing codes. *Ophthalmic Surg Lasers Imaging Retina.* 2020;51(5):S26–S34.

20. Whited JD, Datta SK, Aiello LM, et al. A modeled economic analysis of a digital tele-ophthalmology system as used by three federal health care agencies for detecting proliferative diabetic retinopathy. *Telemed J E Health.* 2005;11(6):641–651.

21. Shaw J. Teleophthalmology: ready for prime time? In: *EyeNet Magazine.* American Academy of Ophthalmology; 2016.

22. van Eijk KN, Blom JW, Gussekloo J, Polak BC, Groeneveld Y. Diabetic retinopathy screening in patients with diabetes mellitus in primary care: incentives and barriers to screening attendance. *Diabetes Res Clin Pract.* 2012;96(1):10–16.

23. Davis FD, Bagozzi RP, Warshaw PR. User acceptance of computer technology: a comparison of two theoretical models. *Manag Sci.* 1989;35(8):902–1028.

24. Woodward MA, Ple-Plakon P, Blachley T, et al. Eye care providers' attitudes towards tele-ophthalmology. *Telemed J E Health.* 2015;21(4):271–273.

25. Horton MB, Brady CJ, Cavallerano J, et al. Practice guidelines for ocular telehealth-diabetic retinopathy, third edition. *Telemed J E Health.* 2020;26(4):495–543.

26. Liu Y, Benkert R. *A Guide to Implementation for Sustained Impact in Teleophthalmology (I-SITE).* HIPxChange; 2020. https://www.hipxchange.org/I-SITE. Accessed 05.01.20.

27. Perry CK, Damschroder LJ, Hemler JR, Woodson TT, Ono SS, Cohen DJ. Specifying and comparing implementation strategies across seven large implementation interventions: a practical application of theory. *Implement Sci.* 2019;14(1):32.

28. McCarty D, Gustafson DH, Wisdom JP, et al. The network for the improvement of addiction treatment (NIATx): enhancing access and retention. *Drug Alcohol Depend.* 2007;88(2–3):138–145.

29. Centers for Medicare and Medicaid Services. *Quality of Care External Quality Review;* 2020. https://www.medicaid.gov/medicaid/quality-of-care/medicaid-managed-care/quality-of-care-external-quality-review/index.html#:~:text=An%20External%20Quality%20Review%20(EQR,contractors%2C%20furnish%20to%20Medicaid%20beneficiaries. Accessed 28.02.21.

30. NIATx. *How to Conduct a Walk-Through.* CHESS/NIATx; 2021. Accessed 28.02.21.

31. Torres Diaz A, Lock LJ, Molfenter TD, et al. Implementation for Sustained Impact in Teleophthalmology (I-SITE): applying the NIATx Model for tailored implementation of diabetic retinopathy screening in primary care. *Implement Sci Commun.* 2021;2(1):74. https://doi:10.1186/s43058-021-00175-0. PMID: 34229748; PMCID: PMC8258481.

32. Maa AY, Wojciechowski B, Hunt KJ, et al. Early experience with technology-based eye care services (TECS): a novel ophthalmologic telemedicine initiative. *Ophthalmology.* 2017;124(4):539–546.

33. Ramchandran RS, Yilmaz S, Greaux E, Dozier A. Patient perceived value of teleophthalmology in an urban, low income US population with diabetes. *PLoS One.* 2020;15(1):e0225300.

CHAPTER 13

Technology Considerations for Implementing an Eye Telehealth Program

GERALD SELVIN, OD, FAAO • APRIL MAA, MD • STEPHANIE J. WEISS, DO

SECTION I: TECHNOLOGY CONSIDERATIONS—BANDWIDTH, INFORMATION SECURITY, TECHNOLOGY SUPPORT

Gerald Selvin, OD FAAO
INTRODUCTION

Like all clinical programs, Eye Telehealth is driven by need. During the COVID-19 pandemic, there was an obvious need to minimize direct exposure between patients and providers and yet still achieve the clinical goals of an in-person exam. However, what the pandemic has revealed to the eye care field is that there is a significant amount of care, initially done mostly by traditional in-person clinics that actually can be delivered

Ocular Telehealth. https://doi.org/10.1016/B978-0-323-83204-5.00013-5

by telehealth. This is consistent with findings across other non-eye care disciplines.[1]

Eye telehealth programs cannot successfully be deployed without strong collaboration and understanding of the technology needs of the program, which is independent of well-established, preferred clinical patterns and guidelines. Without the appropriate technological support, it is not possible to provide remote care outside of a limited synchronous telehealth to home encounter.

The majority of ocular telehealth encounters operational in 2021 have been "store and forward" or asynchronous. This means that the patient encounter and the provider evaluation occur at different times. The patient site encounter with the imager or other telehealth facilitator gathers imaging and important patient history and demographic information along with an important risk assessment. All of this information, including applicable images, must be accessible to the provider reviewing the case regardless of their location. The challenge for decades has been the movement of information. Over the past 20 years, broadband has become more available allowing for a larger amount of information to travel the "information highway" and be accessible to any provider logged onto a system network—whether it is a large nationwide system like the Department of Veterans Affairs (VA) or sprawling academic medical center; or a smaller rural hospital system. Once the availability of high-capacity transmission is verified, issues such as security, encryption, and continuous vigilance against attacks from outside of any network or system must be established and maintained. These features are widely recognized as a critical step to bringing eye telehealth to a wider cohort of at risk patients. Furthermore, the availability of broadband and cloud computing storage methods now allows a much greater ability to transmit increasingly larger and more complex images, increasing the capability of telehealth programs to bring high-resolution images to providers. In turn, this increases the readability and quality of studies and further focuses the eye telehealth program's ability to provide high-quality care through accurate risk assessment, along with the ability to refer to in-person clinic at the clinically appropriate time. The value of in-person clinics in reducing unnecessary appointments versus a schedule filled with an array of subspecialty patients cannot be overstated!

Important components to launching any eye telehealth program include prioritization of the information technology (IT) needs for all stakeholders. Here the authors utilize a case study, the VA diabetic teleretinal imaging program, to illustrate important points related to IT.

IMPORTANT IT INFRASTRUCTURE CONSIDERATIONS

In an ocular telehealth program, there has to be a commitment to developing simple yet relevant systems that are capable of meeting the clinical needs of both patients and providers. Strong collaboration among eye and non-eye providers, IT personnel, and biomedical or clinical engineers is extremely critical in the early planning stages and will most assuredly contribute to a telehealth program's ultimate success and rapid acceptance. These groups should collectively determine what would be an ideal workflow for image acquisition, transfer, interpretation, and results reporting. Some key aspects, or "best practices," for asynchronous ocular telehealth IT infrastructure include reading list and bandwidth speed.

Technology Needs Assessment

When beginning an ocular telehealth program, assessing the technology needs is important. The assessment identifies gaps in technology and knowledge before the program is implemented and solutions to address the problems can be found and executed. The following is a reasonable list of questions to consider as part of a comprehensive technology needs assessment:

1. What are the clinical needs of the program (e.g., synchronous video versus asynchronous images) and has this been discussed in depth with the eye team including readers, imagers, IT personnel, and other patient site personnel?

2. What equipment is being chosen for the telehealth program and how will this equipment be networked, what characteristics of the images/system will facilitate secure information transfer?

3. What is the required bandwidth to carry out the ocular telehealth program, and can there be an eye care dedicated bandwidth to accommodate the transmission of complex and large images or direct video?

4. How will remote providers, who are providing the results of the eye telehealth study log in and access the study and supporting information? How will results be sent back to the referring provider or conveyed to the patient?

5. Is there a "closed" system whereby readers resolve a study and hit "send" by either signing in a system's EMR or similar pathway?

6. What is required to ensure information security? What recommendations are present from IT?

7. Are patients able to achieve the advantages of eye telehealth from their homes? (broadband, proper equipment, private space) and how can the program help support this effort?

A few specific examples answering these questions are listed here, using the VA diabetic teleretinal screening program as a case study.

Clinical Needs and the Development of a Reading Worklist

First, using the development of the VA diabetic teleretinal imaging program as an example, the largest recognized obstacle was how to create a system to allow for seamless image transfer from one VA to another? The clinical need of the program was the ability to capture a retinal image from any location in the country, send that image securely to a reading station, and then have the report sent back to the referring provider. Moreover, it was desired to have multiple readers working at the same time. The providers, biomedical engineers, and IT experts ended up developing a "modality worklist" concept utilizing the VA's electronic medical record (EMR), Computerized Patient Record System (CPRS), to route studies from any location to the reading center, and to use that same method to route results back to the referring providers. Software to enable seamless image viewing for any discipline (e.g., radiology studies, dermatology photos) was developed in a 2006 software patch that complemented and integrated into the pre-existing image storage system of the VA, Vista Imaging. Included as part of the patch was the development of a "worklist" that put the oldest imaging study at the top, so it would be addressed first by the reading team (in the VA it was called Tele-reader). In order to avoid redundancy in the case of multiple readers accessing the worklist at the same time, the study is "locked" once one reader opens it. For a study to appear on the "read list," it must be complete with the order number and demographic information as well as the images received by the provider site. This is part of the Digital Imaging and Communications in Medicine (DICOM) process which is described later in this chapter.

The work to develop the system in the earliest days has allowed millions of patients with diabetes to be risk assessed and triaged from anywhere within the VA enterprise, arguably saving thousands from potential major vision loss.[2,3] Of perhaps even greater importance is the fact that this patch not only accelerated the deployment of eye telehealth but also enabled all providers from all disciplines to view radiology and clinic images from any hospital in the nationwide system. Providers were able to filter images that would automatically download to local servers, and that reduced slowing from too much data (most of it extraneous) using the available bandwidth. In addition, eye telehealth providers could download non-eye images as necessary based on the clinical presentation.

Bandwidth Speed

Image download speed with inadequate bandwidth significantly slows the process and negatively impacts the reading provider, rendering them inefficient. Unfortunately, there is still a large disparity in the availability of reliable broadband technology across the United States with the rural areas being the most underserved. While the United States, in general, is considered to have strong broadband across the land, there is a high degree of disparity. As more complex imaging becomes well suited for eye telehealth, the ability to use high speed regardless of location becomes even more critical.[4,5]

Again using the VA as a case example, in 2006, it became quickly apparent that lack of bandwidth in some primary care imaging locations significantly slowed image downloads. Within urban VA communities, download speed was adequate. However, imaging in a rural location with reading at an urban VA center illustrated the limitations of bandwidth in many cases. To address this issue, the VA built out infrastructure to accommodate the needed bandwidth across their domain. The lesson learned is the importance of an IT needs assessment before the actual deployment of a program.

In 2021, systems are much more likely to have adequate bandwidth to accommodate eye images from complex devices. If a hospital system or a collaborative consortium of providers deploys an eye teleheath system, then attention to bandwidth must be a prerequisite. Ensure adequate bandwidth exists before the program begins if possible.[5] Recommended minimal bandwidth speeds for image transmission vary from 4 Mbps in a solo practice to 1000 Mbps in an Academic Medical Center.[6] Furthermore, dedicated, discipline-specific bandwidth is strongly encouraged, e.g., Eye Care Local Area Network (Eye Care LAN) with enough space sequestered for the eye care needs of the organization. This should ensure minimization of slow download times which reduce efficiency as described earlier. Eye telehealth population screening as well as advanced screening is mainly asynchronous. However, as discussed in other chapters, there are synchronous eye telehealth programs as well, and the bandwidth needs of synchronous video telehealth to home or a healthcare setting should also be considered. Synchronous telehealth bandwidth requirements may be higher than that needed for image transmission as the provider is, by definition, "live" interacting with the patient during the telehealth encounter.

Luckily the current digital age with cloud computing, fiberoptic networks, and cellular data networks makes the issue of obtaining adequate bandwidth less of a problem even for small, private clinics.

Digital Imaging and Communication in Medicine (DICOM)

The essential part of any technology which permits a provider to review a study remotely from a patient in a secure manner is DICOM. DICOM is a worldwide standard and provides a standard protocol that stores both text and pixel data in different formats (e.g., the pixels of the fundus images and the patient's name). DICOM was used initially in 1992.[7] Many systems for eye telehealth in the ensuing 14 years did not have the ability to have DICOM-capable eye imaging devices—they were few and far between. This limited reading capability to small, local groups. Software could be loaded to interpret images for a particular location but evaluating systemwide images using the same network is not yet possible.

By the time the VA deployed the diabetic teleretinal imaging program, DICOM became the difference on what was acceptable technology versus that which was not. If the technology chosen for telehealth included only DICOM-capable devices, then the ocular telehealth program will have the ability to transfer images from any location to any location. In 2021, many high-quality ocular imaging devices have achieved DICOM capability and are now routinely used. Today, with such a wide array of ophthalmic imaging devices for so many ocular modalities, a common practice is to use a consolidated picture archiving and communication system (PACS) to bring all technology together and enable seamless image transfer for remote providers to access.[8]

The requirement of DICOM-capable devices is complex. The typical modality is to use JPEG format with lossless compression.[10] Each study must have unique identifiers which include the demographics of the patient. Devices must have a system of unlimited access numbers. With limited access numbers, the possibility of overwriting a prior study can result in the incorrect images for a given patient transferred to the medical record. Bandwidth must be adequate to transmit from patient site to server and then from server to provider on demand. Fortunately, there is strong impetus to equalize bandwidth across the United States.[11,12]

The goal of telemedicine, in general, is to provide the right care in the right place at the right time. What could be more patient-centric than that mantra? But in order to achieve this goal, society must make broadband ubiquitous throughout the United States in order to at least achieve 100 Mbps download speeds. Hospital systems, large and small, must have enough bandwidth to achieve rapid transmission of images and be fast enough for live, real-time video visits, whether to a patient's home or to a clinic setting. Prioritizing these speeds for all may well be among the most important health care priorities in the public domain.[13]

Information Security

Assurance of information safety and security must have the highest priority. There have been multiple hacks into medical systems given a large amount of information for hackers to glean.[9] While 100% assurance is probably not possible, strong encryption and constant monitoring of activity into and out of servers is critical. All providers at the patient and remote site should work within the firewall of the system and observe all applicable rules of engagement. The data servers and computers should have malware protection, and encouraging and enforcing strong cybersecurity practices such as strong passwords, adhering to security rules (e.g., not sharing passwords), using Health Insurance Portability and Accountability Act (HIPAA) compliant methods to transmit and store information. Keep in mind that HIPAA and privacy violations can pause operations and, in the worst case scenario, bring down a entire program.

CONCLUSION

Since technology changes constantly, the need for continuous support either with smaller private setting EHRs or with larger hospital systems is extremely important. What is perfect today is soon rendered obsolete as newer, more efficient ways of doing the same things emerge. The future of eye care, and indeed, all of telehealth is bright. It is now well accepted by patients and increasingly more providers. It is better and better understood by IT personnel and other supporting staff members. With current and emerging technology, particularly with the emerging field of artificial intelligence, the landscape of all eye care over the coming years will continue to change. Providers and patients are "riding the train" together with the ultimate destination being the best possible care delivered, regardless of where and how.

SECTION II: OCULAR TELEHEALTH EQUIPMENT FOR NON-POSTERIOR SEGMENT EXAMINATION—VISION, REFRACTION, PUPILS, IOP, AND FUNCTIONAL TESTING

April Maa, MD

INTRODUCTION

This section provides information about non-fundus camera equipment that could be utilized for an ocular telehealth program. Note that examples mentioned throughout this chapter are meant to be examples and do not constitute an exhaustive list. None of the authors have any financial conflict of interest regarding the equipment discussed and inclusion in this chapter does not signal endorsement by any of the authors.

There are a few important and practical considerations when choosing equipment to include in an ocular telehealth program. One guiding principle is to evaluate the "big picture" and consider the "value add." First, what is/are the goal(s) of the program, and does the equipment accurately gather the information required to achieve the goal(s)? How much time does it take to acquire the information, and how much does that equipment cost? Also consider ease of use, ease of training, and type of personnel required to operate the equipment (and whether that level of personnel is readily available to conduct the program). Finally, if there are space constraints, then combination equipment or portable/handheld devices may be preferred.

VISION MEASUREMENT TOOLS

An important vital sign in eye examinations is visual acuity. Depending on the goals of the ocular telehealth program, visual acuity measurements may need to be incredibly precise and refined by refraction versus obtaining an estimated vision for triage purposes. Visual acuity can be measured by a simple printed wall chart, a printed near card, a formal electronic or mirror-based visual acuity projection chart, or with smartphone applications. Since many readers are familiar with the traditional vision charts, this section focuses on smartphone applications.

There are hundreds of smartphone apps[14,15] to measure both distance and near visual acuity but very few of these apps are validated compared to the gold standard eye charts.[14] Past literature reviews of smartphone applications in eye care[16,17] recommended more validation studies before clinical use. In Samanta et al.'s systematic review, only 10 apps were found to have validation studies.[15] Some of them tested in the literature were found to be inaccurate.[18,19] Others, including PEEK (Portable Eye Examination Kit) Acuity,[20] Paxos

Check up,[21] and EyeChart app,[22] were found to be comparable to vision obtained on an Early Treatment Diabetic Retinopathy Study (ETDRS) chart.

If a smartphone-based eye chart is going to be used to measure visual acuity, the vision tester should be aware that contrast and brightness levels of the screen will impact accuracy, potentially overestimating vision.[23] In addition, optotype size on the smartphone-based applications vary in accuracy (from 4 to 39% difference) compared to Snellen charts[19] and may further change depending on phone screen size. Therefore, users have to adjust the distance the smartphone is held for optotype display size unless the app automatically calculates this factor.[14]

There are also vision checking apps that are meant to be used direct to home, for example, Vision at home,[24] which was found to correlate well with ETDRS charts for distance and near vision. Samanta et al. performed a recent review on apps for home and found that Peek Acuity[25] had the strongest studies supporting its accuracy, especially for home-based visual acuity testing.[15]

REFRACTION TOOLS

Uncorrected refractive error is a significant cause of visual impairment in the world with high societal cost.[26–29] The World Health Organization (WHO) has challenged the eye field to find quick, accurate ways to screen and correct refractive errors. This problem is complex to solve because screening and correcting refractive error requires special equipment, skill, and is time-intensive—resources that may not be readily available to the global population.

If an ocular telehealth program is designed to screen and provide eyeglass prescriptions to patients (see Chapter 2), the measurement of refractive error and the process of subjective refraction is paramount. When considering technologies for measuring and correcting refractive error for ocular telehealth, one may consider factors such as patient demographics (e.g., age, presence of ocular disease), accuracy, speed, equipment expense, space needed, and skill of telehealth facilitator. Several devices are available to estimate a patient's refractive error and to assist with manifest refraction. This section focuses specifically on autorefractors and phoropter technologies.

Tabletop Autorefractors

There are a multitude of commercially available handheld and tabletop autorefractors that many eye providers are familiar with already. Any of these devices can be used for telehealth. Some of the tabletop autorefractors contain additional tools that may be helpful for a telehealth program (depending on the goal). For example, the Marco ARK 1S and Topcon KR-800S contain a built-in visual acuity chart and the Topcon model also contains an Amsler grid (Figs. 13.1–13.3).

Marco makes another autorefractor that contains a noncontact tonometer, ARK Tonoref II.

Traditional autorefractors are based on the ray deflection principle.[30] These autorefractors work by having the machine project an image into the eye and when the light beams hit the retina, a small amount of light reflects back from the retina toward the autorefractor. The machine is then capable of sensing the distortion and defocus of these light rays is then corrected by software/internal lenses. When these corrections by the image eventually allow the autorefractor to make one clear image, the result yields the estimated refractive error (Fig. 13.4).

Studies show that various traditional autorefractors may differ from each other. Kinge et al. in 1996 compared two autorefractors in 448 patients and found the Nidek to be better than the Humphrey,[31] however, Wang et al. found in 886 children that the Topcon KR-800 and Grand Seiko WAM were similar in accuracy to each other.[32] The varying results may be due to the different populations tested, and also consider that the technology for traditional autorefraction has advanced considerably in the intervening 24 years.

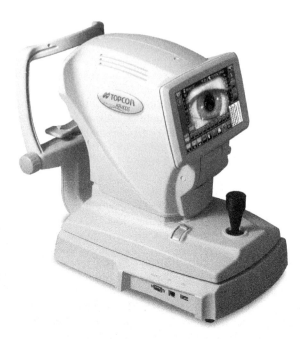

FIG. 13.2 Topcon KR-800S Autorefractor. (Credit: used with permission from Topcon.)

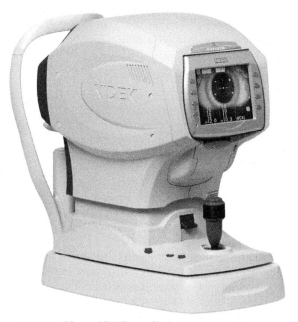

FIG. 13.3 Marco ARK Tonoref II Autorefractor with tonometer. (Credit: used with permission from Marco.)

Wavefront Aberrometry Technology and Handheld Autorefractors

A newer development in autorefractor technology, found in several handheld autorefractors, utilizes wavefront aberrometry. Instead of using a reflected ray

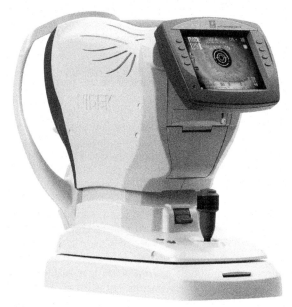

FIG. 13.1 Marco ARK 1S Autorefractor. (Credit: used with permission from Marco.)

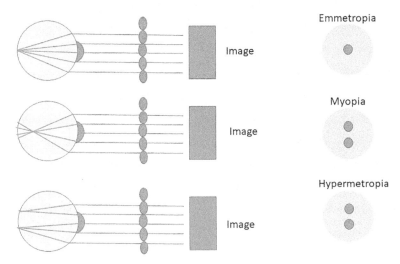

FIG. 13.4 Ray deflection principle of traditional autorefractors. (Credit: Line drawing by April Maa, MD.)

of light, wavefront aberrometry measures how light passes through the cornea and lens and how the light wave is distorted. As the light wave passes through the eye, distortions are measured by a specialized optical sensor called the Shack–Hartmann wavefront sensor. These distortions, or aberrations, are captured by the sensor and translated into a refractive error measurement (Fig. 13.5).

Several devices have arisen utilizing wavefront aberrometry, especially smaller, handheld autorefractors,

and multiple studies have been done to assess the accuracy of these devices.[33–38] A recent systematic review found that the Quicksee and the SVone were the most accurate handheld wavefront aberrometers when compared to subjective refraction, and both were better than EyeNetra and Retinomax, even though Retinomax was the fastest (Fig. 13.6).[26]

With the increased adoption of telehealth and the huge global need for refractive error screening, there is a goal to find inexpensive, portable autorefractors that

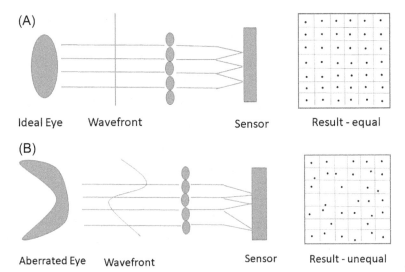

FIG. 13.5 (A) and (B) Wavefront Aberrometry of newer, handheld autorefractors. (A) shows the ideal state and (B) shows the aberrated state. (Credit: Line drawing by April Maa, MD.)

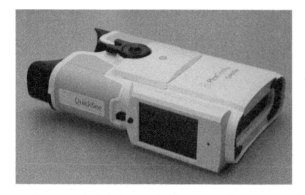

FIG. 13.6 Quicksee, one example of a handheld autorefractor utilizing wavefront aberrometry technology. (Credit: Photo taken by Jennifer Damonte, MA.)

can produce accurate enough measurements to prescribe eyeglasses with minimal manifest refraction. This aim is more applicable for resource-poor and highly rural populations in the world, where patients may not have access to skilled refractionists or eye providers, and therefore an alternative solution is necessary. Therefore, it is not surprising that several studies have been done to evaluate the patient acceptance of eyeglasses from autorefraction alone[39–41] and have generally concluded that autorefractors should be used as starting points but **not** as a replacement for manifest refraction. The most recent study conducted by Durr et al. still found similar data, however, the differences were less than in the previous reports.[42] Seven hundred and eight patients were enrolled and their glasses from a wavefront autorefractor prescription were compared to glasses from retinoscopy-based subjective refraction. Forty-two percent of patients preferred their glasses obtained from subjective refraction, 33% liked the autorefraction prescription (statistically significant difference), and 25% had no preference. Despite patient preferences, autorefractor prescriptions averaged a visual acuity difference in patients of only 1 letter worse. Interestingly, if the patients were less than 40 years old, 96% had no preference between the prescriptions.

The very best results for refraction and eyeglass prescriptions occur when an autorefraction is complementing a subjective refraction. Tabernero et al. compared a wavefront autorefractor Visual Adaptive Optics (VAO) with/without subjective refinement versus standard autorefractor versus a manifest refraction and found that the best accuracy was when the VAO autorefractor was utilized in conjunction with subjective refraction. They also stratified the results by age, refractive error type, and presence of an ocular condition. The presence of

an ocular condition significantly deteriorated the accuracy of all refraction methods.[43]

The findings from the papers discussed earlier highlight several important points regarding refraction technology. Patient factors (age, neural plasticity, likelihood of eye disease) clearly appear to impact acceptance of eyeglass prescriptions and the target population of the ocular telehealth programs should take the following factors into account:

- Accuracy of the autorefractor device may vary depending on the type of technology used.
- Manifest refractions are still considered the gold standard, especially if one has the ability to do them. In Durr et al., note that refractions here were done by highly trained technicians but not eye providers.

Phoropters, Algorithms, and Refraction Suites

Given that subjective manifest refraction is the best method for patients but generally requires a highly trained individual or an eye provider, industry has developed machines that render manifest refraction easier to accomplish in a shorter period of time. Many companies have developed digital phoropters which contain algorithms that make the manifest refraction process semiautomated. Recent articles have investigated the accuracy of an algorithm-based approach to refraction—the "digital" phoropter.[44–46] These studies consistently report that the algorithm-driven phoropters are similar to the standard manual refraction process but are much faster. Of note, in these reports, a wavefront autorefractor is often used to obtain the objective refractive starting point.

Currently, there are multiple companies selling digital refraction systems, many designed to fit in a small space. A digital refraction suite includes a vision chart, automated lensometer, autorefractor, and digital phoropter with motorized lens movement and algorithms to support the individual completing the manifest refraction. Each component can be substituted (i.e., lensometer and autorefractor could be different manufacturers) but if the components are all the same brand, then the system is able to seamlessly transfer data over and therefore reduces time spent and reduces error associated with data entry. Some examples of refraction systems include: Topcon CV-5000, Marco Epic, Phoropter VRx (Reichert), Visuphor (Zeiss), and Vx55 (Visionix) (Figs. 13.7 and 13.8).

There are also smaller tabletop models such as the Marco TS-310 or 610, and VASR (Vmax Vision). In an optometric review article, VASR was felt to be incredibly accurate and help patients see even better than 20/20[47] (Fig. 13.9).

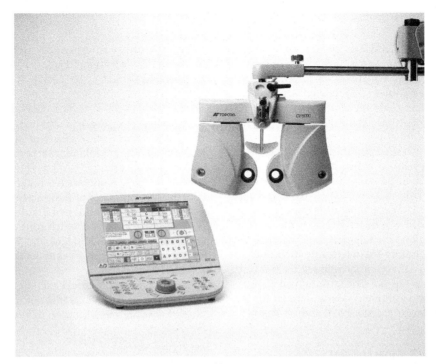

FIG. 13.7 Topcon CV-5000, automated phoropter. (Credit: used with permission from Topcon.)

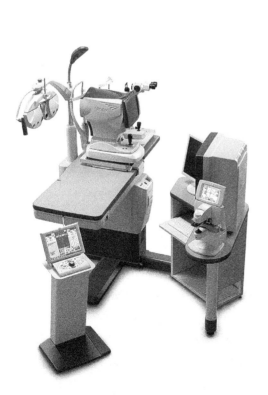

FIG. 13.8 Marco Epic Refraction Suite. (Credit: used with permission from Marco.)

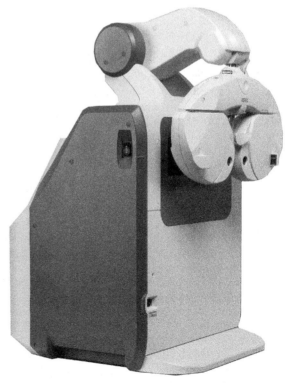

FIG. 13.9 Marco TS 610, smaller Refraction Suite. (Credit: used with permission from Marco.)

Other features to consider include split prism, which allows the patient to simultaneously view a proposed change (e.g., + 0.50D sphere), and the current baseline. The ability to remotely refract (e.g., operator separate from the patient) is also a desireable feature for many ocular telehealth programs. The largest detractor to the use of these refraction suites is usually cost and ease of portability. Several companies have also developed software that allows these digital phoropters to be controlled through a web-based program, (e.g., Topcon RDx, Marco Infinity, Eye Refract from Luneau) thus allowing the refractionist or eye provider to be remote from the patient. This would also allow the tele-presenter who may be in the room facilitating the telehealth encounter to not be trained in refraction techniques. At the time of this chapter writing, the Chronos did not have remote refraction capability but this is planned for the future per the company (Figs. 13.10 and 13.11).

OTHER OCULAR MEASUREMENTS: PUPILS/APD, IOP, PACHYMETRY

Several ocular telehealth programs may also want additional data aside from vision and refraction including the presence of APD, IOP, and corneal thickness.

Pupils, RAPD, and Oculomotor Testing

A penlight or Finoff transilluminator is commonly used to evaluate pupil size and the presence of a relative afferent pupillary defect. Studies in the neurosurgical literature have demonstrated that automated pupillometry is far superior to manual methods,[48–50] and automated pupillometry is increasingly used to monitor critically ill patients such as trauma victims with increased intracranial pressure. NPi-200 (Neuro-Optix) is, per Zafar et al., the only automated pupilometer currently sold in the United States.[49] Konan Medical has a promising product, EyeKinetix,[51–53] an infrared pupillometer that can determine the presence or absence of an APD which NPi-200 does not do. EyeKinetix, however, is listed as CE Mark Pending and FDA listed; at the time of this book writing (Fig. 13.12). Another company, Neuroptics RAPiDo makes a machine capable of providing log unit measurement of rAPD with a 25-s test. Neurolign[54] produces diagnostic equipment that assesses oculomotor, vestibular, and cognitive tests through a headset (used for comprehensive neurologic assessment) that then links to their online platform. Neurolign

is currently utilized more in the field of Neurology, but the technology may be applicable or adapted to ocular telehealth.

IOP

Ocular telehealth programs routinely check eye pressure and there are a wide variety of portable devices to measure IOP. The gold standard is considered Goldman Applanation Tonometry (GAT) but the portable version of this, the Perkins tonometer, is difficult to use and requires the instillation of fluorescein. Most telehealth programs utilize the tonopen (multiple companies), or a rebound tonometer, which currently only has one manufacturer, iCare (Fig. 13.13 and 13.14). Key differences to note between iCare and the Tonopen are listed in Table 13.1.

One can also use a noncontact tonometer, however, in the era of the pandemic, it is not recommended because of possible aerosolization of virus[60,61].

Pachymetry

In published studies, the majority of the time, central corneal thickness (CCT) was gathered for a glaucoma telehealth program. CCT can be measured by a handheld pachymeter or by an imaging device, for example, an OCT. The third section of this chapter reviews posterior segment equipment. If there is a concern regarding sterilization of the pachymeter tip, Micro Medical Devices makes a pachymeter that has a disposable cover (PalmScan P2000) (Figs. 13.15 and 13.16).

VISUAL FIELD EQUIPMENT

Several ocular telehealth programs utilize visual field testing equipment for screening or following glaucoma. When deciding on a visual field device, important factors to consider include ability to connect to network, availability of testing algorithms, and standardization with in-person clinic equipment. For example, if the ocular telehealth program intends to alternate visits between telehealth and a traditional clinic follow-up, then the perimeter at the telehealth location will need to be the same as the clinic to ensure that the visual fields obtained are comparable between the telehealth sites and the in-person clinic sites.

Possible perimetry devices include frequency doubling technology (FDT) devices (Welch Allyn, Humphrey Matrix (Zeiss)), standard tabletop

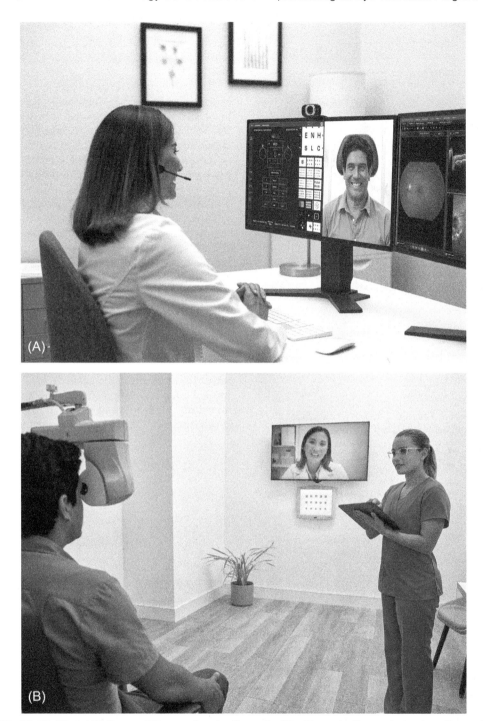

FIG. 13.10 (A) and (B) Topcon RDx, remote refraction suite. (Credit: used with permission from Topcon.)

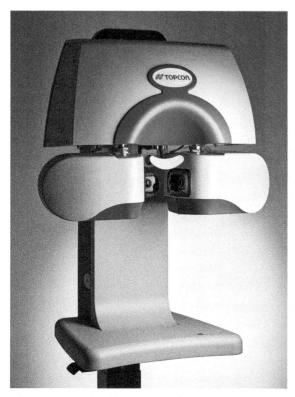

FIG. 13.11 Topcon Chronos 3-in-1 refraction suite. (Credit: used with permission from Topcon.)

perimeters (Zeiss HFA, Octopus Field Analyzer), and recently, more portable visual field tests utilizing an app on a tablet or a virtual reality headset[62] (Figs. 13.17 and 13.18).

Razeghinejad et al. compared the VisuALL virtual reality headset to the Humphrey Sita-Standard protocol and found that it took 3 min longer than the standard test but was able to separate healthy from glaucomatous patients and did not require a technician to monitor the patient.[63] Furthermore, the VisuALL is more portable and therefore could be mailed to the patient's home. The VisuALL is one of the few head-mounted devices for visual field testing that utilizes the same strategy as the Humphrey, and the results look promising. However, even though the technology is advancing, the more portable perimetry options are not mainstream and more data is necessary about reproducibility and accuracy compared to the standard perimeters.

In terms of tablet-based perimetry testing, a couple of examples include the Visual Fields Easy (VFE) and Melbourne Rapid Fields (MRF).[62] Accuracy compared to the gold standard perimeters is better for the MRF. VFE was not very accurate for early glaucoma with a low area under the curve (AUC)[64] whereas MRF showed good correlation to the Sita-Standard protocol over time.[65,66] Even though these portable apps show good correlation, they are still not used in mainstream

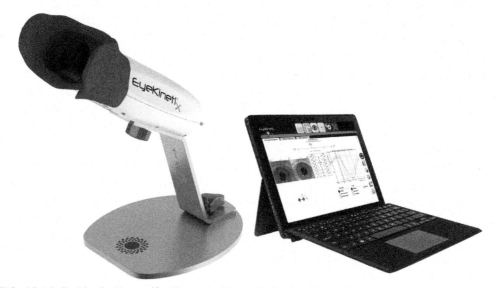

FIG. 13.12 EyeKinetix, Konan. (Credit: used with permission from Konan.)

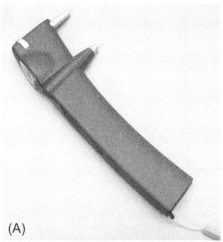

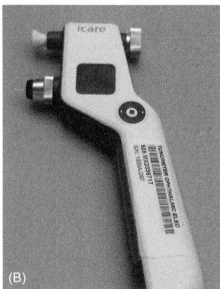

(A)

(B)

FIG. 13.13 (A) and (B) Rebound tonometers, TA01 (*top*) and ic400 (*bottom*). (Credit: Photo taken by Jennifer Damonte, MA.)

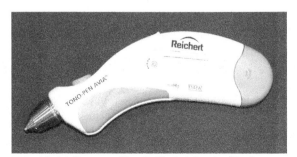

FIG. 13.14 Tonopen. (Credit: Photo taken by Stephen Herman, COT.)

TABLE 13.1
Characteristics of the Rebound Tonometer and Tonopen

Characteristic	Rebound Tonometer	Tonopen
Portable	Yes	Yes
Easy to Use/Train	Yes	Yes
Sterile tip/cover	Yes	Yes
Require drops before use	No	Yes
Comparable to GAT	Yes[55,56]	Yes[57,58]
Has in-home version	No	Yes[59]

Credit: April Maa, MD

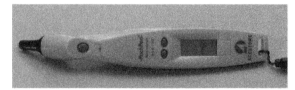

FIG. 13.15 Pachymeter. (Credit: Photo taken by Jennifer Damonte, MA.)

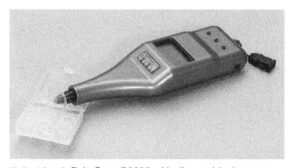

FIG. 13.16 PalmScan P2000 with disposable tip covers. (Credit: Photo taken by Jennifer Damonte, MA.)

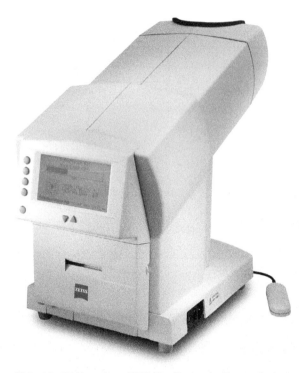

FIG. 13.17 Humphrey FDT. (Credit: used with permission from Zeiss.)

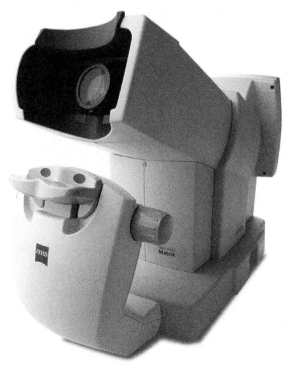

FIG. 13.18 Humphrey Matrix, smaller tabletop visual field analyzer. (Credit: used with permission from Zeiss.)

care and the lack of eye tracking limits its reliability. Newer apps like EyeCatcher have an inexpensive eye-tracking clip-on, attached to the tablet or smartphone device, to accompany the app and have a reported AUC of 0.97. Most patients reported that their experience with the app was preferable to standard automated perimetry.[67–70]

Another portable solution for field testing is virtual reality headsets, with several companies manufacturing these devices (e.g., Micro Medical, CFA). Mees et al. tested the C3 Field Analyzer (CFA). Even though the virtual reality headset tested the same locations as an HVF 24–2, it fell short of identifying some of the early 24–2 deficits that HVF found.[71] Other companies install a smartphone into the head-set[72] and during the pandemic a team at University of California San Francisco (UCSF) reported a successful use case study on an elderly gentleman using the virtual reality headset remotely.[72] While many exciting new technologies are on the horizon that will render visual field testing more portable and less reliant on expensive, immobile tabletop perimeters, the newer devices need more research to ensure accuracy and correlation with the Sita-Standard protocols. See Chapter 5, Glaucoma Telehealth, for additional information.

ANTERIOR SEGMENT EXAMINATION

Multiple devices are capable of taking an external photograph including tabletop fundus cameras or a smartphone. Paxos, a completely smartphone-based device has a secure phone app where a user can enter information (e.g., vision) and attach a smartphone adapter to take both external and fundus photographs of the eye.

Given the relative ease to obtain an external photograph of an eye and almost any camera (e.g., cell phone) is capable of doing this, the remainder of this section instead focuses on technologies that allow for slit-lamp imaging and/or slit-lamp video. The accuracy of slit lamp versus external photographs is covered in both Chapter 3, Anterior Segment Telehealth and Chapter 17, Ocular Triage.

Slit-Lamp Cameras

Several companies make true slit-lamp cameras. Benefits to this type of equipment include the fact that the eye provider has the full functionality of a true slit lamp and the photos and videos taken are of the highest quality (Fig. 13.19).

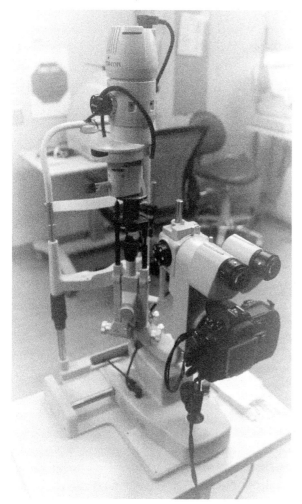

FIG. 13.19 Slit-lamp camera. (Credit: Photo taken by Stephen Herman, COT.)

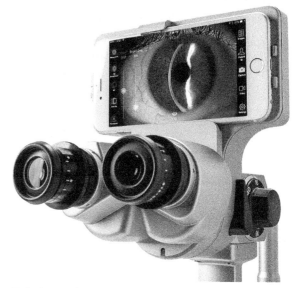

FIG. 13.20 Marco Ion, slit-lamp camera. (Credit: used with permission from Marco.)

Slit-Lamp Adapters

Other companies make slit-lamp adapters. Some of these utilize a variation of smartphone technology. These devices are either integrated into the whole slit lamp, replace an ocular, or stabilize the smartphone as it takes photos through an ocular of a standard slit lamp. One important consideration when evaluating this equipment is to consider how images or videos would be downloaded and transferred in a Health Insurance Portability and Accountability Act (HIPAA)

compliant manner. This equipment again allows for the eye provider to have gold standard equipment and may be less expensive for the Emergency Room (ER) or Urgent Care (UC) clinic to buy an attachment as opposed to a full slit-lamp camera (Fig. 13.20). However, the slit lamp attachment does require that the clinic site own a 'regular' slit lamp.

Additionally, there are companies that make portable attachments for telehealth carts that provide anterior segment views and can support both asynchronous and synchronous telehealth modalities. While these attachments are more limited than a true slit lamp, they may be beneficial because they are generally less expensive than a full slit lamp and utilize equipment that the ER/UC is likely to already own, e.g., the telehealth cart. JedMed makes two types of anterior segment attachments, one which is simpler and only takes 2D external photos and the second which has more complex features and has more slit-lamp functions (Fig. 13.21).

Stability of the patient's head is important for getting high-quality video or slit-lamp images, therefore, a "stand" or chin rest is also helpful and can be purchased at additional cost for these telehealth cart attachments (Fig. 13.22).

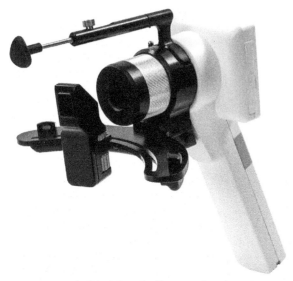

FIG. 13.21 JedMed, Anterior Segment Attachment on Horus Handle. (Credit: used with permission from JedMed.)

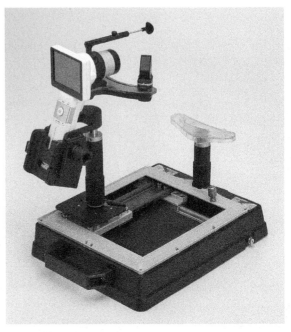

FIG. 13.22 JedMed chin rest (with anterior segment attachment inserted into the holder). (Credit: used with permission from JedMed.)

SECTION III: OCULAR TELEHEALTH EQUIPMENT FOR POSTERIOR SEGMENT EXAMINATION—FUNDUS PHOTOGRAPHY AND OPTICAL COHERENCE TOMOGRAPHY

Stephanie J. Weiss, DO
INTRODUCTION

This section provides information regarding posterior segment imaging equipment that can be used for an ocular telehealth program. As with the anterior segment imaging equipment in Section II, examples mentioned throughout this section do not constitute an exhaustive list and none of the authors have any financial conflict of interest regarding the equipment discussed. Inclusion in this chapter does not signal endorsement by any of the authors.

When considering posterior segment imaging options for an ocular telehealth program, there are several factors that come into play: image quality, field of view, space, cost, ease of use, and portability. In recent years, significant technological advances have allowed imaging equipment to meet more of the desired qualities for a telehealth program. However, each piece of equipment will also have its limitations and one must prioritize and sometimes compromise when selecting the best imaging equipment for each setting.

FUNDUS CAMERAS
Traditional tabletop fundus camera

Traditionally, true color digital fundus cameras were a mainstay of ophthalmic imaging, capable of capturing high-quality images of the retina with a 30–45-degree field of view. Montage or composite images, created using multiple internal fixation targets to capture images of different regions of the retina, can be utilized to widen the field of view. However, these images can be technically challenging for minimally trained personnel to acquire and often require a high level of patient cooperation. Traditionally, mydriasis was also required to capture retinal images well. More recently, nonmydriatic options have become more popular. Despite nonmydriatic capabilities, imaging equipment often still requires mydriasis to achieve an optimal field of view. Commonly, a nonmydriatic camera will be capable of capturing an image with a limited field of view with a minimum pupil size of 3.3 mm while a full field of view will require a minimum pupil size of 4 mm. Even with cameras designed to be nonmydriatic, mydriasis will often also improve the quality of the image.

When used as part of a telehealth program, non-mydriatic fundus cameras can prove an effective screening tool. Chin et al. found that a single 45-degree fundus image taken with a nonmydriatic fundus camera was effective in screening for diabetic retinopathy in both rural populations with limited access to eye care providers and urban populations who were nonadherent to screening recommendations.[73] This study found this single image to be highly effective not only in diagnosis of diabetic retinopathy but also in grading.[73]

Automated tabletop nonmydriatic fundus camera

Automated nonmydriatic fundus cameras have become a popular option in telehealth programs over recent years, owing to the minimal training and ease of use typically required for operation. This type of camera is defined by the ability to automatically focus on the retina and capture an image. They can also automatically produce stereo photos of the optic disc and can automatically produce montage photos using multiple internal fixation points and software to fit the images together (Figs. 13.23 and 13.24).

These cameras can even automatically switch between the two eyes without assistance. While this level of automation can make a camera like this ideal for untrained staff to capture high-quality images, for personnel previously trained in or familiar with fundus imaging, it can actually become more time-consuming

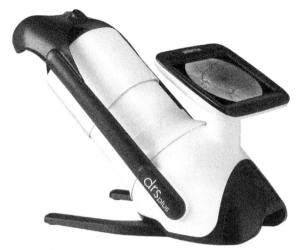

FIG. 13.24 Centervue DRSplus. (Credit: used with permission from iCare.)

and be viewed negatively.[74] Of note, most automated fundus cameras do have a manual mode that can be utilized by highly trained personnel or when image acquisition is particularly difficult.

One popular automated nonmydriatic fundus camera is the Topcon NW 400.[75] This is a traditional tabletop camera that features autofocus, autocapture, and automated movement between eyes. As with many nonmydriatic cameras, it has a 45-degree field of view with a 4.0 mm or larger pupil and has a "small pupil mode" that is capable of capturing a 30-degree field of view with a minimum 3.3 mm pupil. Nine internal fixation targets can be used to create a wide-field montage image. Automatic pairing for stereo disc photos is also featured on this model. For space savings considerations, this camera is entirely controlled via a rotating touchscreen, allowing the camera to be oriented in any direction necessary for the available space (Fig. 13.25).

The Marco AFC 330[76] is another popular nonmydriatic automated fundus camera. It features similar automated focusing, capture, and stereo pairing as the Topcon model, and has a similar small pupil mode to allow for image acquisition with a minimum pupil size of 3.3 mm. Both of these models feature a low flash intensity to improve patient comfort. Additionally, both of these models are capable of capturing high-quality 2D anterior segment images, an important consideration when performing a complete ocular telehealth screening examination. Some fundus cameras are also designed to transmit directly to a cloud, such as the Konan Nexy (Fig. 13.26).

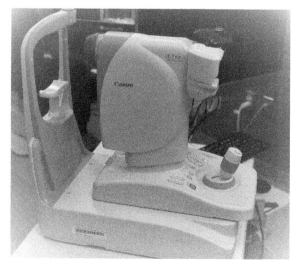

FIG. 13.23 Canon Fundus Camera. (Credit: Photo taken by Stephen Herman, COT.)

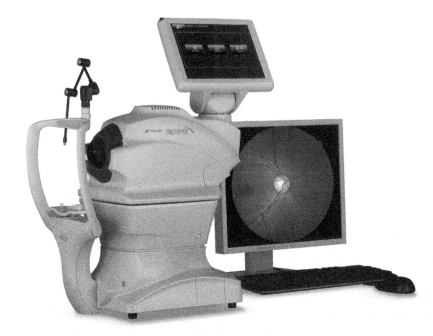

FIG. 13.25 Topcon NW400. (Credit: used with permission from Topcon.)

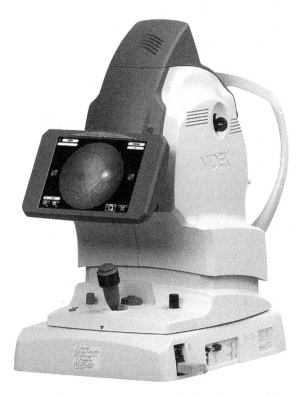

FIG. 13.26 Caption: Marco AFC 330. (Credit: used with permission from Marco.)

Ultra-widefield fundus imaging

In recent years, the development of ultra-widefield devices has revolutionized the ability to image the fundus. It is well established that ultra-widefield devices allow for superior detection of peripheral retinal pathology and vitreous pathology including retinal tears, lattice degeneration, and posterior vitreous detachment when compared to traditional digital fundus cameras with or without dilation.[77,78]

Confocal scanning laser ophthalmoscope (SLO) imaging

An SLO utilizes a system of rotating mirrors to drive laser illumination across the fundus in a raster pattern and an objective lens to gather the reflected light. A confocal aperture positioned in front of the image detector blocks nonimage-forming light. This is advantageous not only in that it allows for an enhanced ability to image the peripheral retina but also in that the SLO system requires lower levels of illumination, is capable of acquiring a high-quality image with a smaller pupil, and is less susceptible to media opacity interference.

The Optos cameras[79] utilize a concave ellipsoidal mirror with two conjugate focal points to image up to a 200-degree field of view in a single image. They are capable of automatically creating a montage image

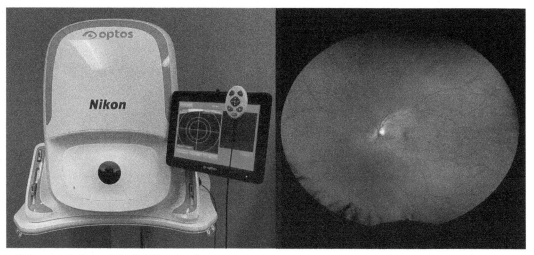

FIG. 13.27 Optos Widefield Fundus Camera and sample image. (Credit: Photo by Stephanie J. Weiss, DO.)

that can capture up to 220 degrees. There are several models within the Optos line that feature different capabilities including fluorescein angiography, indocyanine green angiography, spectral-domain OCT, and/ or swept-source OCT in addition to the standard red-green pseudocolor images, autofluorescence images, stereo disc images, and central pole images (to provide a more detailed view of the macula). In a direct comparison between the Optos and a conventional digital fundus camera, the Optos was found to be comparable in evaluating the macula, and superior in evaluating peripheral retinal pathology (Fig. 13.27).[80]

The Eidon[81] is another example of a confocal SLO widefield fundus imaging device. However, this device utilizes white LED light, including the entire visible light spectrum in its images. Sarao et al. found that the Eidon produced images more in the center of the chromatic space when compared to conventional digital flash fundus photography that tended to shift toward the red spectrum at the expense of the blue and green spectrums, suggesting that Eidon actually produced a more balanced color image.[82] This same study suggested that this color quality can provide better diagnostic capabilities for readers more accustomed to the typical color fundus photographs.[82] While it does not capture the peripheral retina to the degree of the Optos devices, a single image with the Eidon device provides a 60-degree field of view but can capture up to 110 degrees when a montage is created. Like the Optos, the Eidon is also capable of performing fluorescein angiography. When comparing Eidon fundus images to traditional digital fundus photos, Olvera-Barrios et al. found

that the Eidon was capable of detecting additional pathology not only in the periphery not imaged in a traditional camera but also in the macula (Fig. 13.28).[83] (See Fig. 13.29.)

Other ultra-widefield technology

While the Zeiss Clarus 700[84] does not rely on confocal SLO, it is still capable of capturing ultra-widefield images of the fundus. With a single image, the Clarus has up to a 133-degree field of view. This can be improved to 200 degrees with a two-image montage and up to 267 degrees with a six-image montage. Like the SLO options, the Clarus has a minimum pupil diameter of 2.5 mm and has the option to perform stereo disc photos and fluorescein angiography as well as fundus autofluorescence. Unlike the SLO options, the Clarus utilizes true color to capture images that appear more similar to the fundus as it is viewed clinically. Additionally, the Clarus is capable of capturing 2D external images of the orbit and anterior segment, a unique feature of an ultra-widefield device not found in Optos or Eidon devices.

Several studies have compared the Clarus to the Optos with each device having its own pros and cons. The Optos is capable of imaging a larger area of the retina than the Clarus with a single image, which improves the detection of peripheral retinal pathology.[85,86] While the Optos was found to capture more pixels in each of the four quadrants, the Optos was also found to have more artifacts (typically lid and lash) obscuring critical areas of the retina when compared to the Clarus.[85,86] The Clarus has been shown to be more

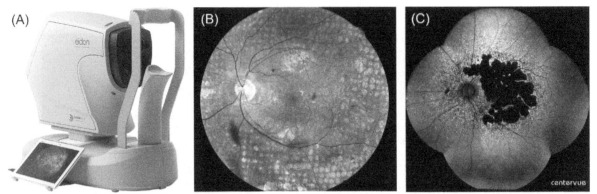

FIG. 13.28 (A) Eidon Fundus Camera. (B) Eidon Fundus Photo Example. (C) Eidon Autoflourescence Mosaic Fundus Photo Example. (Credit: used with permission from iCare.)

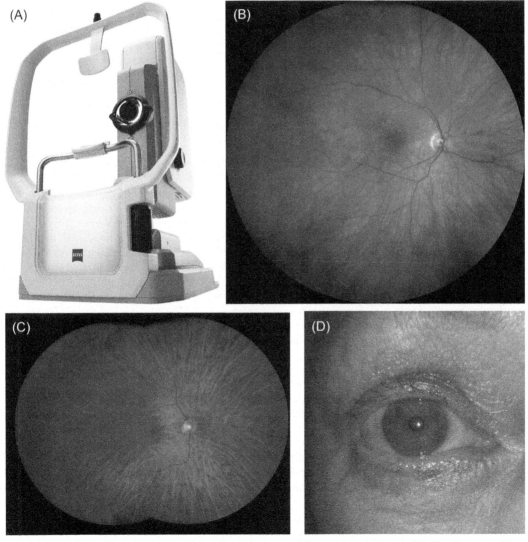

FIG. 13.29 Zeiss Clarus (A), single photo (B), photomontage (C), and external image (D). (Credit: used with permission from Zeiss.)

sensitive in detecting retinal hemorrhage and choroidal neovascular membrane (CNVM) in patients with diabetic retinopathy and neovascular age-related macular degeneration, possibly owing to the fact that the Clarus has a 7-μm resolution compared to the 14-μm resolution of the Optos.[85,87] The Clarus has also been shown to outperform the Optos and traditional fundus imaging in eyes with media opacity such as cataract.[87]

Handheld fundus cameras

Traditionally, fundus imaging devices have relied on tabletop equipment. This means that the equipment must remain stationary and requires a certain degree of space to perform image acquisition. While tabletop devices have the advantage of stability during image acquisition, they also tend to be larger and more costly. In recent years, the development of handheld fundus cameras has allowed a significant degree of mobility, often at a much lower price point. While cost-effectiveness and portability can provide significant advantages when establishing an ocular telehealth program, the trade-off with these devices is often in image quality and field of view. Additionally, the lack of stability can prove a significant challenge when aligning the camera and the patient to get useful images, but slit lamp and chin rest attachments can help mitigate this obstacle.[88] Handheld cameras can be extremely helpful for community screening and rural programs, including international programs.[88,89] They have also proven helpful in examining geriatric and pediatric populations, instances when patients are not capable of positioning at traditional imaging devices.[88] While traditional fundus cameras have been shown to produce superior image quality, image quality with handheld devices can be improved with mydriasis and experienced technicians.[90,91] Several studies have found that handheld cameras can produce images of acceptable quality (especially for screening programs) even without dilation or experienced photographers.[90–92] Zapata et al. tested several handheld fundus imaging devices for screening in an occupational health setting and, while their patient population skewed younger than the average eye clinic, they found only 0.7% of images were insufficient to be used for screening.[93] They also found a high satisfaction rate (owing to the cost-effectiveness and convenience) and were able to detect a variety of retinal pathology including choroidal nevi, glaucoma, and macular signs of high myopia.[93]

While there are many handheld fundus cameras currently available, one option is the Volk Pictor Series.[94] The Pictor Plus option has a 40-degree field of view while the Pictor Prestige has a 50-degree field of view

and is designed for a small pupil. Both Volk options can capture red-free images, video as well as still images, and external/anterior segment images. An additional feature is a cobalt blue light to capture fluorescein anterior segment images. Zhang et al.[95] evaluated the ability of the Pictor to screen for referrable diabetic retinopathy in dilated and undilated eyes and found that successful image acquisition rates were similar among the dilated and undilated groups but image acquisition was more efficient in those that were dilated. When compared to an in-person dilated clinical exam, the Pictor had high sensitivity and acceptable specificity, suggesting this was a sufficient screening method for diabetic retinopathy (Fig. 13.30).

The Welch Allyn RetinaVue 700 Imager[96] is another example of a handheld fundus camera. It features automated alignment, focusing, and image capture and is designed to be used by primary healthcare providers. It has a minimum pupillary diameter of 2.5 mm and has a 60-degree field of view, making it a more widefield option than most handheld devices. It is also capable of external imaging but one must obtain and put the "anterior segment" attachment on before it can be used for 2D external images. The RetinaVue also has an optional pedestal that can convert the unit to a tabletop device which can help with stabilization challenges.

The JedMed Horus Portable Fundus Camera[97] is also a nonmydriatic handheld fundus camera that is capable of capturing single images as well as videos of the fundus. It has a 45-degree field of view and features seven internal fixation points to assist with imaging other more peripheral areas of the retina. One advantage of this device is that it has an optional anterior segment attachment to facilitate external images as well as a portable chin rest to assist with stabilization during image acquisition. It is also capable of connecting to a telehealth cart (Figs. 13.31 and 13.32).

Smartphone-based fundus cameras

As the field of ocular telehealth has grown dramatically to include more rural- and community-based screening programs, the demand for portable and cost-effective fundus camera options has grown significantly. Among the significant advantages of smartphone-based fundus cameras are the extreme mobility and cost-effectiveness even when compared to the more traditional handheld fundus cameras. This can be attributed to the smartphone-based camera's ability to capitalize on the already sophisticated and high-quality camera that comes standard in almost every smartphone currently on the market. Additionally, many of these cameras rely on

(A)

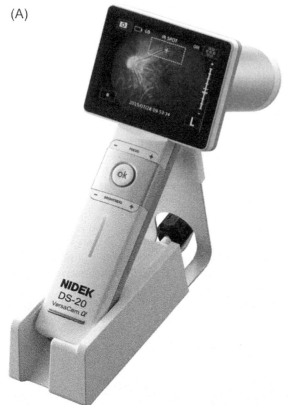

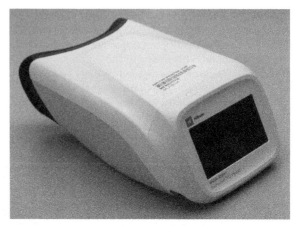

FIG. 13.31 Welch Allyn RetinaVue. (Credit: Photo taken by Jennifer Damonte, MA.)

(B)

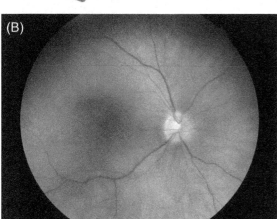

FIG. 13.30 (A) and (B) Versacam Handheld Fundus Camera and a sample photo. (Credit: used with permission from iCare.)

connectivity to a paired smartphone application specially designed to comply with patient privacy standards while providing efficient and effective image acquisition and transfer of information. Studies have established that smartphone-based fundus camera systems are ca-

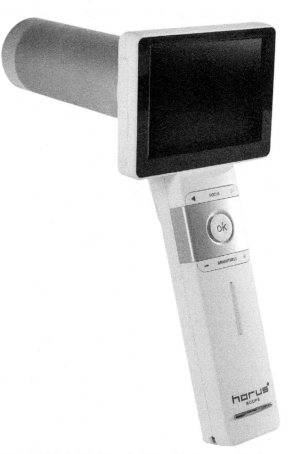

FIG. 13.32 JedMed Handheld Fundus Camera. (Credit: used with permission from JedMed.)

pable of detecting referable diabetic retinopathy among other retinal pathology.[98] Perhaps to a higher degree than with more traditional handheld fundus cameras, smartphone-based fundus cameras are limited by a narrower field of view and reduced image quality.

The Digital Eye Center D-Eye[99] is an FDA-approved smartphone-based fundus camera based on direct ophthalmoscopy principles that can produce up to a 20-degree field of view and capture single images or videos. It pairs with its own unique app to maximize effectiveness. This device exploits the smartphone camera's autofocus feature and uses the app to dim the camera's flash to a more optimal level. The device, which magnetically attaches to a smartphone, utilizes a cross-polarization technique to minimize artifact and reflection from the cornea, improve image detail and contrast, and minimize reflectivity to improve visualization of the nerve fiber layer (Fig. 13.33).[100]

The Welch Allyn Panoptic Ophthalmoscope and iExaminer attachment[101] are capable of capturing a 25-degree field of view while relying on the iPhone camera for image resolution and quality. The attachment aligns the optical axis of the ophthalmoscope with the iPhone capture to enable the camera to effectively image the fundus. LaMonica et al. found this device to be helpful in screening for glaucoma by accurately allowing cup-to-disc ratio measurement in an international screening program based in the Independent Nation of Samoa.[102] This camera system was also found to be useful in a pediatric emergency room in which images were successfully acquired in over 91% of children aged 2–18 years (though image acquisition was limited in children under 2 years of age).[103] This device is not capable of capturing external or anterior segment photos.

The DigiSight Paxos Scope has also been shown to have a high success rate in screening for anterior segment and retinal pathology with high levels of patient satisfaction and cost-effectiveness. The Paxos Scope is capable of capturing anterior segment photos as well as fundus photos. Hong et al.[104] compared the Paxos Scope with remote ophthalmologists reading the images to screening technicians performing an in-person exam in a clinic in Nepal and found that remote ophthalmologists with access to the images were able to detect significantly more pathology than the in-person technician. In this case, the scope was paired with an iPod touch camera instead of a smartphone for enhanced cost-effectiveness. When compared to a traditional digital fundus camera, the ability to capture images by the Paxos Scope was found to be comparable to the traditional camera.[105] When compared to OCT, the Paxos Scope was found to be comparable in enabling evaluation of a vertical cup-to-disc ratio in a glaucoma screening program.[106]

OPTICAL COHERENCE TOMOGRAPHY (OCT)

In clinical practice, OCT has become a mainstay of glaucoma and retinal evaluation for the eye care provider. Traditional ocular telehealth programs have focused on fundus imaging. However, several studies have shown that the addition of OCT is preferable to fundus imaging alone in eye screening exams, particularly for diabetic screening exams.[107,108] The OCT is more sensitive in detecting diabetic macular edema as well as other macular pathology that can be easy to miss based on fundus imaging alone. While the addition of OCT imaging can be helpful in the detection of more subtle

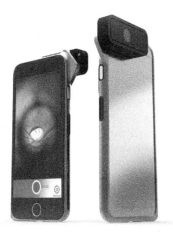
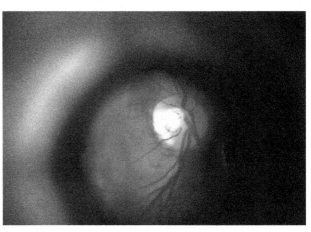

FIG. 13.33 D-eye smartphone-based fundus camera and sample fundus image. (Credit: used with permission from D-eye.)

macular pathology, traditional spectral-domain OCT devices including Heidelberg Spectralis, Zeiss Cirrus, Topcon, and Optovue can be large and costly.

Handheld OCT

Traditional OCT devices are cumbersome and lack the portability of the handheld and smartphone-based fundus camera options. While no widely available handheld OCT options are available at this time, mechanisms for handheld and smartphone-based OCT devices have been proposed. Mehta et al.[109] proposed a smartphone-mounted OCT probe that can be wirelessly controlled by a remote user. Meanwhile, Nankivil et al. proposed a handheld swept-source OCT capable of imaging the anterior and posterior segments.[110] These developments show promise for the future possibilities of integration of OCT into more rural- and community-based ocular telehealth programs.

COMBINATION OCT/FUNDUS CAMERA

While handheld and smartphone-based OCT devices have yet to be developed to the point where they are in mainstream use, combination OCT and fundus cameras have become a popular option for integrating OCT into ocular telehealth programs. These devices have the advantage of space savings, requiring only one machine to simultaneously acquire OCT and fundus photos. The Topcon Maestro[111] is a fully automated model featuring automatic alignment, focusing, image capture, and montage. This device is also capable of performing OCTA scans and anterior segment OCT scans. The Zeiss Cirrus Photo[112] is another example of a combination OCT and fundus photo device. This device has a maximum 45-degree field of view and is capable of capturing fundus autoflourescence, fluorescein angiography, indocyanine green angiography, and anterior segment images in addition to high-quality, spectral-domain OCT images. Additionally, the Optovue i-Fusion[113] is capable of capturing spectral-domain OCT images as well as fundus images with a 21-degree field of view through a minimum 2.5 mm pupil diameter as well as external images. Recently, Optos[79] has developed an ultra-widefield fundus camera with simultaneous ultra-widefield swept-source or spectral-domain OCT as well. All of these options are capable of capturing high-quality images of the entire eye with one device, making them an ideal option for ocular telehealth screening programs looking to perform comprehensive eye evaluations (Figs. 13.34 and 13.35).

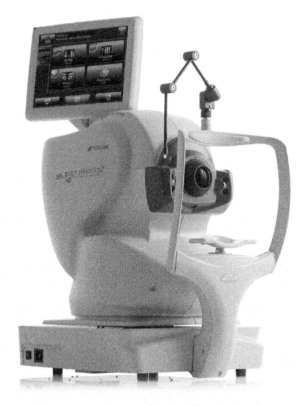

FIG. 13.34 Topcon Maestro Combination Fundus/OCT Camera. (Credit: used with permission from Topcon.)

SUMMARY

Recent significant improvements in multimodal fundus imaging have revolutionized the ability of ocular telehealth programs to effectively capture the fundus with excellent options for ultimate quality, field of view, portability, and cost-effectiveness.

CONCLUSION

When considering the best technology options for each ocular telehealth program, one must consider the goals of the program, assess the technology needs, collaborate with IT, Biomed, and clinicians, and determine what equipment will fit the parameters required to carry out the telehealth process.

The authors of this chapter recommend selecting specific eye telehealth equipment that (1) meets the needs/goals of the overall program, (2) is appropriate for the IT infrastructure, telehealth facilitator, and patient population, and finally, (3) fits into the telehealth program's workflow and adds value.

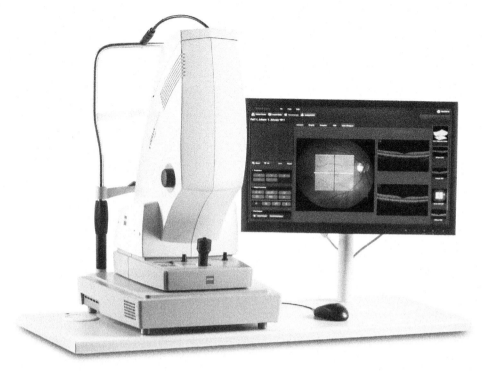

FIG. 13.35 Zeiss Cirrus Photo Combination Fundus/OCT Camera. (Credit: used with permission from Zeiss.)

REFERENCES
Section I

1. Wilson LS, Maeder AJ. Recent directions in telemedicine: review of trends in research and practice. *Healthc Inform Res.* 2015;21(4):213–222. Published online October 31, 2015 https://doi.org/10.4258/hir.2015.21.4.213.
2. Sabanayagam C, Banu R, Chee ML, et al. Incidence and progression of diabetic retinopathy: a systematic review. *Lancet Diabetes Endocrinol.* 2019;7(2):140–149.
3. Cavallerano AA, Cavallerano J, Katalinic P, et al. Joslin vision network telemedicine eye health care model for diabetic retinopathy in a veterans health administration medical center. *Am J Ophthalmol.* 2005;139(4):597–604.
4. https://en.wikipedia.org/wiki/List_of_countries_by_Internet_connection_speeds.
5. https://broadbandmap.fcc.gov/#/.
6. https://www.healthit.gov/faq/what-recommended-bandwidth-different-types-health-care-providers.
7. https://www.extrahop.com/company/blog/2016/introduction-to-dicom-protocol/.
8. https://en.wikipedia.org/wiki/Picture_archiving_and_communication_system.
9. https://healthitsecurity.com/news/the-10-biggest-healthcare-data-breaches-of-2019-so-far.
10. https://www.acr.org/-/media/ACR/Files/Practice-Parameters/elec-practice-medimag.pdf.
11. Wilcock AD, Rose S, Busch AB, et al. Association between broadband internet availability and telemedicine use. *JAMA Intern Med.* 2019;179(11):1580–1582.
12. https://mhealthintelligence.com/news/new-telehealth-bill-seeks-funding-for-broadband-expansion-programs.
13. Tan IJ, Dobson LP, Bartnik S, Muir J, Turner AW. Real-time teleophthalmology versus face-to-face consultation: a systematic review. *J Telemed Telecare.* 2017;23(7):629–638. https://doi.org/10.1177/1357633X16660640. Epub 2016 Jul 20 27444188.

Section II

14. Brady CJ, Eghrari AO, Labrique AB. Smartphone-based visual acuity measurement for screening and clinical assessment. *JAMA.* 2015;314(24):2682–2683.
15. Samanta A, Mauntana S, Barsi Z, Yarlagadda B, Nelson PC. Is your vision blurry? A systematic review of home-based visual acuity for telemedicine. *J Telemed Telecare.* 2020. Nov 22:1357633X20970398.
16. Hogarty DT, Hogarty JP, Hewitt AW. Smartphone use in ophthalmology: what is their place in clinical practice? *Surv Ophthalmol.* 2020;65(2):250–262.

17. Charlesworth JM, Davidson MA. Undermining a common language: smartphone applications for eye emergencies. *Med Devices (Auckl)*. 2019;12:21–40.

18. Tofighi B, Chemi C, Ruiz-Valcarcel J, Hein P, Hu L. Smartphone apps targeting alcohol and illicit substance use: systematic search in in commercial app stores and critical content analysis. *JMIR Mhealth Uhealth*. 2019;7(4), e11831.

19. Perera C, Chakrabarti R, Islam FM, Crowston J. The eye phone study: reliability and accuracy of assessing Snellen visual acuity using smartphone technology. *Eye (Lond)*. 2015;29(7):888–894.

20. Bastawrous A, Rono HK, Livingstone IA, et al. Development and validation of a smartphone-based visual acuity test (peek acuity) for clinical practice and community-based fieldwork. *JAMA Ophthalmol*. 2015;133(8):930–937.

21. Pathipati AS, Wood EH, Lam CK, Sales CS, Moshfeghi DM. Visual acuity measured with a smartphone app is more accurate than Snellen testing by emergency department providers. *Graefes Arch Clin Exp Ophthalmol*. 2016;254(6):1175–1180.

22. Ansell K, Maconachie G, Bjerre A. Does the EyeChart app for iPhones give comparable measurements to traditional visual acuity charts? *Br Ir Orthopt J*. 2020;16(1):19–24.

23. Tofigh S, Shortridge E, Elkeeb A, Godley BF. Effectiveness of a smartphone application for testing near visual acuity. *Eye (Lond)*. 2015;29(11):1464–1468.

24. Han X, Scheetz J, Keel S, et al. Development and validation of a smartphone-based visual acuity test (vision at home). *Transl Vis Sci Technol*. 2019;8(4):27.

25. https://www.peekvision.org/en_GB/peek-solutions/peek-acuity/. Accessed 30.01.21.

26. Samanta A, Shetty A, Nelson PC. Better one or two? A systematic review of portable automated refractors. *J Telemed Telecare*. 2020; 1357633X20940140.

27. Durr NJ, Dave SR, Lage E, Marcos S, Thorn F, Lim D. From unseen to seen: tackling the global burden of uncorrected refractive errors. *Annu Rev Biomed Eng*. 2014;16:131–153.

28. Naidoo KS, Leasher J, Bourne RR, et al. Global vision impairment and blindness due to uncorrected refractive error, 1990–2010. *Optom Vis Sci*. 2016;93(3):227–234.

29. Fricke TR, Holden BA, Wilson DA, et al. Global cost of correcting vision impairment from uncorrected refractive error. *Bull World Health Organ*. 2012;90(10):728–738.

30. Lebow KA, Campbell CE. A comparison of a traditional and wavefront autorefraction. *Optom Vis Sci*. 2014;91(10):1191–1198.

31. Kinge B, Midelfart A, Jacobsen G. Clinical evaluation of the Allergan Humphrey 500 autorefractor and the Nidek AR-1000 autorefractor. *Br J Ophthalmol*. 1996;80(1):35–39.

32. Wang D, Jin N, Pei RX, et al. Comparison between two autorefractor performances in large scale vision screening in Chinese school age children. *Int J Ophthalmol*. 2020;13(10):1660–1666.

33. Ciuffreda KJ, Rosenfield M. Evaluation of the SVOne: a handheld, smartphone-based autorefractor. *Optom Vis Sci*. 2015;92(12):1133–1139.

34. Agarwal A, Bloom DE, de Luise VP, Lubet A, Murali K, Sastry SM. Comparing low-cost handheld autorefractors: a practical approach to measuring refraction in low-resource settings. *PLoS One*. 2019;14(10), e0219501.

35. Gil A, Hernandez CS, Perez-Merino P, et al. Assesment of the QuickSee wavefront autorefractor for characterizing refractive errors in school-age children. *PLoS One*. 2020;15(10), e0240933.

36. Durr NJ, Dave SR, Vera-Diaz FA, et al. Design and clinical evaluation of a handheld wavefront autorefractor. *Optom Vis Sci*. 2015;92(12):1140–1147.

37. Rubio M, Hernandez CS, Seco E, et al. Validation of an affordable handheld wavefront autorefractor. *Optom Vis Sci*. 2019;96(10):726–732.

38. Jeganathan VSE, Valikodath N, Niziol LM, Hansen S, Apostolou H, Woodward MA. Accuracy of a smartphone-based autorefractor compared with criterion-standard refraction. *Optom Vis Sci*. 2018;95(12):1135–1141.

39. Bullimore MAAC, Fusaro RE, Bauman M, et al. Acceptance of auto-refractor and clinician prescriptions: a randomized clinical trial. *Invest Ophthalmol Vis Sci*. 1996;37(3):S704.

40. Strang NC, Gray LS, Winn B, Pugh JR. Clinical evaluation of patient tolerance to autorefractor prescriptions. *Clin Exp Optom*. 1998;81(3):112–118.

41. Sun JK, Aiello LP, Cavallerano JD, et al. Visual acuity testing using autorefraction or pinhole occluder compared with a manual protocol refraction in individuals with diabetes. *Ophthalmology*. 2011;118(3):537–542.

42. Durr NJ, Dave SR, Lim D, Joseph S, Ravilla TD, Lage E. Quality of eyeglass prescriptions from a low-cost wavefront autorefractor evaluated in rural India: results of a 708-participant field study. *BMJ Open Ophthalmol*. 2019;4(1), e000225.

43. Tabernero J, Otero C, Pardhan S. A comparison between refraction from an adaptive optics visual simulator and clinical refractions. *Transl Vis Sci Technol*. 2020;9(7):23.

44. Otero C, Aldaba M, Pujol J. Clinical evaluation of an automated subjective refraction method implemented in a computer-controlled motorized phoropter. *J Optom*. 2019;12(2):74–83.

45. Venkataraman AP, Sirak D, Brautaset R, Dominguez-Vicent A. Evaluation of the performance of algorithm-based methods for subjective refraction. *J Clin Med*. 2020;9(10):1–8.

46. Ohlendorf A, Leube A, Wahl S. Steps towards smarter solutions in optometry and ophthalmology-inter-device agreement of subjective methods to assess the refractive errors of the eye. *Healthcare (Basel)*. 2016;4(3):41.

47. Cole J. *Your Phoropter on Steroids? High-tech Refraction Systems Tout Greater Accuracy, Comfort and Time Savings. Skeptics Ask If Such Gains Justify Choosing This Over Other Practice-Enhancing Investments*; 2017. September 15 https://www.reviewofoptometry.com/article/ro0917-your-phoropter-on-steroids.

48. Olson DM, Stutzman S, Saju C, Wilson M, Zhao W, Aiyagari V. Interrater reliability of pupillary assessments. *Neurocrit Care*. 2016;24(2):251–257.

49. Zafar SF, Suarez JI. Automated pupillometer for monitoring the critically ill patient: a critical appraisal. *J Crit Care*. 2014;29(4):599–603.

50. Omburo L, Stutzman S, Supnet C, Choate M, Olson DM. High variance in pupillary examination findings among postanesthesia care unit nurses. *J Perianesth Nurs*. 2017;32(3):219–224.

51. Satou T, Goseki T, Asakawa K, Ishikawa H, Shimizu K. Effects of age and sex on values obtained by RAPDx((R)) pupillometer, and determined the standard values for detecting relative afferent pupillary defect. *Transl Vis Sci Technol*. 2016;5(2):18.

52. Ali M, Lu L, Martinez P, et al. Pupil-based detection of asymmetric glaucomatous damage—comparison of the Konan RAPDx pupillograph, swinging flashlight method, and magnifier-assisted swinging flashlight method. *Invest Ophthalmol Vis Sci*. 2013;54(15):4811.

53. Cohen LM, Rosenberg MA, Tanna AP, Volpe NJ. A novel computerized portable pupillometer detects and quantifies relative afferent pupillary defects. *Curr Eye Res*. 2015;40(11):1120–1127.

54. Neurolign home page. https://neurolign.com/. Accessed 28.03.21.

55. Bao B, Diaconita V, Schulz DC, Hutnik C. Tono-pen versus Goldmann applanation tonometry: a comparison of 898 eyes. *Ophthalmol Glaucoma*. 2019;2(6):435–439.

56. Christoffersen T, Fors T, Ringberg U, Holtedahl K. Tonometry in the general practice setting (I): Tono-Pen compared to Goldman applanation tonometry. *Acta Ophthalmol*. 1993;71(1):103–108.

57. Stoor K, Karvonen E, Ohtonen P, Liinamaa MJ, Saarela V. Icare versus Goldmann in a randomised middle-aged population: The influence of central corneal thickness and refractive errors. *Eur J Ophthalmol*. 2021 May;31(3):1231–1239, 1120672120921380.

58. Jose J, Ve RS, Pai HV, et al. Agreement and repeatability of Icare ic100 tonometer. *Indian J Ophthalmol*. 2020;68(10):2122–2125.

59. Rodter TH, Knippschild S, Baulig C, Krummenauer F. Meta-analysis of the concordance of Icare((R)) PRO-based rebound and Goldmann applanation tonometry in glaucoma patients. *Eur J Ophthalmol*. 2020;30(2):245–252.

60. Guo H, Li W, Huang Y, et al. Increased microbial loading in aerosols produced by non-contact air-puff tonometer and relative suggestions for the prevention of coronavirus disease 2019 (COVID-19). *PLoS One*. 2020;15(10), e0240421.

61. Lai THT, Tang EWH, Chau SKY, Fung KSC, Li KKW. Stepping up infection control measures in ophthalmology during the novel coronavirus outbreak: an experience from Hong Kong. *Graefes Arch Clin Exp Ophthalmol*. 2020;258(5):1049–1055.

62. Prager AJ, Kang JM, Tanna AP. Advances in perimetry for glaucoma. *Curr Opin Ophthalmol*. 2021 Mar 1;32(2):92–97.

63. Razeghinejad RS, Aakriti G. *In the Field*; 2021. www.the-ophthalmologist.com. Accessed 16.05.21.

64. Johnson CA, Thapa S, George Kong YX, Robin AL. Performance of an iPad application to detect moderate and advanced visual field loss in Nepal. *Am J Ophthalmol*. 2017;182:147–154.

65. Kumar H, Thulasidas M. Comparison of perimetric outcomes from melbourne rapid fields tablet perimeter software and humphrey field analyzer in glaucoma patients. *J Ophthalmol*. 2020;2020:8384509.

66. Prea SM, Kong YXG, Mehta A, et al. Six-month longitudinal comparison of a portable tablet perimeter with the Humphrey field analyzer. *Am J Ophthalmol*. 2018;190:9–16.

67. Jones PR, Smith ND, Bi W, Crabb DP. Portable perimetry using eye-tracking on a tablet computer-a feasibility assessment. *Transl Vis Sci Technol*. 2019;8(1):17.

68. Jones PR, Lindfield D, Crabb DP. Using an open-source tablet perimeter (Eyecatcher) as a rapid triage measure for glaucoma clinic waiting areas. *Br J Ophthalmol*. 2020.

69. Jones PR. An open-source static threshold perimetry test using remote eye-tracking (Eyecatcher): description, validation, and preliminary normative data. *Transl Vis Sci Technol*. 2020 Jul 13;9(8):18.

70. Kong YX, He M, Crowston JG, Vingrys AJ. A comparison of perimetric results from a tablet perimeter and Humphrey field analyzer in glaucoma patients. *Transl Vis Sci Technol*. 2016;5(6):2.

71. Mees L, Upadhyaya S, Kumar P, et al. Validation of a head-mounted virtual reality visual field screening device. *J Glaucoma*. 2020;29(2):86–91.

72. Deiner MS, Damato BE, Ou Y. Implementing and monitoring at-home virtual reality oculo-kinetic perimetry during COVID-19. *Ophthalmology*. 2020;127(9):1258.

Section III

73. Chin EK, Ventura BV, See K-Y, Seibles J, Park SS. Nonmydriatic fundus photography for teleophthalmology diabetic retinopathy screening in rural and urban clinics. *Telemed J E Health*. 2014;20(2):102–108. https://doi.org/10.1089/tmj.2013.0042.

74. Ogunyemi O, Moran E, Patty Daskivich L, et al. Autonomy versus automation: perceptions of nonmydriatic camera choice for teleretinal screening in an urban safety net clinic. *Telemed J E Health*. 2013;19(8):591–596. https://doi.org/10.1089/tmj.2012.0191.

75. TRC-NW400. *Topcon Healthcare*. Accessed 14.02.21 https://topconhealthcare.com/us/products/trc-nw400/.

76. AFC-330 Automated Fundus Camera. *Marco Ophthalmic*. Accessed 14.02.21 https://marco.com/product/afc-330-automated-fundus-camera/.

77. Silva PS, Horton MB, Clary D, et al. Identification of diabetic retinopathy and ungradable image rate with ultrawide field imaging in a national teleophthalmology program. *Ophthalmology*. 2016;123(6):1360–1367. https://doi.org/10.1016/j.ophtha.2016.01.043.

78. Silva PS, Cavallerano JD, Haddad NMN, et al. Comparison of nondiabetic retinal findings identified with nonmydriatic fundus photography vs ultrawide field imaging in an ocular telehealth program. *JAMA Ophthalmol.* 2016;134(3):330–334. https://doi.org/10.1001/jamaophthalmol.2015.5605.

79. Optos.com. *Optos Homepage.* Accessed 14.02.21 https://www.optos.com/.

80. Byberg S, Vistisen D, Diaz L, et al. Optos wide-field imaging versus conventional camera imaging in Danish patients with type 2 diabetes. *Acta Ophthalmol.* 2019;97(8):815–820. https://doi.org/10.1111/aos.14118.

81. *iCare EIDON Widefield TrueColor Confocal Fundus Imaging System.* Accessed 14.02.21 https://www.icare-world.com/us/product/icare-eidon/.

82. Sarao V, Veritti D, Borrelli E, Sadda SVR, Poletti E, Lanzetta P. A comparison between a white LED confocal imaging system and a conventional flash fundus camera using chromaticity analysis. *BMC Ophthalmol.* 2019;19(1):231. https://doi.org/10.1186/s12886-019-1241-8.

83. Olvera-Barrios A, Heeren TF, Balaskas K, et al. Comparison of true-colour wide-field confocal scanner imaging with standard fundus photography for diabetic retinopathy screening. *Br J Ophthalmol.* 2020;104(11):1579–1584. https://doi.org/10.1136/bjophthalmol-2019-315269.

84. ZEISS. *Retinal Cameras.* Accessed 14.02.21 https://www.zeiss.com/meditec/int/product-portfolio/retinal-cameras/zeiss-clarus-700.html.

85. Hirano T, Imai A, Kasamatsu H, Kakihara S, Toriyama Y, Murata T. Assessment of diabetic retinopathy using two ultra-wide-field fundus imaging systems, the Clarus® and Optos™ systems. *BMC Ophthalmol.* 2018;18(1):332. https://doi.org/10.1186/s12886-018-1011-z.

86. Chen A, Dang S, Chung MM, et al. Quantitative comparison of fundus images by two ultra-wide field fundus cameras. *Ophthalmol Retina.* 2021 May;5(5):450–457. https://doi.org/10.1016/j.oret.2020.08.017. Epub 2020 Aug 29.

87. Maruyama-Inoue M, Kitajima Y, Mohamed S, et al. Sensitivity and specificity of high-resolution wide field fundus imaging for detecting neovascular age-related macular degeneration. *PLoS One.* 2020;15(8). https://doi.org/10.1371/journal.pone.0238072, e0238072.

88. Editor CL Associate. *Retinal Imaging On the Go.* Accessed 13.02.21 https://www.reviewofophthalmology.com/article/retinal-imaging-on-the-go.

89. Das T, Pappuru RR. Telemedicine in diabetic retinopathy: access to rural India. *Indian J Ophthalmol.* 2016;64(1):84–86. https://doi.org/10.4103/0301-4738.178151.

90. Davila JR, Sengupta SS, Niziol LM, et al. Predictors of photographic quality with a handheld nonmydriatic fundus camera used for screening of vision-threatening diabetic retinopathy. *Ophthalmologica.* 2017;238(1–2):89–99. https://doi.org/10.1159/000475773.

91. Gosheva M, Klameth C, Norrenberg L, et al. Quality and learning curve of handheld versus stand-alone non-mydriatic cameras. *Clin Ophthalmol.* 2017;11:1601–1606. https://doi.org/10.2147/OPTH.S140064.

92. Lin T-C, Chiang Y-H, Hsu C-L, Liao L-S, Chen Y-Y, Chen S-J. Image quality and diagnostic accuracy of a handheld nonmydriatic fundus camera: feasibility of a telemedical approach in screening retinal diseases. *J Chin Med Assoc.* 2020;83(10):962–966. https://doi.org/10.1097/JCMA.0000000000000382.

93. Zapata MA, Martín R, Garcia-Arumí C, et al. Remote screening of retinal and optic disc diseases using handheld nonmydriatic cameras in programmed routine occupational health checkups onsite at work centers. *Graefes Arch Clin Exp Ophthalmol.* 2021;259(3):575–583. https://doi.org/10.1007/s00417-020-04860-z. Epub 2020 Jul 29.

94. Pictor Plus™ Fundus Camera. *Volk Optical.* Accessed 14.02.21 https://www.volk.com/products/pictor-plus-fundus-camera.

95. Zhang W, Nicholas P, Schuman SG, et al. Screening for diabetic retinopathy using a portable, noncontact, nonmydriatic handheld retinal camera. *J Diabetes Sci Technol.* 2017;11(1):128–134. https://doi.org/10.1177/1932296816658902.

96. Allyn W. *RetinaVue 700 Imager|Welch Allyn.* Accessed 14.02.21 https://www.welchallyn.com/en/products/categories/physical-exam/eye-exam/retinal-cameras/retina-vue-700-imager.html.

97. JEDMED. *Portable Fundus Camera.* JEDMED; 2021. Accessed 14.02.21 https://www.jedmed.com/collections/portable-fundus-camera.

98. Queiroz MS, de Carvalho JX, Bortoto SF, et al. Diabetic retinopathy screening in urban primary care setting with a handheld smartphone-based retinal camera. *Acta Diabetol.* 2020;57(12):1493–1499. https://doi.org/10.1007/s00592-020-01585-7.

99. D-Eye Portable Ophthalmoscope; 2015. Accessed 14.02.21. Published online August 9 https://www.digitaleyecenter.com/product/d-eye-portable-ophthalmoscope/. https://plus.google.com/u/1/116096663910200322498.

100. Russo A, Morescalchi F, Costagliola C, Delcassi L, Semeraro F. A Novel device to exploit the smartphone camera for fundus photography. *J Ophthalmol.* 2015;2015:823139. https://doi.org/10.1155/2015/823139.

101. iEXAMINER. Accessed 14.02.21 https://www.welchallyn.com/en/microsites/iexaminer.html.

102. LaMonica LC, Bhardwaj MK, Hawley NL, et al. Remote screening for optic nerve cupping using smartphone-based nonmydriatic fundus photography. *J Glaucoma.* 2021;30(1):58–60. https://doi.org/10.1097/IJG.0000000000001680.

103. Day LM, Wang SX, Huang CJ. Nonmydriatic fundoscopic imaging using the pan optic iExaminer system in the pediatric emergency department. *Acad Emerg Med.* 2017;24(5):587–594. https://doi.org/10.1111/acem.13128.

104. Hong K, Collon S, Chang D, et al. Teleophthalmology through handheld mobile devices: a pilot study in rural Nepal. *J Mob Technol Med.* 2019 Jun;8(1). https://doi.org/10.7309/jmtm.8.1.1.

105. Ludwig CA, Murthy SI, Pappuru RR, Jais A, Myung DJ, Chang RT. A novel smartphone ophthalmic imaging adapter: User feasibility studies in Hyderabad, India. *Indian J Ophthalmol.* 2016;64(3):191–200. https://doi.org/10.4103/0301-4738.181742.

106. Idriss BR, Tran TM, Atwine D, Chang RT, Myung D, Onyango J. Smartphone-based ophthalmic imaging compared to spectral domain optical coherence tomography assessment of vertical cup-to-disc ratio among adults in Southwestern Uganda. *J Glaucoma.* 2021 March;30(3):e90–e98. https://doi.org/10.1097/IJG.0000000000001779. Publish Ahead of Print.

107. Sanborn GE, Wroblewski JJ. Evaluation of a combination digital retinal camera with spectral-domain optical coherence tomography (SD-OCT) that might be used for the screening of diabetic retinopathy with telemedicine: a pilot study. *J Diabetes Complicat.* 2018;32(11):1046–1050. https://doi.org/10.1016/j.jdiacomp.2018.08.010.

108. Boucher MC, Qian J, Brent MH, et al. Evidence-based Canadian guidelines for tele-retina screening for diabetic retinopathy: recommendations from the Canadian Retina Research Network (CR2N) Tele-Retina Steering Committee. *Can J Ophthalmol.* 2020;55(1 Suppl. 1):14–24. https://doi.org/10.1016/j.jcjo.2020.01.001.

109. Mehta R, Nankivil D, Zielinski DJ, et al. Wireless, web-based interactive control of optical coherence tomography with mobile devices. *Transl Vis Sci Technol.* 2017;6(1):5. https://doi.org/10.1167/tvst.6.1.5.

110. Nankivil D, Waterman G, LaRocca F, Keller B, Kuo AN, Izatt JA. Handheld, rapidly switchable, anterior/posterior segment swept source optical coherence tomography probe. *Biomed Opt Express.* 2015;6(11):4516–4528. https://doi.org/10.1364/BOE.6.004516.

111. Maestro2—OCT Camera. *Topcon Healthcare—Global.* Accessed 14.02.21 https://topconhealthcare.com/products/maestro2/.

112. ZEISS. *CIRRUS Photo—Optical Coherence Tomography With Fundus Imaging.* Accessed 14.02.21 https://www.zeiss.com/meditec/int/product-portfolio/optical-coherence-tomography-devices/cirrus-photo-family.html.

113. iVue & iFusion. *The Complete Retinal Imaging Solution.* Accessed 14.02.21 https://www.optovue.com/products/ivue-ifusion-80.

CHAPTER 14

Billing, Coding, and Reimbursement in Eye Telehealth Programs

CHARLES F. PALMER, MD

INTRODUCTION TO BILLING AND CODING

Before this author enters into the details of telehealth coding, a brief overview of good coding practices is an excellent starting point. The Center for Medicare and Medicaid Services (CMS) identified the goal of best coding with the Correct Coding Initiative. The general idea is that there should be a one best Current Procedural Terminology (CPT) code used for each medical encounter. This one code should be the code that best describes the complexity and nature of the visit. More than one code can be utilized, as codes should be combined when procedures or testing are performed at the same visit. Therefore, a single encounter may include multiple codes and modifiers. However, the general idea still applies that there should be one best code to describe the appropriate part of the exam.[1] This chapter will expand the correct coding initiative idea specifically into the realm of telehealth where services are provided synchronously via telephone or video, or asynchronously through remote data review. Regardless of the telehealth modality, the same concept applies. Providers should pick the best code that describes the type or mechanism of care delivery, and then choose the most appropriate level of a code that describes the care given. The key idea is that telehealth encounters "...are considered the same as in-person visits...."[2]

CMS allows services that have normally been furnished in-person to be provided via telemedicine.[1] The guiding principle to keep in mind moving forward is that one does not code to a Relative Value Unit (RVU), instead, one needs to understand the codes used for each format of telemedicine care delivery and then also understand the levels of the codes that describe the care delivered. Providers should also be aware that certain insurance coverages may assign somewhat different RVU amounts to each code and that these codes need to be periodically reassessed to know if and when there are changes.[3] For instance, there are times a certain coverage may allow greater RVU for a certain code to incentivize the use of a particular type of care delivery. There also are certain waivers from CMS and commercial payers that impact technology requirements, time factors from other appointments, and new or established patient criteria. Furthermore, many of the nuances present when this chapter was written are related to the current Public Health Emergency (PHE), with the anticipation of further changes after the PHE is over.[4]

BILLING AND CODING SPECIFICALLY FOR OCULAR TELEHEALTH

For telehealth (TH) in eye care, there are three primary modalities of care delivery that will be used: synchronous video (clinic- or home-based), asynchronous, and telephone. While telephone care is different from the other types of care, it is included in this review as it will be used in addition to the actual telemedicine codes. It is up to the provider to determine which format of care will best meet the needs of the patient.[2] There may be times where more than one modality of care delivery could be chosen by the provider. Also, the circumstances of the healthcare system may lead a specific institution or payer to encourage a certain modality if a specific payer feels that will best serve the patient population. Ultimately, however, the provider decides which format to use and it is also the provider's responsibility to adjust the coding chosen when multiple formats of care delivery are utilized in the same encounter. For example, it is up to the provider to choose which codes to use if a telehealth encounter is initiated as a synchronous video encounter and, due to equipment failure, is completed as a telephone encounter.[1] The accompanying chapters in this textbook expand in more detail these different telehealth modalities of care delivery, how these could be medically useful and how they can be applied. For the coding discussion, the author will look at the nuts and bolts of how to code each of these encounters once the initial decision has already been made. Another consideration to keep in mind is that for generalized discussion, this chapter will focus on CMS/ Medicare structure. As it is likely that each institution will have coding differences in modifiers and assigned RVU,[3] it is critical that each provider maintains current review of the nuances of each insurance carrier as to any different provider unique codes or modifiers, and especially any nuances in assigned RVU for each code. Moreover, it is always safest to document the process spent deciding which codes a provider or clinic is using. The provider or an appropriate entity in the practice or facility should perform periodic reviews of assigned RVU for each code, required modifiers, as well as specific chart documentation requirements by each insurance carrier as these may vary from each insurance carrier and may change over time. This will make certain that any nuances by any particular insurance carrier are known and taken into account.[5] As a general rule of thumb these forms of care now apply to both new and established patients.[3]

The types of telemedicine (including encounter formats other than in-person clinic encounters) that the subsequent sections will discuss are as follows:

- E-communication (including methods of communication with patients such as secure messaging)
- Telephone
- Asynchronous, aka Store and Forward (e.g., diabetic teleretinal screening)
- Synchronous video encounter direct to home (e.g., Zoom call with patient)
- Synchronous video encounter to clinic-based or other healthcare setting (e.g., low-vision ocular telehealth)

Please refer to the appropriate chapters for full details on how each of these care modalities are employed. These options apply variably to both new and established patients, and with current PHE waivers include nearly all new and established patients.

No matter what telehealth modality is utilized, apart from audio-only phone visits which do not require documentation of consent, the provider must document patient consent for telemedicine, at least once annually and this can be done on the same day of the first evaluation.[1] It would be a good practice to include this documentation on all telemedicine encounters, in case the format of the exam changes once the encounter begins depending on what information comes to light to guide treatment. Once that decision has been made, the coding is as follows below.

E-Communications

E-communications are not in-person evaluations. The examples of this include secure messaging. Secure messaging is an online digital service with an established patient regarding a non-urgent issue. These are patient-initiated, associated with a triage team, are non-emergent, not related to a visit in the preceding 7 days, not within a postoperative period, and require some form of medical question to the provider. To answer the question, the provider needs to do a record review and perform some type of medical decision-making. This code would not allow for appointment scheduling or review of testing results but would apply if any medical decision-making takes place during the contact. These must have appropriate documentation in order to bill the codes listed below.[5] For "… Physicians, Nurse Practitioners, Advance Practice Nurses, and Physician Assistants…" the CPT codes 99421-99423 are for "… qualified nonphysician healthcare professionals (nurses, dieticians, pharmacists, etc.)…" Healthcare Common Procedure Coding System (HCPCS) codes G2061-G2063 can be used as applicable.[2,5]

The following codes in Table 14.1 should be used for Established Patient for up to 7 days with cumulative time during the 7 days. These codes should NOT

TABLE 14.1
E-Communication or E-visit for a medical question

Code	Time Required	Modifier	Place of Service
99421	5–10 min	No modifier	11
99422	11–20 min	No modifier	11
99423	21 or more min	No modifier	11

be used for e-communications regarding scheduling appointments or simply conveying test results.

Proper documentation for a billable e-communication requiring provider medical record review includes:
- Documentation of chief complaint
- Working diagnosis
- Working treatment plan
- Time spent in encounter.

The CMS criteria is vague beyond time spent however, for example, most coding auditors want to see medical decision-making (MDM) with at least the above elements documented. It is important to stress that "time spent" begins the moment the provider opens the chart and begins the chart review. It concludes when the provider has completed documentation and billing of the e-communication telehealth encounter.

Clinicians who may not independently bill for Evaluation/Managsement (E/M) visits can use the following HCPCS codes in Table 14.2. "(for example, physical therapists, occupational therapists, speech language pathologists, clinical psychologists)...."[2] These should be established Patients and may be rural or urban. These should be initiated by the Patient, however, "... practitioners may educate beneficiaries on the availability of the service prior to Patient initiation...."[2]

In eye telehealth, the practitioners will be able to bill E/M so those will likely be the predominant codes. A recommended best practice is to check with the specific payer for coding and billing preferences.

TABLE 14.2
HCPCS Codes for E-Communications

Code	Time Required	Cumulative Time
G2061	5–10 min	7-day period
G2062	11–20 min	7-day period
G2063	21 or more min	7-day period

Telephone Care

Telephone care is when the provider interacts with the patient via telephone or when synchronous telehealth video connection is lost, and the encounter is completed via telephone. In cases where the telephone is not the primary telehealth modality, the rule of thumb is that if the video component is lost before a vision is assessed via synchronous video, then the provider should strongly consider billing a telephone encounter. Telephone visits can be used with both new or established patients.[1] The phone encounter would be in place of what would normally be a synchronous video to home encounter.

For this type of encounter, the provider should document the time spent in the actual medical interaction with the patient (dialing phone, leaving messages, and additional attempts to call are not included in the time).

Note that the codes in Table 14.3 include up to 7 days cumulative time and the phone call by the provider is NOT to be used for scheduling appointments or simply conveying test results.

Also, these codes are not to be used when related E/M services have been given within the last 7-day period or the telephone visit will lead to an E/M services or procedure within next 24 h or soonest available appointment. In addition, these codes cannot be used for post-operative visits.

Required documentation for these notes include (similar to the e-communication): chief complaint, working diagnosis, treatment plan, and time spent in encounter.

TABLE 14.3
Return patient messages on the phone

Code	Time Required	Modifier	Place of Service
99441	5–10 min	No modifier	11
99442	11–20 min	No modifier	11
99443	21 or more min	No modifier	11
G2012 (HCPCS code)	5–10 min	No modifier	11

Asynchronous Telehealth Aka Store and Forward (e.g., Diabetic Teleretinal Screening)

Asynchronous, or store and forward telehealth, is a modality in which a telehealth facilitator gathers exam information and testing from the patient site that is stored in a computerized record, and then the eye provider reviews this data at a later time (either the same day or a future day). Traditionally this modality of telehealth was not well reimbursed, therefore, despite these types of programs being the most common form of ocular telehealth, they were not widely used pre-pandemic. Of note, during the PHE caused by the pandemic, these visits are currently billable similar to an in-person exam and include both new and established patients. These appointments can be either non-consult encounters or consult encounters. In a non-consult encounter, the patient is not referred by a provider—they may be self-referred or "walk in." In a consult encounter the patient is referred by a provider—usually primary care. The coding for these visits will consist of two separate encounters and coding. The patient-side encounter will have specific coding and the provider-side encounter will have specific coding. Depending on the coverage, either the HCPCS code G2010 for "...certain practitioners such as physical therapists, occupational therapists, speech language pathologists, licensed clinical social workers, and clinical psychologists, who do not report E/M codes..."[1] or the 99091 (non-consult) or 99451 (consult) code for practitioners who bill E/M codes may be used for store and forward evaluations. It is important to verify with each separate payer what is required for that particular payer.

HCPCS code G2010 can be utilized for established patients. This code includes interpretation of data and follow up with the patient (either via telephone or video visit to convey test results) within 24h. This code can only be used if the telehealth encounter is not originating from a related E/M service within the previous 7 days or not leading to an E/M service or procedure within the next 24 h or soonest available appointment[2,3] "... G2010 and G2012 may be billed...on the same day...."[1,3]

These HCPCS codes would likely not be utilized in ocular telehealth as the practitioners involved are ones who typically bill E/M codes. It is good to verify with any payer regarding any nuances to the use of these codes. Practitioners who bill E/M codes should more accurately use E/M codes 99091 (non-consult) and 99451 (consult). 99091 is defined as collection and interpretation of physiologic data (requiring a minimum of 30 minutes of time each 30 days, which is cumulative time spent by the telehealth facilitator plus the time spent by the provider), and 99451 is defined as greater than or equal to 5 min spent in electronic medical record review to answer question(s) for referring provider.

Furthermore, with asynchronous telehealth methods, one should consider having the patient-side (where a telehealth facilitator is present) code sequentially the parts of the eye exam they perform, and then the provider side bills the interpretation code, either 99091 or 99451.

On the patient side, the codes a telehealth facilitator may bill, depending on what services are performed in the ocular telehealth program, include the following below.

Some payer programs may use a diagnosis code for purposes of reimbursement. Each provider should check with each payer entity to determine if Z codes are accepted. Typically, if a Z code for screening is utilized, which Z code used is decided by the presence or absence of ocular disease. Note that the Z code does not consider the sight threatening risk or severity of disease, but instead focuses on whether known ocular disease is present or absent. Z01.00 is coded if there is no known ocular disease. This should be determined based on the last eye exam note that the telehealth facilitator can find and/or by patient report (the patient states no eye problems). Z01.01 is coded if there is known ocular disease at the time of technician work up. The medical condition can be noted on previous exam notes, available outside records, or by patient report and documented by the telehealth facilitator. Any medical ocular diagnosis applies here—cataract, pinguecula, dry eye syndrome, diabetic or hypertensive retinopathy, etc. For example, if a patient reports a history of glaucoma, then the telehealth facilitator on the patient side may code Z01.01, the presence of ocular disease (since it was gathered during the history part of the exam). Additionally, refractive error, diabetes, or hypertension without retinopathy do not constitute eye disease from this coding standpoint.

The telehealth facilitator should document if the patient was sent for an evaluation by another provider (chart notation, patient report, are all appropriate ways to document the intent of a consult). This will later allow the provider to select the correct type of code for the provider encounter. The telehealth facilitator will next code any known medical eye diagnosis after the Z code for payers that use the Z code.

The imager or telehealth facilitator then codes the testing and exam portions completed by the technician. Examples of this testing include:

Refraction:
- 99174 Autorefraction, Bilateral
- 92015 Refraction

It is not necessary to code for the autorefraction if a manifest refraction is performed. The telehealth facilitator should always code the highest/best representative code for the work done.

Glasses fitting:
- 92340 Glasses Fitting, Monofocal
- 92341 Glasses Fitting, Bifocal
- 92342 Glasses Fitting, Multifocal

The telehealth facilitator should code any appropriate glasses fitting if this was done as part of the encounter.

Imaging codes

92227—Remote imaging for screening with no retinal pathology.

If the imager chooses 92227, it includes the following other codes: 92250 (fundus photo), 92185 (external photo), meaning that the telehealth facilitator cannot code 92227 and any of the other above listed codes at the same time.

There is no technical component modifier or other modifier with 92227.

92228—management of active retinal disease.

If the imager chooses 92228, it includes the following other codes: 92250 (fundus photo), 92185 (external photo), 92134 (Optical Coherence Tomography—OCT— Macula). The same principle applies as above in that the telehealth technician cannot code 92228 and any of the other listed codes at the same time.

There is no technical component modifier or other modifier with 92228.

The advent of artificial intelligence and FDA approval of computer-assisted algorithms has led to the development of another CPT code, 92229—Retinal imaging with automated point of care. This would have a role with AI image interpretation. As with the other two retinal imaging codes, if the imager chooses 92229, it includes the following other codes: 92250 (fundus photo), 92185 (external photo), 92134 (OCT Macula). 92229 should not be combined with 92227 or 92228. Furthermore, one should not simultaneously code both 92227, 92228, or 92229 at the same encounter.

Additional ancillary testing such as visual fields

Typically, the telehealth facilitator or the provider, but not both, could code the ancillary testing 92083 for Visual Field and 92133 for Optic Nerve OCT. Note that 92228 should not be used by the telehealth facilitator on the patient side if they are gathering information for a glaucoma telehealth program because glaucoma is not considered a retinal disease from the coding perspective (i.e., unlike Age-Related Macular Degeneration—AMD or Diabetic Retinopathy—DR).

92134 Macular OCT

If this is done as a stand-alone test without retinal fundus images, then on the patient-side encounter the telehealth technician can code just 92134 for the OCT. However, if retinal images (92228) are performed, then 92134 should not be coded as 92228 includes 92134 as described above. 92134 would be used for the patient seen for Macular OCT only such as in an asynchronous tele-follow up with no fundus images taken.

Asynchronous Telehealth—Provider Coding

The provider will code sequentially the parts of the telehealth encounter related to interpretation of the images. The provider should check with each payer entity to determine if Z codes are used. If they are, first, code for the presence or absence of ocular disease— Z01.00 or Z01.01. Remember that this Z code does not take into account the sight-threatening risk or severity of disease, but just whether known ocular disease is present. Refractive error, diabetes or hypertension without retinopathy do not constitute eye disease.

- Z01.00 is coded if there is no ocular disease/diagnosis. This should be determined based on the sum total of review of the data (past records, images, testing) available at the time of interpretation by the provider.
- Z01.01 is coded if there is known ocular disease. This should be determined based on the sum total of review of the data (past records, images, testing) available at the time of interpretation by the provider. Remember that any medical ocular diagnosis applies here; cataract, pinguecula, dry eye, diabetic or hypertensive retinopathy, etc.).
- This Z code does not have to match the telehealth facilitator's encounter as there may have been no known history of ocular diagnosis at the time of technician assessment, but disease noted by the provider on review of the data. Technicians and providers are able to code this differently at this step because this exam is asynchronous.
- The provider will next code any known medical eye diagnosis after the Z code (when applicable per payer).

After the diagnosis codes are selected, the asynchronous telehealth provider will then choose the type of exam, non-consult or consult based on the documentation in the chart. Subsequently the provider will determine the appropriate level of exam of the correct type.

For a Non-consult Encounter

99091—This code requires a minimum of 30 minutes of cumulative time, telehealth facilitator time plus provider time in a 30 day period. This code includes, but does not require, a call to the patient. This code can be used in conjunction with a telephone call to the patient at provider discretion if provider feels that this code 99091 or the medical record review most accurately reflects this encounter. If the practitioner feels that the phone contact with the patient best reflects the telehealth encounter, then only the phone encounter code would be used for this encounter. (Refer to phone encounter portion above for that review).

For Consults

- Intent of consult must be documented in note. Report to consulting provider must take place and be documented in the record. This inter-provider communication can be done in any form whether it is a written note, letter, or electronic medical record (EMR) reporting mechanism, to the referring provider.
- For consults with no phone contact or minimal phone component 99451 without a modifier can be used if 5 min or more is spent on record review. 99452 can also be used if the time spent is greater than 20 min but this is rare. 99453 and 99454 are not applicable to eye care as these include monitoring of physiologic parameters.
- As long as the provider clearly documents "greater than 5 min spent in encounter," then the time documentation requirements for 99451 will be satisfied. 99451 should not be reported if a transfer of care or request for in-person consult occurs as a result of the consultation within the ensuing 14 days.

As there is not a separate "phone only consult"—telephone codes should be applied only when the provider feels that the phone encounter best describes the encounter. See the telephone encounter section for review.

A noteworthy nuance to the use of these asynchronous telehealth codes is detailed below:

Consider the following situation: After the asynchronous telehealth interpretation, the provider tries to call the patient to discuss findings of the exam but cannot reach the patient. Later, the patient calls back—how should a provider code this encounter?

The provider should initially code 99091 or 99451 for the asynchronous telehealth encounter as he/she did not speak with the patient. Then, if the patient calls back in less than 7 days, if the provider communicates with the patient via synchronous video home based telehealth, the provider can go back and change the prior 99091 or 99451 to the appropriate E/M or consult code with modifier 95 and document total time spent after speaking with the patient. The provider may do this because they may perform medical counseling or modify treatment/management plan after a synchronous video encounter with the patient.

However, if the patient calls back after the 7-day criteria has passed, then the provider would enter a new, separate phone note and code a phone encounter

after speaking with the patient if 99451 was used. This would not apply if 99091 was used as this code includes cumulative time over 30 days.

Other special considerations in asynchronous coding apply:

- The TC (technical component) modifier is no longer required because the workload is not being split into components. Splitting the work into components would be unbundling of the codes and should be avoided.
- If the telehealth facilitator is performing the refraction, image testing, OCT, visual field, they should code for it on the patient side encounter. The provider is using 99091 or 99451, which describes the collection and interpretation of physiologic data. Therefore, 99091 or 99451 will include provider review of all the work the telehealth facilitator has done. TC is not required as it is the telehealth technician who is providing the whole testing service. The provider has a different code for their review/interpretation of all data.

Synchronous telehealth direct to patient is a modality used when the eye provider connects in real-time with the patient, who is either in a non-facility location, such as his/her home, or a healthcare setting, such as a clinic. The key difference here compared to asynchronous is that the eye provider establishes a video connection with the patient. The examination is either conducted by the provider directly with the patient (who may or may not have a family member or helper on the patient end) or a telehealth facilitator is present with the patient in a clinic-based setting.

The provider coding is the same in both types of synchronous telehealth encounters. However, when the patient is in a medical facility with a telehealth facilitator who is a staff member of the medical facility, there will be two encounters billed, one for the provider and one for the telehealth facilitator. The provider codes for his/her care provided regardless of whether the patient is in the clinic or at home. However, if the patient is receiving synchronous telehealth inside a facility, the staff member present acting as the presenter will *also* code an encounter for their work done as the facilitator. For example, the telehealth facilitator may be an eye technician who assists with the exam at the direction of the provider. The eye provider needs to make sure they have appropriate contact information to reestablish phone contact if the video component is lost. CMS allows these synchronous visits (whether to home or to a healthcare setting) to be treated like in-person traditional visits, with the use of modifier 95 (synchronous remote care) for location of services. Of note, during the PHE, this applied to new and established patients.[1]

TABLE 14.4
New Patient E/M ad Eye Codes for Synchronous Telehealth Encounters

E/M or Eye Code	Time Spent	Medical Decision-Making	Place of Service
99201 (Modifier 95)	10 min	Straightforward	11
99202 (Modifier 95)	20 min	Straightforward	11
99203 (Modifier 95)	30 min	Low	11
99204 (Modifier 95)	45 min	Moderate	11
99205 (Modifier 95)	60 min	High	11
92002 (Modifier 95)	n/a for Eye codes	New patient, intermediate exam	11
92004 (Modifier 95)	n/a for Eye codes	New patient, comprehensive exam	11

TABLE 14.5
Established Patient E/M and Eye Codes for Synchronous Telehealth Encounters

E/M or Eye Code	Time Spent	Medical Decision Making	Place of Service
99211 (Modifier 95)	5 min	n/a doesn't qualify	11
99212 (Modifier 95)	10 min	Straightforward	11
99213 (Modifier 95)	15 min	Low	11
99214 (Modifier 95)	25 min	Moderate	11
99215 (Modifier 95)	40 min	High	11
92012 (Modifier 95)	n/a for Eye codes	Established patient, intermediate exam	11
92014 (Modifier 95)	n/a for Eye codes	Established patient, comprehensive exam	11

TABLE 14.6
Synchronous Consult Codes for New or Established Patients

Code	Time spent	Service Rendered
99446	5–10 min	Verbal and written report to consulting provider
99447	11–20 min	Verbal and written report to consulting provider
99448	21–30 min	Verbal and written report to consulting provider
99449	31 or more min	Verbal and written report to consulting provider

For proper documentation, include in note: patient consents to a telehealth visit, patient identification verified by two different identifiers, time spent in encounter, and the appropriate factors, for example, history elements, and physical exam elements;

essentially the same as an in-person visit (Tables 14.4, 14.5, and 14.6).

Note that in Table 14.6, use of any of these consult codes requires *both* a verbal and written report to consulting provider. The consulting provider also needs to have a written consultation request in the medical record and reason for consult documented (the mechanism of the request can be any form of communication—provider-to-provider written, via phone, or electronic or reported by patient and documented in record, but the intent of the consult needs to be documented in the record). More than 50% of time spent must be consultative rather than time spent reviewing data.[6]

DOCUMENTATION GUIDELINES

Documentation required to meet the threshold to use these codes can be existing problems assessed for stability versus change (e.g., glaucoma suspect follow-up) or can be new presenting problem with possible worsening (e.g., possible conversion to wet AMD from previously dry AMD). Any diagnostic tests ordered or reviewed (lab, radiology, or clinical ancillary eye tests such as OCT), and review of past records from old notes or history from patient should be written.[3] Moreover, provider documentation should indicate both new and existing problems and whether these are stable or changing, review of appropriate testing to assess stability versus change, and medical assessment and treatment plan including any over-the-counter or prescription medications, non-pharmaceutical treatment management, any lab, radiology, or clinical testing ordered, and the resultant treatment plan.[3]

If the video component is lost and the practitioner finishes the encounter via the phone only, then the practitioner must decide which exam type best describes this encounter.[1] The practitioner should not bill both an E/M or an Eye code (with Modifier 95) in conjunction with a phone code. The practitioner should choose one or the other. The practitioner should document the time spent in each modality. The level of code is based on this time. There are no strict criteria based on time in each modality that mandates the use of one code or the other. However, the code used should represent the nature of the exam which will most likely reflect the time spent in each modality to some extent. As mentioned earlier, a reasonable rule of thumb would be to consider when vision is assessed. If the video component is present through the vision check, then it might be reasonable to consider the encounter best represented by the synchronous codes listed above. If the video component is lost before the vision is checked, then it might be reasonable to consider the phone code to best represent the encounter. As there is not a clear demarcation to make this decision, this is also a scenario in which it is reasonable to include the clinic or facility coding entity regarding any "rule of thumb" approach that is utilized by the practitioners when making this decision.

Modifications Using HCPCS Codes

Clinicians who may not independently bill for E/M visits can use the following HCPCS codes. "(for example - physical therapists, occupational therapists, speech language pathologists, clinical psychologists)...."[2] These should be established patients and may be rural or non-rural. These should be initiated by the patient, however, "... practitioners may educate beneficiaries on the availability of the service prior to patient initiation...."[2]

- G2061 established patient, up to 7 days, cumulative time during this 7-day period; 5–10 min
- G2062 established patient, up to 7 days, cumulative time during this 7-day period; 11–20 min

- G2063 established patient, up to 7 days, cumulative time during this 7-day period; 21 or more min

Again, in eye telehealth, the practitioners will be able to bill E/M so HCPCS codes are much less likely to be used.

Recall that if the patient is participating in a synchronous clinic-based encounter, the telehealth facilitator also codes the patient-side visit. If the telehealth presenter is working with a clinical provider that does not typically use E/M codes, the telehealth facilitator on the patient side will code Q3014. Additionally, the telehealth facilitator will code for any testing done on the patient side. The clinic testing can include any testing within the scope of care of the telehealth technician as directed by the provider. The technician should document if the patient was sent for an evaluation by another provider (chart notation, per patient report, are all appropriate ways to document the intent of a consult). This will allow the provider to later select the correct type of code for the provider encounter.

When the telehealth technician codes the testing and exam portions completed by him/her, these services will be coded using the same guidelines for testing services administered by the telehealth facilitator, that were described earlier. See the section earlier in this chapter that outlines how the testing services will be coded such as refraction, fundus images, OCT's, visual fields.

RELATIVE VALUE UNITS

It is worth a brief review of RVU, or Relative Value Units. CMS has guidelines of criteria and the numeric RVU worth. Each institution has the leeway to arbitrarily assign values that may not exactly match Medicare RVU values. The amount of RVU assigned can be for different reasons, but during the PHE, it included the goal to facilitate access to care. When a patient could be seen with more than one modality of care, it is worthwhile for a provider to understand what his/her particular institution has assigned for the RVU and if there is an RVU assignment to encourage use of that modality of care (for instance, to facilitate and encourage the use of one form of telehealth over another in order to facilitate access of care for more acute patients).

It is reasonable for providers to understand which modality is preferred by their healthcare facility, so long as the care rendered is high-quality and appropriate. An example of this is the change in RVU value of telephone encounters during the PHE to allow improved access to care without requiring an in-person visit to facilitate social distancing. CMS has increased the RVU of each level of phone code to the next higher comparable

E/M code during the PHE.[1,3] The practitioner may want to take this into consideration when deciding which telehealth modality of care to choose and which modality will best reflect the complexity of the work done. For this reason, it is important to periodically check the institution's RVU assignments. This is particularly important as the RVU generated often has an impact on clinic resource availability, since that may directly be based on provider and clinic productivity.

Using the above coding guidelines, it is important to document thoroughly and correctly and code the appropriate level of care for each modality. Some nuances during the PHE change some of the restrictions for the use of these codes. These nuances may vary from Medicare to other institutions and payers, so it is important to verify any special considerations or exemptions with the institutions with which a practitioner works. For example, Health and Human Services will not conduct audits to distinguish new versus established patients during the PHE.[3]

While writing this chapter, the PHE from COVID-19 was still applicable. Therefore, a brief review of the atypical changes during the PHE is worth consideration. Due to limited clinic access and social distancing, certain requirements have been relaxed or suspended during the PHE. The goal is to best facilitate access to care in a time that clinic access is limited. The flexibilities are expected to last as long as the PHE. It is unknown what will occur after the PHE subsides. Furthermore, practitioners are allowed to inform their patients about the available telehealth options.[1] Other examples of payer specific nuances are the Veterans Administration (VA) decision to waive the requirements of the patient initiating the E/M telephone encounter and the decision to waive the time factors such as visit in the last 7 days.[7] The VA also requires additional documentation when using telephone code in place of an in-person encounter (beyond the CMS required time documentation) including chief complaint, mode of care, pertinent review of history and review of pertinent systems, evidence of medical decision making (MDM), and the actual time interacting with the patient.[7]

When considering the options for the modality of care delivery, a general guideline is to think of the medical telehealth services as encounters that would have normally taken place in-person at the clinic setting. E-communications, some telephone services, and remote evaluation reflect services that would not normally be in-person visits. This is reflected in the RVU structures and therefore, the reimbursement of each.[1] Another nuance is when the provider and the patient are in different locations in the same medical facility. This should not be billed as telemedicine, but as in-person services.[1] The clinic setting for care will guide the decision of which code or type of care delivery is the best code to describe the care given.

CONCLUSION/SUMMARY

In summary, ocular telehealth coding is approached in the same way as coding for any medical care. While this often makes it more straightforward to code for telehealth encounters, telehealth billing and coding is complicated by the nuances that each commercial payer may have somewhat different requirements.[3] The author recommends that telehealth eye providers try to think of the one best code that best describes the care provided. As a provider, consider what options one can choose to deliver the care. Consider what time and complexity is anticipated to address the medical question at hand. Consider any special nuances of facility assigned RVU[8] that is in place to facilitate care. If a particular form of care delivery is encouraged by RVU assignment, then consider if that form of care delivery is an appropriate care modality.

The provider has the ability to choose which format that he/she feels is best or most appropriate to employ for each particular encounter.[2] Always remember, as in all of medicine, document, document, document. Document thoroughly and address the care question at hand. Code appropriately to the level of the care provided. The well-documented chart will always clearly support the code chosen.[1]

REFERENCES

1. COVID-19. *COVID-19 Frequently Asked Question (FAQ) on Medicare Fee-for-Service FSS Billing (Updated 2/8/21)*; 2021.
2. Medicare. *Medicare Telemedicine Health Care Provider Fact Sheet*; 2021.
3. V1.0 April 20, 2020 Office of Connected Care 1 US Dept of Veterans Affairs. *Provider Coding and Reference Sheet Telephone and VA Video Connect*; 2020.
4. CMS.gov Newsroom. *Trump Administration Issues Second Round of Sweeping Changes to Support U.S. Healthcare System During COVID-19 Pandemic.* April 30; 2020.
5. Health Information Management Office of Informatics and Analytics. *Secure Messaging Workload Credit*; January 2020.
6. AAP. *2 New Codes Developed for Interprofessional Consultation. From the AAP Division of Health Care Finance.* January 4; 2019.
7. Health Information Management Office of Informatics. *HIM Practice Brief—Guidelines for Coding Clinical Care.* May 1; 2020.
8. *Coding for Phone Calls, Internet, and Telehealth Consultations. V2. Updated May 4*; 2020.

FURTHER READING

9. Medicare Update Webinar. *The Financial Impact of the CMS Final Fee Schedule Rule on Ophthalmic Practice.* Updated Aug 12; 2020.

10. *CMS Regulatory Relief Bolsters Telehealth Service Payments During COVID-19. April 30;* 2020.

11. Coding for Telemedicine Phone calls, Internet and Telehealth Consultations; American Academy of Ophthalmology; American Academy of Ophthalmic Executives; Contributing Director Sue Vicchrilli, Academy Director of coding and reimbursement. *Coding for Telemedicine Toolkit.* 6-18-2020; 2020.

12. Coding for Phone Calls, Internet and Telehealth Consultations. *American Academy of Ophthalmology 4-16-2021;* 2021.

CHAPTER 15

Ethical and Legal Considerations in Eye Telehealth Programs

DANIEL LEE, BA • APRIL MAA, MD

INTRODUCTION

Telehealth care delivery models have changed how patients interact with their healthcare providers and ocular telehealth is no exception. Even though care can happen across distance and time, the professional and ethical responsibilities of eye providers toward their patients remain unchanged.

As an emerging area of medicine, ocular telehealth presents novel clinical practice issues and challenges, just like other innovations in medicine and healthcare delivery have done in the past. For example, with advancements in genomic sequencing, ethical issues have emerged regarding how results should be disclosed and protected and whether insurance payers can discriminate or limit benefits for patients with a higher risk for medical conditions, like breast cancer.

Thus, eye providers practicing in the ocular telehealth space should know the ethical and medico-legal infrastructure that is in place to protect the patient–provider relationship and ensure high-quality patient care delivery. Eye providers should also continue to be actively engaged in researching and developing evidence-based clinical guidelines, ethical standards, and position statements on best practices.

This chapter focuses on current ethical and legal considerations of ocular telehealth. Although this chapter mainly focuses on practicing eye care in the United States (U.S.), certain principles are universal, and therefore applicable to the U.S. and non-U.S. eye providers alike. It is highly recommended that all eye care providers should review and abide by the ethical and legal requirements of their local region, institution, professionally affiliated associations, and licensing organizations. Additionally, as questions emerge with the continued development of ocular telehealth, it is important for eye providers to stay up to date with new policies and keep track of any changes.

Ocular Telehealth. https://doi.org/10.1016/B978-0-323-83204-5.00015-9

SECTION I: ETHICS IN TELEMEDICINE
The Stance of the American Medical Association, American Optometric Association, and American Academy of Ophthalmology

Since its conception in 1847, the American Medical Association (AMA) has played a crucial role in advancing medicine, including developing and publishing the AMA code of ethics, which articulates the values that physicians should commit themselves to.[1] AMA physician members need to abide by the AMA's Code of Medical Ethics,[2] which is widely accepted as an authoritative source of medical ethics.

The AMA has been regularly publishing telehealth policies, which undergo required review and adoption by the AMA House of Delegates, Board of Trustees, and leadership councils, such as the Council on Ethical and Judicial Affairs (CEJA). CEJA Report 1-A-16 titled "Ethical Practice in Telemedicine" was adopted during the 2016 annual House of Delegates meeting and included in the AMA's Code of Ethics as Code of Medical Ethics Opinion 1.2.12 (Ethical Practice in Telemedicine).[3] This opinion serves as the ethical foundation for healthcare providers practicing telehealth.

Both the American Optometric Association (AOA) and the American Academy of Ophthalmology (AAO), the most prominent eye-provider professional associations, have also published information statements regarding telehealth ethics. The AOA discussed ethical principles in telemedicine in their 2020 *Position Statement Regarding Telemedicine in Optometry*[4] and in a published case study[5] by the AOA's Ethics and Values committee. AAO has created an evidence-based code of ethics that is enforceable and applies to all AAO members.[6] In April 2020, AAO's ethics committee published an information statement for ethics in telemedicine.[7] AAO also described numerous practical applications of these ethical principles in a prior 2018 information statement titled *Telemedicine for Ophthalmology*.[8]

The AMA, AOA, and AAO publications all agree that the provider's standard of care and fundamental professional and ethical responsibilities do not change when providing care through telehealth means.[3,4,7] AAO further requires following the Academy's code of ethics and adhering to applicable laws that govern the practice of telemedicine.[7] Both the AOA and AAO organizations outline similar ethical principles specifically relevant for the unique patient–provider relationship and interactions during a telehealth visit.

Ethical principles that govern telehealth can largely be divided into two categories: (1) the provider's responsibility for providing eye care and (2) the

provider's obligation to the patient. The ethical tenets under these two categories and their corresponding table subsection that summarizes findings are as follows:
(1) **Provider's responsibility for providing eye care:**
   - Competence (Table 15.1)
   - Conflict of Interest (Table 15.2)
   - Confidentiality (Table 15.3)
   - Preservation of Data (Table 15.4)
   - Quality Improvement & Equitable distribution of care (Table 15.5)
(2) **Provider's obligation to the patient:**
   - Informed Consent (Table 15.6)
   - Continuity of Care (Table 15.7)

SECTION II: LEGAL CONSIDERATIONS

Disclaimer: Please note, eye care providers should not consider the following legal information to be completely comprehensive or guaranteed. This chapter was intended for informational and educational purposes only, and its content was based on what was available during the time of publication. Providers are responsible for abiding by state and federal laws in addition to familiarizing themselves with the ongoing changes. State-by-state information on telehealth legal and regulatory issues, including licensing, can be found at a website developed by the Center for Connected Health Policy (CCHP).[11] Additionally, it is appropriate for providers to consult legal experts and their state's health professional licensing boards/organizations for guidance or clarification. Furthermore, working with a reputable telemedicine company could better ensure up-to-date compliance with credentialing and licensure policies.

Basics of Telehealth and Licensing—State Licensing

In the U.S., medical licensure is the jurisdiction of the individual states. Each state determines credentialing requirements of health professionals, thus, providers must be credentialed and licensed by the state before being able to practice.

To provide ocular telehealth services, eye care professionals are typically required to be licensed in the state where the patient is located at the time of care. For example, for an eye provider located in California to provide telehealth care to a patient who resides in Texas, the eye care provider must be licensed with Texas. However, if the patient travels to Alabama, the eye care provider must also be licensed with Alabama to provide telehealth services while the patient is traveling to this state. Otherwise, the provider could be exposed to legal risk and liability, even if the breach was

TABLE 15.1
Provider's Responsibility for Providing Eye Care—Competence

AMA[3]	AOA[4]	AAO[7,8]	Examples
• Be proficient in using the relevant telemedicine technologies • Be comfortable interacting with patients and surrogates electronically • Recognize and appropriately address the limitations of telemedicine technologies • Ensure the adequacy of gathered information to make well-grounded clinical recommendations • Be prudent with diagnostic evaluations and online prescribing by: (i) confirm the patient's identity (ii) confirm that telehealth/telemedicine services are appropriate for the patient's individual and medical needs (iii) follow best practice guidelines and any formulary limitations that apply to prescribing electronically (iv) document the prescription and clinical evaluation	• Ensure that patients are aware of limitations of telemedicine and when clinically appropriate, promptly refer or provide in-person care • Maintain documentation of training programs and proof of competency for any technician or clinician who is capturing clinical data or providing optometric telemedicine • Provide or participate in an ongoing training program in telemedicine and • Have a list of criteria for both the distant and receiving sites • Have a good understanding of the culture, healthcare infrastructure, and resources available to the patient at the originating site	• Only perform procedures that the ophthalmologist is competent in via specific training or experience. Alternatively, be assisted by one who is • Do not misrepresent credentials, training, experience, ability, or results • Be sufficiently proficient in using telemedicine platforms to comfortably interact with patients electronically • Consulting ophthalmologists at the distant site should receive initial training and periodic re-evaluation to meet quality standards • Confirm medical malpractice liability coverage for telemedicine activities from their insurer. • Meet the state licensure requirements in the state where the patient resides	• When ocular telehealth management requires a physical examination to ensure the adequacy of the gathered information, have another health care professional at the patient's site conduct the exam—also, obtaining vital information through remote technologies[3] • Many aspects of a slit lamp exam may not be possible or severely limited with current telemedicine platforms, especially if an anterior segment problem is suspected. The eye provider should recognize and appropriately plan for these limitations[6]

Consulting ophthalmologists must review and abide the laws and regulations pertaining to the practice of telemedicine across state borders. Additional details can be found in this chapter's section on licensing.

TABLE 15.2
Provider's Responsibility for Providing Eye Care—Conflict of Interest

AMA[3]	AOA[4]	AAO[7]	Examples
• Disclose any financial or other interests in telemedicine application or service • Proactively manage or eliminate conflicts of interest	• In alignment with AMA	• In alignment with AMA	• Eye care providers should disclose to patients any incentives, investments, intellectual property, and any relationships or activities that may be perceived as a conflicting interest to their care, for example, if they owned significant stock in the telehealth platform they are using.

TABLE 15.3
Provider's Responsibility for Providing Eye Care—Confidentiality

AMA[3]	AOA[4]	AAO[7]	Examples
• Secure appropriate protocols for telemedicine services to prevent unauthorized access • Protect the security and integrity of patient information: (i) at all stages of the electronic encounter (ii) among all professionals and personnel who participate in the telehealth/telemedicine services in accordance to their roles	• Ensure that all protected health and personal information is held in confidence • Provide HIPPA-compliant care • Encrypt all electronic transmissions • Ensure reasonable authentication protocols for clinicians who have electronic access to records	• Provide HIPPA-compliant care • Transmit video and images with proper security protocols, including encryption • Inform patients of the unique, inherent risks to telemedicine and discuss steps that the patient can take to protect confidential information	• Note in the consent form at the point of service and the HIPAA notice of privacy practice that the patient's information will be traveling by electronic means to another site for consultation[4]

Due to international privacy laws and HIPAA in the U.S., the ethical principle of confidentiality is also a legal requirement. Furthermore, when the patient's data is being evaluated by someone outside of a physician's practice, **"business associate" agreements** are necessarily in order to comply with HIPPA requirements.[8]

TABLE 15.4
Provider's Responsibility for Providing Eye Care—Preservation of Data

AMA[3]	AOA[4]	AAO[7]	Examples
• See AOA and AAO columns	• Properly document any eye, health, or vision services provided by telemedicine • Ensure the availability of these health records to the remote site, originating site, and patient	• Record and preserve any gathered clinical data to facilitate continuity of care (just like one would for an in-office interaction) • Consider and address how the data will be stored at the end of the encounter and will be recovered in case of system failure, keeping in mind that telemedicine providers may not have an ongoing relationship with the patient and the unique risks of storing information online	• Ensure information gathered from a telehealth visit is stored properly in the electronic medical record. • Ensure information is transmitted in HIPPA compliant manner; password protected.

TABLE 15.5 Provider's Responsibility for Providing Eye Care—Quality improvement & Equitable Distribution of Care			
AMA[3]	**AOA**[4]	**AAO**[7]	**Examples**

Collectively, through their professional organizations and health care institutions, physicians should:
• Support the continuous refinement of telehealth/telemedicine technologies
• Support the improvement and implementation of clinical and technical standards ensuring patient safety and quality
• Advocate for policies and initiatives to promote access for all patients who could benefit from receiving telehealth/telemedicine services
• Routinely monitor the evolution of the telehealth/telemedicine technology and landscape to:
  (i) identify and address adverse consequences
  (ii) identify and disseminate both positive and negative outcomes
	• Assure that remote monitoring devices are being utilized in a clinically appropriate manner
	• Weigh the risks and benefits of medical devices in an evidence-based approach to ensure efficacy and quality and to protect the public health
		• Periodically evaluate equipment, personnel, and clinical outcomes to ensure compliance with established quality control metrics
		• Assess program quality by specifying the metrics for processes and workflow
		• Continually address technological failures and support advances to improve quality and access to care
			• Incorporate re-reads in addition to inter- and intra-reader variability of readings as part of quality assurance programs[7]
			• When assessing screening services, one quality metric is the rate of referred patients completing any follow-up referrals for examination or treatment[7]

Connectivity Gap/Digital Divide: Although patients in remote areas or those who are socioeconomically disadvantaged may be most at need and benefit the most through access to telemedicine, they may not have access to this type of technology.[9]

TABLE 15.6 Provider's Obligation to the Patient—Informed Consent.			
AMA[3]	**AOA**[4]	**AAO**[7]	**Examples**
• Inform patients regarding the limitations of the relationship and services provided by telemedicine • Modify the informed consent to inform patients about the distinctive features of telehealth/telemedicine in addition to medical issues and treatment options	• In alignment with AMA • Inform patients of their right to choose in-person eye, health, and vision services at any time	• In alignment with AMA • Ensure that patients understand how telemedicine will be used in their care, the technology's limitations, and expectations of patients when using these technologies.	• The Ophthalmic Mutual Insurance Company (OMIC) provides a sample consent to treatment via telehealth form for ophthalmologists.[10]

Some states require a separate informed consent for the use of telemedicine in addition to a general informed consent for providing care.[8] Additional details can be found in this chapter's section on licensing.

TABLE 15.7
Provider's Obligation to the Patient – Continuity of Care

AMA[3]	AOA[4]	AAO[7]	Examples
• Consider how information can be preserved and accessible for future episodes of care and how follow-up care can be provided when needed • Advise users how to arrange for follow-up care when indicated • Encourage users with primary care physicians to inform them about the online health consultation, even if in-person care is not immediately needed • Assure how information will be communicated to the patient's primary care physician and other physicians currently caring for the patient	• Ensure protocols to facilitate and refer for follow-up care, in addition to urgent and emergent services, in the patient's local geographical area	• Advise the patient on follow-up care and next steps after completing the consultation • When possible and with the patient's permission, provide results from the telemedicine consultation to the patient's local primary care provider and/or local eye care provider.	• Arrange follow-up care for patients that would be no different than if they were examined through a traditional in-person clinic visit.

In addition to alerting the patient's primary care provider of acute or urgent findings, **timely reporting** (within applicable medically-defined guidelines and any local, state, or federal regulatory standards) is necessary, with a goal to expedite interpretation as appropriate to the circumstances.[8] Failure to communicate test results is the foundation of numerous malpractice suits and adverse awards.[8] Additional details in legal/liability section.

an unintended mistake. The risks include but are not limited to violating state law, receiving sanctions, and losing malpractice insurance coverage. The AOA and AAO both urge providers to review the laws and state board regulations in their state and the patient's state and abide by all licensing and legal requirements.[4,8]

Despite telehealth's ability to easily provide care in remote locations, the states' credentialing and licensing requirement can pose significant limitations and barriers for both providers and patients. This situation creates an administrative and cost burden to providers in procuring additional licenses. As a result, a provider's ability to provide care via telehealth may be limited geographically. The licensing requirement also creates barriers for patients, who need to find specialized providers licensed in their home state to receive telehealth care. Moreover, patients who travel across state lines for leisure or business may be unable to see their home eye care provider that is most familiar with the patient's conditions, needs, and treatments if their telehealth encounter occurs in a state where their normal provider is not licensed.

Recognizing that state-by-state licensure laws limit healthcare professionals and patients from providing and receiving care, several states have adopted exceptions to the state licensure requirement. These exceptions outline scenarios where a healthcare provider is licensed in one state to deliver care in another state where the provider is not licensed. In addition, health professional organizations have created licensure compacts to facilitate interstate collaboration and to expedite out-of-state licensing, which can be utilized by both telemedicine and non-telemedicine practitioners alike.

As state licensure laws and health professional licensing models adapt to the rapid advancement of telemedicine, being able to practice interstate ocular telehealth should become more convenient over time. The following sections describe the current landscape of these exceptions and licensure compacts.

Point of clarification for providers
Unless legal exceptions or waivers for specific scenarios are applicable, if one of the eye provider's regular

patients is on vacation or business travel in another state, to provide care via telemedicine, the eye provider is generally required to be licensed where the patient is during the encounter. Additionally, suppose the provider has patients who regularly come for care from out of state. In that case, the eye provider must be licensed in their home state to provide medicolegally defined care via telemedicine if they reach out to the provider from their home residence. Although this might seem like a too-rigid interpretation and may be a common occurrence for some providers, eye pracitioners should review applicable state laws or consult a trusted legal source to identify exceptions and practice within legal, licensing requirements. Another solution is to ensure providers who may routinely see patients from neighboring states to obtain additional licenses in relevant states. In this scenario, if telemedicine care needs to be provided and the regular eye provider is not licensed in the state where the patient happens to be located at the time, the provider should identify and direct out-of-state patients to alternative sources to obtain care, as necessary. According to the Ophthalmic Mutual Insurance Company (OMIC), confirming the patient's location should become a vital process in telemedicine practice protocols.[12]

Exceptions to The State Licensing Requirement

The general rule of thumb is that providers must be licensed by the state where the patient is located at the time of service. However, several states have implemented exceptions for telemedicine or eased the restrictions by allowing license portability.

Examples include:

- *Licensure portability and bordering state reciprocity:* Currently, the states of New York, Virginia, Maryland, and the territory of Washington D.C. allow licensure reciprocity from bordering states. In more rare cases, like in South Dakota, states may allow medical license reciprocity from any state, but providers must meet specific requirements.

- *Issuance of telemedicine license:* Several states, including Minnesota, Louisiana, New Mexico, Texas, and Georgia, will issue telemedicine licenses for physicians who are licensed out of state.

These exemption policies and the state allowed exemptions have changed over time. Currently, the interactive map created by the Center for Connected Health Policy (CCHP) tracks the most up-to-date information (Fig. 15.1).

States may also temporarily waive state licensure requirements during a natural disaster or state of emergency. The state usually declares the exemption in the form of an executive order to meet the state's healthcare needs. Notably, during the time of writing and publication of this textbook, state regulations governing telemedicine were relaxed in response to the COVID-19 pandemic and the increased need for rapid implementation of care modalities that allowed

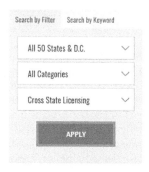

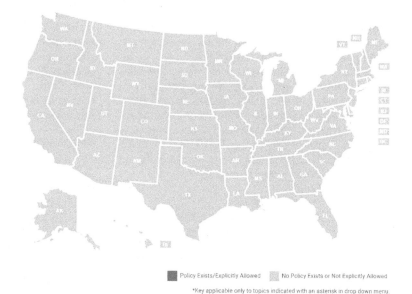

FIG. 15.1 The Center for Connected Health Policy's interactive map of state-by-state policies (as of February 2021).[13] (Credit: From the Center for Connected Health Policy; used with permission.)

for social distancing. More than 40 states and U.S. territories, like Washington D.C., instituted a temporary licensure waiver during the pandemic. The Federation of State Medical Boards published and maintained an updated collection of states and territories with waivers for licensure requirements for telehealth adopted for COVID19.[14] Some of them may opt to continue relaxed laws indefinitely, and some states may eventually expire the waivers. Given the ever-changing nature of waived licensure requirements in response to the pandemic, it is best to consult a trusted source to determine the most current state laws and regulations governing telemedicine.

Aims to address the telehealth barrier has been made at the federal level as well. In 2018, the United States Department of Veterans Affairs (VA) expanded their telehealth services by overriding state licensing restrictions and allowing VA telehealthcare providers to provide care to VA patients in states where the provider is not licensed.[15]

However, not all large health systems provide licensing exceptions. For example, Kaiser Permanente can capitalize on the benefits of telehealth through better coordination of care through its large, integrated system. However, Kaiser providers are still required to follow state licensing requirements. Kaiser Permanente supports legislation in states where they operate to implement compacts, like the Interstate Medical Licensure Compact (IMLC), so physicians could expedite their licensing process.[16]

In addition to the reasons listed above, some other examples of exceptions include when the health professional is a military spouse, or an employee of a federal government agency or facility. Exceptions could also be provided when health professionals consult another peer or provide temporary, infrequent consultation to a patient. Finally, in some states, there is a limited number of remote patient visits per year that a physician without that state's license can respond to when a pre-existing patient-provider relationship exists.

A comprehensive and complete list of exceptions is outside the scope of this textbook. For additional details and lists of exceptions, eye care providers should consult the licensing board of their state and their potential patients' states.

Health Professional Compacts—Expediting the Out-of-state Licensing Process

Recognizing that physicians (MD/DO) will practice across different states more often than before with the advancement of telemedicine, the Interstate Medical Licensure Compact (IMLC) was created. The IMLC is an agreement between participating states to streamline the licensing process for physicians who want to practice in multiple states. It offers an expedited pathway to qualifying physicians through participating compact states.

A growing number of states and the U.S. territories have joined the compact since its inception in April 2017, especially with the advancement and widespread adoption of telemedicine. In February 2021, the compact included 29 states, the District of Columbia, and the territory of Guam. The IMLC compact is represented by the map in Fig. 15.2.

The IMLC substantially reduces the administrative and financial burden on providers and increases access to care for patients. Physicians only need to apply with one common application to join the compact, and they can use the common application to qualify for licensure in any compact state of their choosing. Costs include the initial application of $700 and the additional cost of licensing in the desired compact state, which ranges from $75 to $700.[18]

At this time, there are no interstate compacts for Optometry. However, a public memo from 2017 between the Federal Trade Commission and the National Association of Optometrists and Opticians regarding occupational licensing reform advocates for adopting interstate compacts or model laws to facilitate licensure mobility in the future.[19] Thus, an interstate compact for Optometry could be established in the near future, especially with the current rapid advancements in telehealth.

Until then, optometrists can still practice out of state but need to follow the licensing requirements for each desired state. Optometrists should acquaint themselves with telemedicine regulations and licensing requirements for each state in which they desire to practice due to their wide variation. For example, optometrists only need to complete an out-of-state telehealth provider registration to practice ocular telehealth in Florida without a Florida state license.[20] In contrast, Oregon requires out-of-state optometrists to be licensed in Oregon, and the licensing process involves a written examination.[21]

Telehealth and HIPAA

The standards of complying with the Health Insurance Portability and Accountability Act (HIPAA) are the same for telemedicine as in office. The goal is to protect sensitive health information and patients' privacy from being inappropriately breached without their consent or knowledge.

In the *Telemedicine for Ophthalmology statement*, AAO outlines specific aspects of telemedicine to ensure HIPAA compliance as follows[8]:

- *Staff*: Everyone involved with telemedicine should be familiar and compliant with HIPAA.
- *Equipment*: All equipment used in ocular telemedicine should be either HIPAA-compliant or used in

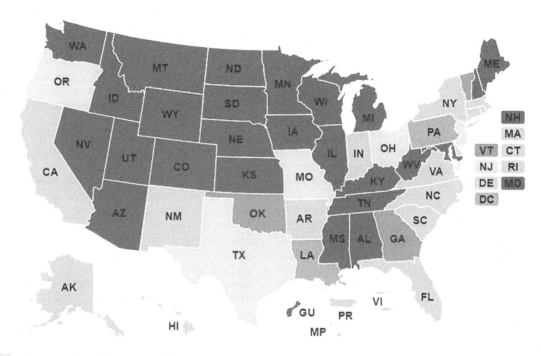

= Compact Legislation Introduced

= IMLC Member State serving as SPL processing applications and issuing licenses*

= IMLC Member State non-SPL issuing licenses*

= IMLC Passed; Implementation In Process or Delayed*

* Questions regarding the current status and extent of these states' and boards' participation in the IMLC should be directed to the respective state boards.

FIG. 15.2 U.S. States and Territories participating in the Interstate Medical Licensure Compact (as of February 2021).[17] (Credit: From the Interstate Medical Licensure Compact; with permission.)

a HIPAA-compliant manner. This applies to information acquisition devices (cameras, tonometers, visual field machines, etc.) and data transmission devices (computers, servers, network devices, etc.).

- *Data security:* In addition to using HIPAA compliant equipment, information technology staff should regularly validate proper security, integrity, and availability of data. Also, all data transmissions, including images and videos, should include appropriate security measures and encryption.
- *Business associate agreements (BAA):* BAAs compliant with HIPAA should be in place between all covered entities involved with telemedicine services.

Additionally, in the *Position Statement regarding Telemedicine in Optometry*, AOA suggests a reasonable authentication process for accessing electronic records and the consent form to disclose that the patient's information will be traveling electronically to another location for evaluation and consultation.[4]

Coverage and Payment: State Level

At the state level, telehealth payment and coverage laws pertain to Medicaid and commercial insurance. Overall, the trend has been to expand the coverage for telehealth services. Details of each category are summarized below. For more details, refer to Chapter 14.

Medicaid

According to the Center for Medicare & Medicaid Services (CMS), telemedicine is considered a cost-effective alternative to in-person services; CMS encourages states to expand telemedicine coverage.[22]

At the time of publication, all 50 states and D.C. reimburse synchronous, live video telehealth services. However, the extent of coverage varies widely among states and depends on the specialty, type of provider, and patient's location (i.e., clinical setting).

Eighteen state Medicaid programs offer coverage for asynchronous, store-and-forward services. However, some state Medicaid programs that do not cover store-and-forward services have exceptions for certain services. For instance, Maryland's program does not reimburse store-and-forward but does not consider the fields of dermatology, ophthalmology, and radiology to fit into the definition of store-and-forward.

Twenty-one state Medicaid programs have some form of coverage for remote patient monitoring, with varying levels of restrictions and specifications. Additionally, 32 states cover transmission fees, facility fees, or both.

Up-to-date information on state-specific Medicaid coverage can be found on the Center for Connected Health Policy's interactive map of state-by-state policies[13].

Commercial Insurance

Significant variations exist among state laws regarding telehealth coverage, but two fundamental concepts, telehealth coverage and telehealth payment parity, have emerged.

Telehealth coverage laws require health plans to provide the same coverage to telemedicine services as in-person services. This law provides patients with the option to decide to see their provider via telehealth or in-office. At the time of publication, 43 states and the district of Columbia expanded laws requiring private payers to cover telehealth.

Telehealth payment parity laws require telehealth be reimbursed at the same rate as an in-person service. This law prevents health plans from only paying a percentage of the in-person rate for telemedicine services. This issue exists in many states that incorporated telehealth coverage law without a payment parity law, effectively nullifying telehealth coverage's legal establishment. Essentially, without a payment parity law, providing telehealth becomes financially disadvantageous and unsustainable, discouraging providers from providing these services. Thus, even if health insurance carriers are obligated to cover telehealth services, patients would not experience the technology's benefits to its full effect due to diminished supply. As of 2019, only 16 states have mandated payment parity for private insurance compared to 28 states with Medicaid payment parity coverage.[23] Therefore, further advancement in payment parity laws is required. Otherwise, the widely established telehealth coverage laws

functionally remain ineffective as providers will be disincentivized to offer telehealth services.

Up-to-date information on state-specific commercial coverage can be found on the Center for Connected Health Policy's interactive map of state-by-state policies[13].

Coverage and Payment: Federal Level

In comparison to the state level, Medicare substantially lags behind telemedicine coverage and payment due to statutory limitations. Eligibility is determined by rural geography, type of originating site, type of distant site practitioner, and telecommunication technology.

The rural geographic restriction is the most limiting. Medicare mandates that patients be at a qualifying originating site in a rural healthcare professional shortage area, rural census tract, or a county outside of a metropolitan statistical area. The vast majority of Medicare patients are ineligible for telehealth services because they live in non-rural communities. As of 2000, the Secretary of Human Health and Services (HHS) made exceptions to geographical restrictions for entities participating in a federal telehealth demonstration project. The HHS created a website called "Medicare Telehealth Payent Eligiblity Analyzer," where one can verify all telemedicine eligible sites.[24]

In addition to the georgraphical restriction, telemedicine services is further limited by all other Medicare imposed restrictions as follows[25]:

- *Eligible originating site:*
  - Physician and practitioner offices
  - Hospitals
  - Critical Access Hospitals (CAHs)
  - Rural Health Clinics
  - Federally Qualified Health Centers
  - Hospital-based or CAH-based Renal Dialysis Centers (including satellites)
  - Skilled Nursing Facilities (SNFs)
  - Community Mental Health Centers (CMHCs)
  - Renal Dialysis Facilities
  - Homes of beneficiaries with End-Stage Renal Disease (ESRD) getting home dialysis
  - Mobile Stroke Units
- *Eligible distant site practitioners:*
  - Physicians
  - Nurse practitioners (NPs)
  - Physician assistants (PAs)
  - Nurse-midwives
  - Clinical nurse specialists (CNSs)
  - Certified registered nurse anesthetists
  - Clinical psychologists (CPs) and clinical social workers (CSWs)
  - Registered dietitians or nutrition professional

- *Eligible telehealth technology:*
  - Real-time visitations with interactive audio and video telecommunication must be used. Store-and-forward is only permitted in Alaska and Hawaii Federal demonstration programs.

Hospital Telehealth Credentialing

Both the Centers for Medicare and Medicaid Services (CMS) and Joint Commission Standard require credentialing and privilege for health practitioners providing services, including telemedicine. This process is an essential component of healthcare to ensure patient safety.

To streamline this process, both organizations offer a streamlined credentialing process called "credentialing by proxy (CBT)." It allows originating sites to rely on the privilege and credentialing of the distant site providing the telehealth services, as long as specific criteria are met.

CBT is far less time-consuming and efficient than the traditional credentialing process. It allows originating site hospitals to utilize telemedicine services more easily without facing the full administrative burden associated with the traditional credentialing process, which would still be undertaken by practitioners at the distant site.

The CBT can only be utilized when the practitioner who provides telemedicine services is located at either a Medicare-participating distant site hospital or a Distant Site Telemedicine Entity (DSTE). A DSTE is an entity that provides telemedicine services, is not a Medicare entity, and provides all contracted services that allow the originating site to meet Medicare Conditions of Participation.

Furthermore, the originating and distant site needs to enter into a written agreement, including specific requirements that enable shared decision-making on credentialing and continued quality assessment and improvement. However, even with an established written agreement, originating sites are not required to use the CBP process for any or all telemedicine practitioners.

Details regarding the contractual agreement and further considerations regarding CBT can be found in the *NAMSS-ATA Credentialing by Proxy Guidebook* created by the National Association Medical Staff Services (NAMSS) and American Telemedicine Association (ATA) in 2019.[26]

Informed Consent

Several states require specific informed consent for the use of telemedicine in addition to general consent requirements. These consent requirements could be incorporated as part of a Medicaid policy, law, or regulation.

OMIC provides a sample consent form for ophthalmologists.[10] It outlines both benefits and risks of using telemedicine, including the risk of a potential delay in medical treatment due to limited or inadequate information gathering, breach of privacy and personal information, and lack of access to full medical records resulting in potential medical errors and adverse drug or allergic reactions. Also, the AOA recommends informing the patient about opting out at any time in favor of in-person visitations.[4]

Providers should ensure that consent forms are compliant with legal and contractual requirements.

Patient–Provider Relationship

A valid patient–provider relationship is critical for the practice of telemedicine. Not only is establishing this relationship an ethical duty, but it is also a legal requirement in most states. Once a patient–provider relationship is established, all in-person requirements of standard of care and legal issues, such as informed consent, prescription, and tort liability, become applicable. In some circumstances, the law has argued that just casual discussion with a patient may establish a doctor-patient relationship, even if the doctor does not intend for this to occur. Therefore, a telehealth visit of any kind (even a telephone visit) may establish a doctor-patient relationship, and eye providers should be mindful of this fact to prevent taking on unintended medical liability.

In most states, a patient–provider relationship can be established through a real-time synchronous audio-visual telemedicine encounter. However, providers need to review and confirm the laws of each applicable state. Some states have specific requirements, such as a prior in-person visitation, a telehealth facilitator being with the patient for the initial telemedicine examination, or the patient being at an established medical site during the initial telemedicine visit. How and when a provider can use telemedicine after establishing a doctor-patient relationship does involve two different and somewhat bifurcating concepts. The first is related to patient-doctor relationship and reimbursement. The state may limit the ability of the provider to practice telehealth without first meeting the requirements of a patient-provider relationship (e.g. having an in-person exam first) and if a provider doesn't meet the state's requirements, they may not be paid for the telemedicine visit. However, the tort system would treat providers as having a doctor-patient relationship for malpractice situations even if the telehealth visit was not reimbursable or a patient care relationship not established from the state's perspective. Eye providers should know the specific state laws regarding required prerequisites to establish a patient-provider relationship for telehealth, ensure they meet those standards, and then treat the telehealth visit equal to a traditional in-office visit from the perspective of patient care and medical liability.

Prescribing Online Via Telemedicine for Ophthalmologists

Most states allow physicians with a valid doctor–patient relationship to prescribe medication after a telehealth examination. The current gold-standard approach is when the provider conducts a synchronous audio-video exam after reviewing that patient's records.[27] However, state law may have more specific requirements, such as an initial in-person examination of the patient. Most states do not consider using only an online questionnaire to establish a patient–provider relationship to be adequate for prescribing medication.

Remotely prescribing controlled substances is a more complex issue. Physicians need to follow both state and federal law. Federal law supersedes state law unless the state law is more strict, which is usually the case.

Up-to-date information on state-specific online prescribing for physicians can be found on the Center for Connected Health Policy's interactive map of state-by-state policies.[13]

Prescribing Online Via Telemedicine for Optometrists—Pharamaceuticals and Corrective Lenses

Online prescribing for optometrists via telemedicine is state-dependent as well. In most states, optometrists have prescription authority to most or all topical and oral medications. Many states also allow the prescription of oral steroids and a short duration of controlled substances. Optometrists should review state law and licensing boards to confirm online prescribing requirements, as regulations on both in-person and online prescribing vary state by state.

For example, in Alabama, optometrists can prescribe medication online with a proper provider–patient relationship established by at least one face-to-face meeting via in-person or online.[28] Also, the provider must confirm the identity of the patient.[28] As another example, California law also allows optometrists to prescribe medication online, including limited duration of controlled substances.[29] Again, most states do not consider using only an online questionnaire to establish a patient–provider relationship to be adequate for prescribing medication.

In terms of offering a prescription for glasses or contact lenses, the AOA has a specific stance regardless of privileges allowed by state law. In the absence of an existing doctor–patient relationship, AOA advises against offering prescriptions for glasses or contact lenses without an in-person comprehensive exam. Crucial elements of the exam cannot be delivered independently through tele-optometry, and the care would not be meet the current standard of care.[4] For instance, visiting the eye doctor for a comprehensive eye exam could result in an earlier diagnosis of asymptomatic conditions such as glaucoma and early diabetic retinopathy. However, the current telemedicine technology involving remote, refraction-only tests, would miss detecting these diseases, and optometrists would not be able to provide the same standard of care via telemedicine as in-person.[5] Given the current limitations of telemedicine, prescribing of corrective eyewear under these circumstances, for both new and existing patients, would be a violation of an optometrist's ethical obligations and duty of care.

Telemedicine Tort Liability—Entering a New Legal Frontier

Tort liability is based on negligence due to a breach of duty within the provider–patient relationship. Generally, it is considered a state-law issue, where states allow patients to make a malpractice claim against a provider, regardless of the provider's state of residence.

Although malpractice lawsuits have existed for a long time, telemedicine is a relatively newer healthcare delivery model. Thus, much less is known regarding telehealth lawsuits and outcomes are less predictable. Also, the majority of malpractice claims, both telemedicine and in-person, are either dismissed or settled via confidential agreements, so claim results are not accessible via public court records.

There is limited legal precedent to fully assess telemedicinal liability exposure. Professional organizations have weighed in on specific circumstances as follows:
- *AAO*[7]:
  - The reading center is liable for errors in reading.
  - If a licensed physician does not perform the interpretation of images, there should be a physician who is ultimately responsible for interpreting the images to avoid charges of unauthorized medical practice.
- *AOA*[4]:
  - If there is no assistance provided by referring site, the consulting doctor bears full responsibility.
  - Given that management recommendation are based solely on the information provided by the patient, liability should be based on the information available at the time of service.
  - In a consultative model (doctor-to-doctor), liability may be shared, but the allocations may vary on a case-by-case and state-by-state basis.

Due to the immature legal landscape of telemedicine tort lawsuits, accurately discerning legal liability may not end up being so black-and-white. The best course of action that eye care providers can take is ensuring appropriate malpractice insurance coverage before providing telehealth services and reducing liability risk within their practice.

Telemedicine malpractice insurance

Providers should ensure that their malpractice insurance carrier provides coverage for telehealth services in all jurisdictions in which they intend to practice, especially if the practice is across multiple states. Many malpractice insurance carriers offer coverage for telehealth services in their original agreement. However, some carriers will not include telemedicine coverage in the original agreement unless specifically requested. Also, coverage may have restrictions such as only covering the state where the insurance company is licensed or only allowing peer-to-peer consultation but not direct telehealth care to patients.

Providers should consult with malpractice carriers and carefully select among the various carriers and plans for adequate coverage of all activities and services. Considerations should include[30]:

- Provides a policy that extends coverage in all states and jurisdictions that the provider will provide services.
- Provides well-defined and extensive telehealth malpractice coverage.
- Provides coverage for claims brought by patient's estate.
- Provides coverage for claims brought by state licensing or health regulatory boards.

Mitigating telemedicine tort liability risk

In addition to ensuring adequate malpractice coverage, providers should take steps to reduce liability risk. Telehealth companies have taken various steps to manage tort liability risk such as[30]:

- Regularly polling patient satisfaction with telehealth services and communication.
- Identifying and addressing telemedicine professionals subject to frequent patient complaints.
- Addressing complaints promptly by contractually requiring telemedicine professionals to notify the provider group within 3 days of the complaint.
- Understanding and following applicable laws and guidance in each state where telehealth services are offered.
- Only providing services in states where the provider is licensed and authorized.

- Incorporating industry practice guidelines and standards, such as practice guidelines published by the American Telemedicine Association.
- Documenting patient understanding of terms of use, limitations, and associated conditions.

Additionally, OMIC has provided several steps to mitigate telemedicine liability risk as follows[12]:

- Stay connected and maintain the physician–patient relationship.
- Do not lose patients to follow-up; do not wait for patients to contact you, especially if the care or communication of test results is urgent.
  - The AAO also emphasizes that the failure to communicate test results has been the foundation of numerous malpractice lawsuits and adverse outcomes[7]
- Contact your medical professional liability insurance company to confirm coverage for telemedicine and to help guide you on complying with state and federal regulations.
- Do not assume blanket exemptions or waivers in states where your patients are located.
  - Monitor state law, as failure to comply can be used by the plaintiff attorney and negatively impact the defense of a professional liability claim.
- Account for the limitations of telemedicine.
- Include specific accommodations for patients with special needs per the Americans with Disabilities Act.
- Proactively manage the patient's expectations regarding telemedicine by utilizing a well-executed informed consent process.
- Document all information obtained in telemedicine just like any other communication with the patient.

CONCLUSION

Telemedicine is the same as an in-person examination in terms of the physician–patient relationship and regardless of the location of the patient, provider, or telehealth modality utilized, the ethics of practicing telemedicine is equivalent to the ethics of practicing medicine. From the perspective of licensure and tort liability, providers should be licensed in the state that the patient is located in, and licensure compacts can help mitigate some of the cumbersome barriers of practicing interstate. Finally, providers should follow best practices in reducing tort liability in both traditional clinic and telemedicine visits by actively maintaining a healthy provider–patient relationship, conducting appropriate informed consent, communicating results timely, verifying that their malpractice insurance will cover telehealth services, and educating themselves on the state specific rules for telemedicine.

Ultimately, by following the principles outlined in this chapter, it is possible to ethically and safely provide care through ocular telehealth programs. The ability to do so allows for a powerful tool to supplement eye care across the world that improves patient quality of life and promotes global healthcare equity.

ACKNOWLEDGMENTS

We would like to gratefully acknowledge the AAO and the AAO ethics committee chair, Dr. Ron Pelton M.D. Ph.D., for reviewing and providing feedback on this chapter. We also thank Dr. Paul Lee M.D. J.D., Director of University of Michigan's Kellogg Eye Center, and Linda Harrison Ph.D., OMIC's director of risk management, for sharing their expertise, feedback, and suggestions.

REFERENCES

1. *Code of Medical Ethics Overview.* https://www.ama-assn. org/delivering-care/ethics/code-medical-ethics-overview. Accessed 24.01.21.
2. *Council on Ethical & Judicial Affairs (CEJA).* https://www. ama-assn.org/councils/council-ethical-judicial-affairs. Accessed 24.01.21.
3. Opinion 1.2.12—Ethical Practice in Telemedicine AMA Code of Medical Ethics Opinion—Chapter 1: Patient-Physician Relationships https://www.ama-assn.org/ delivering-care/ethics/ethical-practice-telemedicine. Accessed 24.01.21.
4. *Position Statement Regarding Telemedicine in Optometry;* 2020. https://www.aoa.org/AOA/Documents/Advocacy/ position%20statements/AOA_Policy_Telehealth.pdf. Accessed 4 February 2021.
5. Kenneth Lawenda OD, Robert Moses OD. *Case Study No. 17: Telehealth Care/Telemedicine;* 2021. https://documents. aoa.org/about-the-aoa/ethics-and-values/ethics-forum/ telehealth-care/telemedicine.
6. Code of Ethics. https://www.aao.org/ethics-detail/code-of-ethics. Accessed 24.01.21.
7. Information Statement. *Ethics in Telemedicine. April 28, 2020.* https://www.aao.org/ethics-detail/information-statement-ethics-in-telemedicine. Accessed 11 March 2020.
8. Force ATT. *Telemedicine for Ophthalmology Information Statement —2018;* 2018. https://www.aao.org/clinical-statement/telemedicine -ophthalmology-information-statement.
9. Claude J, Pirtle KLP, Brian C. Drolet. telehealth: legal and ethical considerations for success. *Telehealth Med Today.* 2019;4. https://telehealthandmedicinetoday.com/index. php/journal/issue/view/14.
10. *Telemedicine Consent Form.* https://www.omic.com/ telemedicine-consent-form/. Accessed 16.02.21.
11. *State Telehealth Laws & Reimbursement Policies. Fall 2019;* 2019.
12. Bruhn HK. Telemedicine: dos and don'ts to mitigate liability risk. *J AAPOS.* 2020;24(4):195–196.
13. *Current State Laws & Reimbursement Policies.* https://www. cchpca.org/telehealth-policy/current-state-laws-and-reimbursement-policies. Accessed 2 April 2021.
14. *U.S. States and Territories Modifying Requirements for Telehealth in Response to COVID-19;* 2021. https:// www.fsmb.org/siteassets/advocacy/pdf/states-waiving-licensure-requirements-for-telehealth-in-response-to-covid-19.pdf. Accessed 5 May 2021.
15. *VA Expands Telehealth by Allowing Health Care Providers to Treat Patients Across State Lines;* 2018. https://www.va.gov/opa/ pressrel/pressrelease.cfm?id=4054. Accessed 2 April 2021.
16. *Fact Sheet: Transforming Care Delivery With Telehealth at Kaiser Permanente.* https://www.kpihp.org/wp-content/ uploads/2020/03/Telehealth_FactSheet_032620_noon_ ba.pdf. Accessed 3 March 2021.
17. *Participating States.* https://www.imlcc.org/participating-states/. Accessed 2 April 2021.
18. *What Does it Cost? .* https://www.imlcc.org/what-does-it-cost/. Accessed 2 April 2021.
19. The National Association of Optometrists and Opticians. *RE: Occupational Licensing Reform. In: Commission FT, ed.* Federal Trade Commission; 2017. https:// www.ftc.gov/system/files/documents/public_com-ments/2017/10/00033-141413.pdf.
20. *Out-of-State Telehealth Provider Registration.* https://flori-dasoptometry.gov/licensing/out-of-state-telehealth-pro-vider-registration/. Accessed 3 January 2021.
21. Oregon Legislature. *Licensing of Applicant Holding License in Another State;* https://www.oregonlegislature.gov/bills_ laws/ors/ors683.html. Accessed 7 September 2021.
22. *Telemedicine.* https://www.medicaid.gov/medicaid/bene-fits/telemedicine/index.html. Accessed 15.02.21.
23. *2019 State of the States Report: Coverage and Reimbursement.* https://www.americantelemed.org/initiatives/2019-state-of-the-states-report-coverage-and-reimbursement/. Accessed 16.02.21.
24. *Medicare Telehealth Payment Eligibility Analyzer.* https://data. hrsa.gov/tools/medicare/telehealth. Accessed 16.02.21.
25. Telehealth Services. *Medicare Learning Network.* Centers for Medicare & Medicaid Services; 2020.
26. *Credentialing by Proxy—A Guidebook.* National Association Medical Staff Services and American Telemedicine Association; 2019. https://www.namss.org/Portals/0/ Policies_And_Bylaws/CBP%20Guidebook%20-%20 NAMSS%20Finalv2.pdf.
27. *Model Policy for the Appropriate Use of Telemedicine Technologies in the Practice of Medicine;* 2014. https://isb. idaho.gov/wp-content/uploads/150402_hea_materials5. pdf. Accessed 16.02.21.
28. Wallace F. *The Alabama Board of Optometry Administrative Code.* 630-X-13-.02; 2015.
29. Optometrists: telemedicine. In: *AB-1224. California Legislative Information;* 2007.
30. Lacktman NM. Chapter 24. Legal and regulatory issues. In: *Understanding Telehealth.* McGraw-Hill; 2021.

CHAPTER 16

Monitoring Quality and Improving Services in Ocular Telehealth Programs

ROBERT MORRIS, OD, FAAO

INTRODUCTION TO QUALITY ASSURANCE AND PROGRAM IMPROVEMENT

Key components of a successful clinical program include comprehensive quality assurance and performance improvement strategies. This is especially valuable for telehealth programs which provide clinical care when time and/or distance separate patient and provider and are heavily dependent on technology. Identifying the important quality indicators at program initiation and clearly defining the mechanism to evaluate these aspects of the program creates a foundation that will ensure regular assessment of the quality of care and the ability of the program to meet established goals. The United States-based National Committee for Quality Assurance (NCQA) Taskforce for Telehealth Policy issued the following findings and recommendations regarding telehealth quality assurance: "hold telehealth to the same quality standards as other settings, adapt, rather than reinvent, quality measures for telehealth."[1]

It is important to assign responsibility to manage the quality assurance and performance improvement aspects of the program to a quality team or individual. The quality team will coordinate critical aspects of the program including defining the quality standards, establishing the process for data extraction, developing reporting mechanisms, as well as managing program improvement activities.

QUALITY ASSURANCE

There are numerous elements to consider when developing a quality assurance program. A valuable initial step is to identify and review established clinical standards and guidelines for the care provided. This process includes researching both established and emerging clinical guidelines from multiple sources. Published reference materials such as textbooks and scientific literature should be an essential component of this initial step. Additionally, medical professional organizations publish specific care guidelines for certain conditions. For an ocular telehealth program, reviewing established guidelines should also include reviewing the American Telemedicine Association guidelines and those of ophthalmic professional organizations.

When the relevant clinical standards for the program are identified, obtain input from providers and key program members with the goal of achieving consensus on clear quality standards. Obtaining this input and agreement has another significant benefit in that it improves program buy-in and will contribute to a strong foundation for success. Once the standards and consensus are established, the next recommended step is to determine the process of identifying and measuring key elements for each standard. To develop an efficient quality assessment tool, each element should be clearly defined, be quantifiable, and be easy to obtain.

Ocular Telehealth. https://doi.org/10.1016/B978-0-323-83204-5.00016-0

Electronic health records (EHR) provide a great opportunity to extract critical elements of a telehealth visit which can be measured and reported to monitor quality. When using an EHR, utilizing existing clinical pathways to record key data should be preserved as much as possible. For example, the introduction of additional, nonclinical steps for the purpose of creating a data object to be extracted for monitoring quality adds inefficiency and may frustrate staff and providers.

The process of and responsibility for data extraction and developing and distributing reports at regular intervals should be clearly established early in the program. The quality team is tasked to execute these actions. Reports illustrating current performance and progress toward quality standard goals should be developed and tested for data validity as soon as possible. Quality reports should be distributed to the quality team, supervisors, and program leadership at established intervals to regularly monitor performance and identify aspects that need attention for improvement or safety.

CASE STUDY: DIABETIC RETINOPATHY SCREENING PROGRAMS

Diabetic retinopathy screening is currently the most established ocular telehealth program and has been implemented around the world. Using diabetic retinopathy screening as a case study, the following examples highlight quality elements of an ocular telehealth program. Daskivich and Mangione shared their recommendations for optimizing a diabetic retinopathy screening program with the goals of substantially reducing blindness and establishing the technology as the expected standard for diagnostic screening programs.[2] Their paper stressed the importance of national standardization in the protocols and workflow including the use of a validated and internationally accepted grading scale used by certified readers with seamless bidirectional communication between primary care and specialty providers through the electronic health record. They emphasized the importance of uniform reporting of results from a recognized grading system which would ensure the accuracy and reliability of the program. They also described the quality goal of identifying the true global need for specialty eye care within a healthcare system and identifying the individual patients with current need for specialty eye care. Accurately identifying these items is critical to provide timely eye care for the individual patient and understanding the eye care needs of a population. Integration of this information through an electronic

health record provides great opportunity to efficiently accomplish these goals.[2]

Another quality goal of diabetic teleretinal programs is efficacy—does the screening program provide a benefit to patients? Does it work? i.e., does it prevent vision loss from diabetic retinopathy? While many studies report short-term benefits of a diabetic retinopathy screening program, Mansberger et al. completed a long-term comparison of diabetic retinopathy ocular telehealth to in-person eye care, following patients for up to 5 years.[3] They randomized 567 individuals with diabetes to ocular telehealth or in-person care in a multicenter clinical trial with an intent to treat analysis. They reported a more frequent examination rate for the telehealth group compared to the in-person group—at the less than 6-month period, 94.6%–43.9%, and the 6–18-month period, 53.0%–33.2%, respectively. They also reported a generally stable diabetic retinopathy severity level during the study period. They concluded primary care-based diabetic retinopathy screening clinics can be used to monitor for disease worsening over a long period.

The value of consistent retinal screening has also been well established. The Four Nations (England, Wales, Scotland, and Northern Ireland) Diabetic Retinopathy Screening Study Group also helps to address the quality metric of efficacy by reporting the significant benefits of timely screening.[4] For individuals not screened in a timely manner, they found an increased rate of developing referable retinopathy and specifically, those with a 3 year or more delay in screening had a 4 times higher risk of developing proliferative retinopathy. The United Kingdom National Health Service reported the National Diabetic Retinopathy Screening program, along with improved glycemic control, has contributed to diabetic retinopathy being replaced by inherited retinal disease as the leading cause of blindness in working age adults for the first time in 50 years.[4]

To maximize efficiency and outcomes of a diabetic retinopathy screening program, high-quality imaging is critically important. High unreadable rates result in increased referrals for in-person care, diminished program efficiency, increased travel burden for the patient, and added demand for eye clinic appointments. Therefore, the "ungradable rate" is an area of focus in quality monitoring programs. Mansberger et al. reported a 3.1%–10.6% nonmydriatic unreadable rate for staging diabetic retinopathy severity and a 12.6%–22.3% unreadable rate for assessing macular edema.[3] Using this data, one proposed option to improve the ability to evaluate macular edema is to incorporate optical coherence tomography testing to the imaging protocol to enhance the effectiveness of unreadable studies for macular edema.[5]

Additional quality metrics recommended by Silva and Aiello include concentrating current efforts on advancing the efficiency, positive outcomes, and sustainability of the program.[5] The specific items they focused on were "quality control, quality assurance, referral guidelines and standards for patient care and safety."

QUALITY ASSESSMENT

The previous examples highlight many quality and clinical outcome aspects of diabetic retinopathy ocular telehealth programs. Quality assessment initiatives can be classified into several categories; some of the more relevant metrics for ocular telehealth include:

- Clinical Quality: evaluating the quality of different aspects of care including image unreadable rate for an asynchronous program, over-reading studies as part of a peer review program, and comparison of clinical findings relative to an in-person exam.
- Access: evaluating the availability of clinical care including scheduling appointments.
- Efficiency: evaluating the efficiency of a clinical process including number of days to complete an asynchronous ocular telehealth study.

Some detailed examples of quality assurance approaches are listed below, with other possibilities in parentheses, including specific items that could be considered and modified as needed for any ocular telehealth quality assurance program.

Clinical Quality Metric:
- Quality standard: *Diabetic retinopathy examination rate (Program Utilization Rate)*
  - ○ Details: Identify baseline diabetic retinopathy examination rate for a target population prior to implementing a screening program. Track rate of exams monthly to measure the effectiveness of the program to improve performance toward established targets.
  - ○ Reporting elements:
    - Identify number of individuals with diabetes in target population.
    - Monthly report on the rate of diabetic retinopathy examination for the target population.
    - Quality team reviews and shares results with program leads and referring providers.
  - ○ Performance improvement: When the rate of diabetic retinopathy exams is below target, the quality team would initiate a review to identify factors related to current performance and determine what actions to take to improve

performance. Examples of action for this standard might include:
- Review process to identify and capture individuals due for exam while in the primary care clinic to minimize the need for additional travel for a future exam.
- Develop and review a report of patients due for retinal screening that have upcoming primary care appointments. Preschedule these patients for retinal screening exams while the patient is in the clinic.
- Marketing the convenience and benefits of the program and the value of same-day retinal screening to clinical and clerical staff to improve capture rate.
- Direct outreach to patients to inform them of the importance of regular retinal evaluations for individuals with diabetes, provide an overview of the screening program and how to schedule an appointment.

- Quality standard: *Image quality: unreadable rate (Also consider Technology Failure Rate)*
  - ○ Details: Identify the number and percentage of unreadable diabetic retinopathy studies for each clinic location and telehealth technician. Measure and report unreadable rates monthly to monitor image quality and identification of potential technical problems impacting image quality. Evaluate image quality performance compared to established targets. Readers will evaluate images for readability and assess quality on reader clinic note.
  - ○ Reporting elements:
    - Identify through electronic health record: telehealth technician identity and location; image unreadable rate for each study and each telehealth technician.
    - Monthly report identifies number of studies per telehealth technician and unreadable rate for that telehealth technician and location.
    - Quality team reviews and shares results with telehealth technicians and supervisor.
  - ○ Performance improvement: When the unreadable rate exceeds target, the quality team would initiate a review to identify factors related to current performance and determine what actions to take to improve performance. Examples of action for this standard might include:
    - Identifying factors related to unreadable studies. Programs may identify specific details which could be used to further distinguish reasons for an unreadable study.

- Patient factors: inability to fixate or properly position for imaging, media opacities, small pupils (for nonmydriatic screening programs).
    - Imaging factors: missing fields, blur or out-of-focus images. These factors would typically be expected to be within the telehealth technician's control. Actions that would be appropriate for this include review of standard imaging protocol, including required fields, to ensure telehealth technician submits all required fields with each study. Review requirements for a readable study with attention to field composition, blur, and focus so telehealth technician can better understand what readers are expecting with the goal that this helps the technician determine if additional images should be taken to improve image clarity on future studies. Further actions may include additional education with a trainer.
        - Frequency of imaging could be a factor if a telehealth technician is not assigned to the diabetic retinopathy clinic on a regular basis. Requiring a minimum number of studies per timeframe (month, year) is a valuable element to maintain skills and knowledge and should be considered as a component of the competency assessment along with unreadable rate.
            - Actions for an elevated unreadable rate due to infrequent imaging could include additional assignments in the clinic with close monitoring of unreadable rates.
- Quality standard: *Reader peer review (also consider accuracy of telehealth screen compared to in-person exam)*
    - Details: Establish process for completed ocular telehealth studies to be reviewed by an ocular telehealth peer to assess quality and consistency. Example: 5% of all studies to be over-read by a peer.
    - Reporting elements:
        - Image quality assessment: was study readability assessment consistent with program guidelines.
        - Review clinical findings: compare peer review findings to original reading findings and referrals, were findings and referrals consistent with program guidelines.
    - Performance improvement: When the peer-review process identifies results that are not consistent with program guidelines the quality team

would initiate a review to identify factors related to current performance and determine what actions to take to improve performance. Examples of action may include:

- Review of program guidelines for image quality assessment including required fields and degree of clarity expected to classify a study as readable.
- Additional peer review overreads for a particular reader to provide additional support and guidance on reading process and program expectations.

Access Metric:
- Quality standard: *Scheduling referrals for an in-person eye examination in a timely manner*
    - Details: Establish target timeline for scheduling an appointment for patient referrals to be completed in a timely manner. Example: 90% of all referrals for an in-person eye appointment from diabetic retinopathy screening should be acted on within 7 days of study completion. Measure and report scheduling rate compared to this target.
    - Reporting elements:
        - Identify through electronic health record: patients with a referral for follow-up eye care, date of study completion and date action was taken to schedule an appointment.
        - Monthly report identifies number of patient referrals per month, calculates the number of days to schedule a follow-up eye appointment and compares to established target.
        - Quality team reviews and shares results with schedulers and supervisors.
    - Performance improvement: When the rate of scheduling a follow-up appointment fails to meet the target, the quality team would initiate a review to identify factors related to current performance and determine what actions to take to improve performance. Examples of action may include:
        - Review outliers, those that were not scheduled within 7 days, to discover contributing factors that lead to not scheduling an appointment within 7 days. Identify common items that can be studied for improvement.
        - Identify opportunities for more rapid identification of referred patients to initiate the scheduling activity as soon as possible.

Efficiency Metric:
- Quality standard: *Image study completion time (also can consider cycle time of visit)*

○ Details: Establish target for studies to be interpreted with a report rendered in a timely manner. Example: 90% of all studies should be completed within 7 days from imaging date. Measure and report study completion rate compared to this target.

○ Reporting elements:
  ■ Identify through electronic health record: date of imaging and date of study completion.
  ■ Monthly report identifies number of studies completed per month, calculates the number of days to complete each study and compares to established target.
  ■ Quality team reviews and shares results with readers and supervisor.

○ Performance improvement: When the rate of completed studies fails to meet the target, the quality team would initiate a review to identify factors related to current performance and determine what actions to take to improve performance. Examples of action may include:
  ■ Review and analysis of current factors leading to underperformance.

○ Ideas for improvement could include:
  ■ Assess reader staffing assignments and coverage for unexpected absences, develop process to notify staff when pending studies are about to exceed target to potentially reassign staff to help complete studies within targeted timeline.
  ■ Provide daily updates for all readers and supervisors of current workload including date and number of studies to be completed.

PERFORMANCE IMPROVEMENT AND STAKEHOLDER SATISFACTION

Several examples of performance improvement actions were discussed above, but without a clear process to review and implement the actions, the ability to effectively and consistently improve on a process will be limited. It is valuable to identify the performance improvement strategy that best meets the needs of the program. Gathering input from key members is again a valuable step to optimize effectiveness of the improvement process. Common components of a strong improvement process include:

1. Identify the problem
2. Gather information and data on the problem including input and improvement suggestions from staff
3. Analyze the problem
4. Identify opportunities for improvement

5. Design a solution for the problem
6. Implement solution
7. Monitor outcomes to determine how the solution impacted performance
8. Repeat cycle

Evaluating stake holder input is an invaluable tool to assess overall satisfaction with a program. This activity typically targets different elements of a program rather than measurement of outcomes or performance toward an established goal such as rate of diabetic retinopathy examinations. This can be accomplished by interviews or satisfaction surveys that drill down to the individual experience. Groups that would be worth surveying include Primary Care providers, referring providers, patient site nursing and support staff, telehealth technicians, schedulers, consulting providers and patients involved in the clinical program. There is significant evidence supporting high levels of satisfaction with ocular telehealth programs.

Kruse et al. analyzed 44 articles to assess the association of asynchronous and synchronous telehealth with patient satisfaction regarding effectiveness and efficiency.[6] Using a consensus approach, they identified the factors listed most frequently by patients to be: improved outcomes (20%), preferred modality (10%), ease of use (9%), low cost (8%), improved communication (8%), and decreased travel time (7%); these six factors accounted for 61% of occurrences. Provider acceptance and interest in exploring innovative methods of providing care utilizing new technology is often a significant challenge for telehealth expansion. Kruse et al. suggested emphasizing to reluctant providers that 20% of the factors of effectiveness were related to improved outcomes, and telehealth can be a successful method of delivering quality care. This, in addition to other factors listed above, provide evidence to support the effectiveness of telehealth and strong patient satisfaction.

A study from Kenya reported 88% of patients with diabetes were completely satisfied with their ocular telehealth examination and 58% preferred to use ocular telehealth, compared to an in-person examination, for their diabetic retinopathy care in the future.[7] They also found 62% of patients reported that the trained nurse explained the indication for ocular telehealth screening. This group of patients rated the most significant benefits of the telehealth program to be visualization of their own retina (85%), convenience (73%) and time savings (58%).

Luzio et al. reported on a European multicenter diabetic retinopathy screening study of 390 patients over a 3-month period.[8] Their study incorporated dilation with 1% tropicamide and found a 99.2% readability rate with only six individual images being unreadable. They also assessed satisfaction of patients and staff. Patient results from two sites reported high levels of comfort with the camera and an overwhelmingly high rate of program satisfaction with 100% at one site and 94% at another site. After some early technical problems were resolved, photographers reported satisfaction with training and data reporting, and high satisfaction with the overall process. The readers described the training as easy and reported satisfaction with image quality and image grading form.

Obtaining satisfaction feedback from patients, technicians, and readers covers most of the parties involved in an ocular telehealth program, but referring providers are another important group to survey. Gensheimer et al. evaluated a secure ocular telehealth mobile phone application at military treatment facilities in Afghanistan.[9] They reviewed 28 consults over a 6-week period requested by 18 different users. User satisfaction surveys were completed for all 28 consults. They used a rating scale of 1–5, with 1 being very dissatisfied and 5 being very satisfied. Results showed high rate of user satisfaction, overall median satisfaction was 5 (range 3–5), median satisfaction with ease of use was 5 (range 3–5), median satisfaction with treatment and management plan was 5 (range 4–5) and median satisfaction compared to other ocular telehealth methods was 5 (range 3–5). This mobile application program also eliminated the need for 4 (14%) aeromedical evacuations.

OTHER QUALITY METRICS TO CONSIDER FOR AN OCULAR TELEHEALTH PROGRAM

The effectiveness of patient education through an ocular telehealth program is also an important aspect to evaluate as patients that understand their condition are more likely to be compliant with treatment and follow-up visits. Court et al. compared both patient acceptance and education at a virtual ocular glaucoma telehealth clinic to an in-person clinic visit.[10] They reported a mean satisfaction score of 4.3 (5-point scale) for both groups. Patients in the virtual clinic demonstrated strong understanding of their condition by correctly identifying their diagnosis: 95% for those with glaucoma, 83% with ocular hypertension and 78% for glaucoma suspects. They concluded the virtual clinic patients did not demonstrate inferior knowledge compared to in-person clinic patients.

Another metric to consider is the equivalence of care between telehealth and in-person exams. Tan et al. completed a systematic review of 12 studies comparing synchronous ocular telehealth to in-person consultation.[11]

They reported the overall ocular telehealth diagnostic accuracy to be comparable to in-person care but identified limitations due to internet transmission speed. They proposed a blend of asynchronous image transmission and synchronous care (hybrid telehealth) as an alternative to overcome slow connectivity rates.

Kumar et al. reported on a remote interactive ocular telehealth consultation program in Western Australia.[12] Over a 12-month period 118 consultations were completed at a remote hospital 940 km from the Perth-based Lions Eye Institute. The majority (94%) of the cases received glaucoma and diabetic retinopathy testing, while 3% were referred for emergency care and 3% for second opinion and postoperative care. A small fraction (3%) of the consultations were referred to the Eye Institute for in-person care and 36% of patients were recommended to follow up by ocular telehealth. Nearly all (98%) of patients reported satisfaction with the program and found it convenient with 74% reporting no concern with the lack of physical contact with an in-person provider.

CONCLUSION

Ocular telehealth programs provide a high-quality method to reach patients that have difficulty accessing eye care for a variety of reasons. A comprehensive ocular telehealth quality assurance program is critical to assess and monitor quality standards and ensure care is consistent, accurate, and timely. The quality standards are established by key members of the program and are based on reference standards and professional guidelines. Development of data reports to efficiently measure performance is an important step to objectively measure the vital processes. Patients report high satisfaction rates with ocular telehealth programs, citing convenience, time savings, and ability to visualize their own retina as many of the factors they appreciate. Ocular telehealth programs would benefit from improved standardization including a consistent grading scale, certified reader training, improved communication with other providers, uniform reporting of results, consistent referral guidelines, and technology advancements that allow for more detailed remote assessment of patients with improved readable rates.

REFERENCES

1. National Committee for Quality Assurance (NCQA). *Taskforce for Telehealth Policy Final Report*; 2021. Accessed 2/15/2021 https://www.ncqa.org/wp-content/uploads/2020/09/20200914_Taskforce_on_Telehealth_Policy_Final_Report.pdf.

2. Daskivich LP, Mangione CM. The promise of primary care-based screening for diabetic retinopathy: the devil will be in the details. *Arch Intern Med.* 2012;172(21):1678–1680.

3. Mansberger SL, Sheppler C, Barker G, et al. Long-term comparative effectiveness of telemedicine in providing diabetic retinopathy screening examinations. *JAMA Ophthalmol.* 2015;133(5):518–525.

4. Sim DA, Mitry D, Alexander P, et al. The evolution of teleophthalmology programs in the United Kingdom: beyond diabetic retinopathy screening. *J Diabetes Sci Technol.* 2016;10(2):308–317.

5. Silva PS, Aiello LP. Telemedicine and eye examinations for diabetic retinopathy: a time to maximize real-world outcomes. *JAMA Ophthalmol.* 2015;133(5):525–526. https://doi.org/10.1001/jamaophthalmol.2015.0333.

6. Kruse CS, Krowski N, Rodriguez B, Tran L, Vela J, Brooks M. Telehealth and patient satisfaction: a systematic review and narrative analysis. *BMJ Open.* 2017;7. https://doi.org/10.1136/bmjopen-2017-016242, e016242.

7. Kurji K, Kiage D, Rudnisky CJ, Damji KF. Improving diabetic retinopathy screening in Africa: patient satisfaction with teleophthalmology versus ophthalmologist-based screening. *Middle East Afr J Ophthalmol.* 2013;20(1):56–60.

8. Luzio S, Hatcher S, Zahlmann G, et al. Feasibility of using the TOSCA telescreening procedures for diabetic retinopathy. *Diabet Med.* 2004;21(10):1121–1128.

9. Gensheimer WG, Miller KE, Stowe J, Little J, Legault GL. Military teleophthalmology in Afghanistan using mobile phone application. *JAMA Ophthalmol.* 2020;138(10):1053–1060.

10. Court JH, Austin MW. Virtual glaucoma clinics: patient acceptance and quality of patient education compared to standard clinics. *Clin Ophthalmol.* 2015;9:745–749.

11. Tan IJ, Dobson LP, Bartnik S, Muir J, Turner AW. Real-time teleophthalmology versus face-to-face consultation: a systematic review. *J Telemed Telecare.* 2017;23(7):629–638.

12. Kumar S, Tay-Kearney ML, Constable IJ, Yogesan K. Internet based ophthalmology service: impact assessment. *Br J Ophthalmol.* 2005;89(10):1382–1383.

Acute Ocular Triage Telehealth

APRIL MAA, MD

INTRODUCTION

Currently, this author is not aware of a widespread, standardized ocular telehealth triage program in the United States. There are several use cases that will be highlighted at the end of this chapter, as this is a growing area of ocular telehealth innovation. More published studies demonstrating the accuracy of a standardized ocular telehealth triage protocol when compared to the gold standard, in-person clinical exam, would be helpful to advance this aspect of ocular telehealth.

The previous chapters of this book discuss important factors for developing an ocular telehealth program: the available types of telehealth, goals of a program, target patient selection (Chapter 1), implementation (Chapter 12), and technology considerations (Chapter 13). Developing an *acute* ocular telehealth triage program considers similar factors. First, it would be important to assess the need and determine the goals of the ocular telehealth program. Second, determine the appropriate form of ocular telehealth: synchronous, asynchronous, or a combination (hybrid). Third, the required equipment and technology to achieve the desired goals of the program needs to be explored. Finally, training, logistics, and billing/coding for the program need to be considered.

CONSIDERATIONS FOR ACUTE OCULAR TRIAGE TELEHEALTH PROGRAMS

Assessment of Need—The Scope of the Problem

The literature highlights that more than 2 million patient visits occur annually for eye complaints to local Emergency Rooms (ER) or Urgent Care (UC) settings across the country.[1] Despite the high number of ER/UC visits for eye complaints, ER providers have low confidence in their ability to examine and diagnose eye diseases.[2] Almost 40% of ER visits for eye complaints result in an ophthalmology consultation.[3] Furthermore, many ER/UC settings lack ophthalmology coverage, especially in the rural hospitals.[4] The inability to meet the demands of eye services for the ER/UC setting with the current available supply of eye providers results in non-eye providers handling most of the eye complaints. The current practice model consequently yields a high rate of diagnostic error related to eye conditions by non-eye providers. For instance, Yip and colleagues conducted a retrospective analysis of 534 cases (1 week worth of referrals) to the Royal Victorian Eye and Ear Hospital. They found 30% of misdiagnoses from general practitioners and 18.8% from outside hospital ER non-eye providers.[5] In contrast, the misdiagnosis rate was 0% when the patient was referred from a private ophthalmologist. The typical misdiagnosis rate for medicine is 10%–15%.[5] The higher rate of eye condition misdiagnosis by non-eye providers raises alarm. Patients could suffer significant vision loss if their care is delayed because their eye problem was previously determined to be less serious than it actually is. In an older study, Statham and colleagues reported a 64% error rate from general practitioners and a 58% error rate from ER doctors.[6] As a result, 11 adverse events (i.e., eye pain, vision loss, or inappropriate therapy) occurred among these misdiagnosed patients. Many of these patients were initially incorrectly diagnosed with "conjunctivitis" by the ER/UC provider, but actually suffered from more serious conditions (i.e., bacterial keratitis, anterior uveitis, glaucoma, or diabetic retinopathy). Several patients experienced delayed follow-up visits from 2 days to 2 weeks. A subset of these patients suffered severe vision loss. These studies emphasize the need for providing enough urgent ophthalmology coverage in the ER/UC settings.

Furthermore, the economic cost of providing ER/UC-based care for eye complaints is much higher than if the care could be given in an eye clinic. Singman et al. found an average annual savings of $580,866 when patients were served in a same day, outpatient eye clinic rather than the ER for their acute eye complaint.[7] Most importantly, up to $3.2 million in ER/UC costs were saved if the patient chose same-day care in the eye clinic because ER/UC settings have additional facility fees. Blackwell et al. estimated costs of transfers for urgent eye complaints to be $100,000 in their study, while simultaneously demonstrating that an ocular telehealth triage program reduced the number of patients transferred from 17 to 4, a cost savings of $1.3 million.[8] In addition, these costs do not factor transit time, ER throughput, patient escort/family member travel and time, or transfer time (if a patient is transferred to higher level facility for further eye evaluation).

It is clear from the literature that there is a need for ocular consultative services to the ER/UC setting. As discussed above, there are millions of visits across the country each year by patients who are experiencing acute ocular complaints, and not enough hospitals have specialty coverage, especially the rural hospitals. With telehealth technology, a specialty eye care provider could cover multiple hospitals or clinics spread over a large area immediately or near-immediately, on demand, and bridge the gap in care.

What Are the Goals of an Acute Ocular Triage Program?

One of the overarching goals of an ocular telehealth triage program should be to reduce the number of unnecessary urgent referrals for eye issues. A second goal

would be to accurately diagnosis and initiate management for the patient to reduce serious visual consequences. Therefore, at minimum, an ocular telehealth triage program should contain the necessary elements for accurate ocular triage and diagnosis, which would then allow for recommendations on the proper time frame for follow up. Critical information to gather toward this goal include: history, vision, eye pressure, anterior segment exam, and posterior segment exam. Published literature illustrates that programs that are able to achieve these goals provide the greatest return on investment. The savings benefit applies to both the healthcare system and the patients. Healthcare systems save costs due to reduction in patient transfers and in consultation time, thereby allowing better throughput and more efficient visits. In Kumar's population in rural Australia, 3% of patients were emergent and they were able to identify and manage serious ocular disorders (corneal ulcer, acute angle closure glaucoma, hyphema).[9] Once the ocular telehealth program was initiated, they had zero patients requiring emergent eye transfers out of the ER, whereas they had seven patients before the initiation of the ocular triage program. This cost savings is significant, as patients requiring emergent evacuation would need a plane flight. In addition, they reduced the time of consultation for the patient from 2 h 45 min to 30 min.[9] Rosengren et al. also found that having an ocular telehealth triage program reduced needs for transfers from the ER.[10]

What Type of Telehealth Modalities Should Be Used and What Type of Equipment Should Be Chosen?

If the goal is to provide accurate diagnoses for ocular triage, it is prudent to examine the epidemiology of eye complaints presenting to the ER/UC setting. Multiple studies have illustrated that the most common complaint in the ER is for "red eye"; with a large proportion involving the anterior segment.[1] Top three diagnoses from patients presenting to the ER include: conjunctivitis, corneal abrasion/foreign body, uveitis/iritis, closely followed by acute vision loss.[6,7] Given the high propensity of anterior segment issues, acute ocular triage programs should encompass a method to accurately assess the anterior segment. Several asynchronous ocular telehealths programs routinely capture external photographs (see Fig. 17.1 and Chapters 2 and 6) as minimally trained personnel can capture these photographs. However, the routine use of a slit lamp for more detailed anterior segment examination is less common. Chapter 4 also provides greater detail on examining the anterior segment with telehealth means.

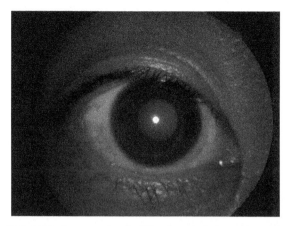

FIG. 17.1 An example of a 2D external photograph used for anterior segment examination. (Credit: Photo taken by Stephen Herman, COT.)

The issue with only using external photographs is that the literature suggests 2D external photos (when used for ER triage)[2,11,12] have large sensitivity ranges: 54%–71% (smartphone application iTouch); 61.3%–81.3% (PictorPlus, Volk, Cleveland Ohio) to 88.9%.[13] The high levels of sensitivity, 88.9%, was achieved only for diagnosis of epithelial defects, and not all ER/UC patients presenting with an eye complaint will have this problem. Another study comparing corneal staining with external photos versus the slit lamp exam and found that the external photos significantly underrepresented the amount of punctate epithelial defects when compared to a slit lamp exam.[14] In addition, cell or flare cannot be directly identified on external photography. These findings highlight that the widespread use of external photos for ocular triage may not provide sufficient accuracy,[15] even when interpreted by ophthalmologists. Using inadequate external photos could pose serious concerns, especially considering the prevalence of iritis presenting to the ER.

Slit lamp photography and slit lamp video offer an alternative solution. They allow for more accurate diagnoses than external photography. Kumar and colleagues showed moderate to excellent kappa using slit lamp photos.[16] Ye's team demonstrated that the slit lamp photos and video were accurate enough for the remote provider to detect a contact lens in the eye and its movement during a blink.[17] The remote provider could not detect the contact lens, however, using the external photography alone. Technological equipment to do a telehealth slit lamp examination is available in a few different forms (e.g., a smartphone mount on a slit lamp, a slit lamp camera).[8,16–19] See Chapter 4 and 13, anterior segment and technology chapters, respectively.

Several researchers studied accuracy and feasibility of ocular telehealth using a slit lamp given the propensity of anterior segment disorders and the benefits of slit lamp examination. Smith and colleagues conducted a remote examination of postoperative cataract surgery patients. They reported that a video transmission for the slit lamp should be at least 384 bits/s and demonstrated that a slit lamp video was better than a slit lamp image.[20] Using only slit lamp images, providers identified zero patients with cell or flare and only 33% of incisions with corneal edema, compared to when providers utilized a slit lamp video.

Additional studies using various combinations of digital portable slit lamp images[9,21,22] or slit lamp videos[23,24] demonstrated even more accurate results than Smith and colleagues'. It is important to note that often, when slit lamp videos were performed in these studies, there was also a synchronous interaction, either by telephone or by video conferencing where the eye provider directed the telehealth facilitator.

In summary, previous studies published on the high accuracy of anterior segment examination with slit lamp equipment, suggest the following points: (1) slit lamp images or video are more accurate than 2D external photos; and (2) live conferencing (either via a synchronous platform or a telephone conversation) is best while the specialist is reviewing the clinical information and slit lamp video.

Once equipment is chosen, the primary telehealth modality should be determined. As discussed in Chapter 1, there are two main categories of telehealth—asynchronous and synchronous. Ocular telehealth has typically utilized asynchronous methods (e.g., diabetic tele-retinal screening), but in an acute ocular triage telehealth program, asynchronous may not be best to achieve the goals outlined above. The literature suggests that the greatest accuracy for anterior segment diagnosis is slit lamp video-based and uses synchronous telehealth modalities.[8–10,19,22–24] For example, a telehealth technician in the ER/UC trained to use a slit lamp facilitates the telehealth encounter while the eye specialist connects remotely and directs/interprets the exam. Blomdahl and Bowman's studies use live slit lamp video, and both showed very high correlation between the telemedicine exam and the in-person eye exam—with only 5% clinically important disagreements.[23,24] It has been recommended by the literature that standard for accuracy for a telemedicine program should be at least 80% sensitive.[25] Since Blomdahl and Bowman's programs far exceed the 80% threshold it suggests using a similar approach will result in an accurate and safe ocular triage telehealth program. Alternatively, one might consider a hybrid-layered model, where, depending on the patient's complaint, discrete data elements such as vision, eye pressure, external and fundus photographs could be sent via asynchronous methods, and when necessary, then utilizing a synchronous portion for a slit lamp exam.

Implementation, Training, Billing and Coding Considerations
Implementation and training aspects
One of the most important aspects of implementing a successful telehealth program is the patient and provider trust in the technology and the process. In the case of an ocular telehealth triage program, one key to high-quality care is the ability of the remote provider to trust the information gathered by the telehealth facilitator. Chief complaint, history, and vision are routinely gathered by non-eye providers and therefore probably do not require focused training. Eye pressure and fundus photography are also important aspects of a telehealth triage program and will require some training, though these devices have become very user-friendly and can quickly be mastered by medical assistants and have automated features (e.g., auto-focus, auto-capture). Chapter 13 discusses this in greater detail. One potential way to obtain training is to determine if the manufacturers of the equipment provide staff training.

The most critical aspect of an ocular telehealth triage program, and the one that is most difficult to carry out, is the adequate training of telehealth facilitators on slit lamp use. While slit lamp images/video yield the most accurate ocular triage using telehealth, there are significant drawbacks. Slit lamp cameras are costly and require significant training to use properly.[10,17,18,23] Very accurate ocular triage programs published in the literature often have an ophthalmology resident[22] or a licensed non-eye provider (e.g., primary care, nurse practitioner) as the telehealth facilitator.[19,24] This poses a challenge for the ER due to the shift-work nature of ER/UC clinics and the baseline lack of knowledge and skill in performing a slit lamp exam of the eye.

With regard to slit lamp training, a basic skill curriculum should be laid out, with competency checks at the end of training, along with "refresher courses" over time when the individual does not utilize the skill set regularly. In addition, multiple individuals need to be trained so that they can cross-cover each other and ensure that there is at least one individual who can carry out the telehealth program on each ER/UC shift. Finally, initial training is likely best carried out by a skilled user of slit lamps, for example, an eye provider or a highly trained ophthalmic technician.

Other important points to consider before the ocular telehealth triage program goes "live" is to increase awareness, both within the system and outside the system, of the availability of the service and appropriate patient candidates. One should do multiple "dry-runs" with different telehealth facilitators so that everyone is comfortable with the platform before using it real time. Contingency plans for technology failure should also be addressed. It is recommended that detailed manuals, with step-by-step instructions, be available to anyone as quick reference.

Billing, coding, and legal aspects
During the time of the COVID-19 pandemic, in the United States, Medicare and Medicaid have agreed to reimburse telehealth services at the rate equivalent to in-person services during the public health emergency (PHE). It is unknown how long these modifications of billing/coding will last and traditionally, Medicare and Medicaid have not reimbursed for asynchronous telehealth services. Synchronous telehealth services, however, have been reimbursed, even before the PHE. One would typically add modifier 95, "synchronous telemedicine service rendered via a real-time interactive audio and video telecommunications system" to the usual code for in-person care. For asynchronous telehealth, CPT codes 92227 (remote imaging for retinal disease without abnormalities) and 92228 (remote imaging for retinal disease with abnormalities) may be used. Chapter 14 discusses billing and coding in greater detail.

From a legal perspective, it is best if these telehealth visits are consultative, where the consulting provider is giving recommendations to the requesting provider, but not assuming care and liability for the patient.

From a licensing perspective, the remote eye provider needs to be licensed in the state that the patient is located in, or in the same state as the ER/UC location. Chapter 15 discusses these principles in greater detail.

CURRENT USE CASES OF OCULAR TELEHEALTH TRIAGE
While writing this book chapter, multiple eye centers and healthcare systems were using a variety of telehealth methods to deliver eye care to the ER/UC setting. Less data was available regarding the accuracy and success of these endeavors. These programs were accelerated by the COVID-19 pandemic, and a few examples (not meant to be an exhaustive list) are included here:
- Banner Health was utilizing a smart phone based solution, Paxos, to transmit information, external, and fundus images to a remote eye provider.[26]

- Several academic centers, including University of Pennsylvania (UPMC),[27] Johns Hopkins,[28] and New York Eye and Ear have ocular telehealth triage programs based on external images transmitted to a remote eye provider.
- EYEmergencyMD is a company that offers multiple solutions for eye care, 24/7, to several different settings, including ERs and UC clinics.[29]
- Moorefields Eye Hospital published results on their retrospective comparison of cohorts of patients who underwent a synchronous, direct to home, video triage program versus a cohort of patients who did in-person triage.[30] Their findings were concerning for the synchronous home-based telehealth modality as a form of ocular triage. They found that patients attending video-based triage were statistically more likely to go back to the ER within a month compared to those who were seen in-person. Moreover, there was poor interrater reliability and more potential harm using video-based triage. Obviously, in the setting of COVID-19, an extreme clinical care circumstance, video triage was probably "better than nothing"; however, this data highlights the need for other modalities to be utilized for ocular triage since video conferencing to home does not appear to be as effective or safe as traditional care.

FUTURE DIRECTIONS

Given the increased uptake of telehealth across the medical field, and the increasing availability and reliance upon technology, telemedicine will likely continue to grow, and the eye care field is no exception. There is clearly a need for specialty eye care to be brought to the ER and UC settings, and the gap in access is possibly best served by telehealth. While current ocular triage telehealth programs are being carried out, this burgeoning field of eye telehealth could be improved by better ways to examine the anterior segment of the eye, using more than just 2D external photographs. A portable, easy-to-use device that would be able to capture slit lamp images or video would be incredibly beneficial, along with more comparative trials between the ocular triage telehealth program and a traditional in-person eye exam. The landscape of ocular telehealth triage may change further if a robotic or remote controlled slit lamp is developed. A remote-controlled slit lamp has been demonstrated[31] but is not commercially available right now. Ocular triage telehealth, however, holds much promise to bridge the access gap for acute eye care in many parts of the world.

REFERENCES

1. Channa R, Zafar SN, Canner JK, Haring RS, Schneider EB, Friedman DS. Epidemiology of eye-related emergency department visits. *JAMA Ophthalmol.* 2016;134(3):312–319.
2. Bursztyn L, Woodward MA, Cornblath WT, et al. Accuracy and reliability of a handheld, nonmydriatic fundus camera for the remote detection of optic disc edema. *Telemed J E Health.* 2018;24(5):344–350.
3. Wang SY, Hamid MS, Musch DC, Woodward MA. Utilization of ophthalmologist consultation for emergency care at a University Hospital. *JAMA Ophthalmol.* 2018;136(4):428–431.
4. Gavin K. *Study: 1 In 4 ER Visits for Eye Problems Aren't Actually Emergencies;* 2017. https://labblog.uofmhealth.org/rounds/study-1-4-er-visits-for-eye-problems-arent-actually-emergencies. Accessed 25.11.19.
5. Yip H, Crock C, Chan E. Diagnostic error in an ophthalmic emergency department. *Diagnosis (Berl).* 2020;7(2):129–131.
6. Statham MO, Sharma A, Pane AR. Misdiagnosis of acute eye diseases by primary health care providers: incidence and implications. *Med J Aust.* 2008;189(7):402–404.
7. Singman EL, Smith K, Mehta R, et al. Cost and visit duration of same-day access at an Academic Ophthalmology Department vs Emergency Department. *JAMA Ophthalmol.* 2019;137(7):729–735.
8. Blackwell NA, Kelly GJ, Lenton LM. Telemedicine ophthalmology consultation in remote Queensland. *Med J Aust.* 1997;167(11–12):583–586.
9. Kumar S, Yogesan K, Hudson B, Tay-Kearney ML, Constable IJ. Emergency eye care in rural Australia: role of internet. *Eye (Lond).* 2006;20(12):1342–1344.
10. Rosengren D, Blackwell N, Kelly G, Lenton L, Glastonbury J. The use of telemedicine to treat ophthalmological emergencies in rural Australia. *J Telemed Telecare.* 1998;4(suppl. 1):97–99.
11. Mines MJ, Bower KS, Lappan CM, Mazzoli RA, Poropatich RK. The United States Army ocular teleconsultation program 2004 through 2009. *Am J Ophthalmol.* 2011;152(1). 126-132 e122.
12. Woodward MA, Bavinger JC, Amin S, et al. Telemedicine for ophthalmic consultation services: use of a portable device and layering information for graders. *J Telemed Telecare.* 2017;23(2):365–370.
13. Maamari RN, Ausayakhun S, Margolis TP, Fletcher DA, Keenan JD. Novel telemedicine device for diagnosis of corneal abrasions and ulcers in resource-poor settings. *JAMA Ophthalmol.* 2014;132(7):894–895.
14. Sorbara L, Peterson R, Schneider S, Woods C. Comparison between live and photographed slit lamp grading of corneal staining. *Optom Vis Sci.* 2015;92(3):312–317.
15. Woodward MA, Musch DC, Hood CT, et al. Teleophthalmic approach for detection of corneal diseases: accuracy and reliability. *Cornea.* 2017;36(10):1159–1165.
16. Kumar S, Yogesan K, Constable IJ. Telemedical diagnosis of anterior segment eye diseases: validation of digital slit-lamp still images. *Eye (Lond).* 2009;23(3):652–660.

17. Ye Y, Wang J, Xie Y, et al. Global teleophthalmology with iPhones for real-time slitlamp eye examination. *Eye Contact Lens.* 2014;40(5):297–300.

18. Barsam A, Bhogal M, Morris S, Little B. Anterior segment slitlamp photography using the iPhone. *J Cataract Refract Surg.* 2010;36(7):1240–1241.

19. Kulshrestha M, Lewis D, Williams C, Axford A. A pilot trial of tele-ophthalmology services in north Wales. *J Telemed Telecare.* 2010;16(4):196–197.

20. Smith LF, Bainbridge J, Burns J, Stevens J, Taylor P, Murdoch I. Evaluation of telemedicine for slit lamp examination of the eye following cataract surgery. *Br J Ophthalmol.* 2003;87(4):502–503.

21. Yogesan K, Henderson C, Barry CJ, Constable IJ. Online eye care in prisons in Western Australia. *J Telemed Telecare.* 2001;7(suppl. 2):63–64.

22. Bar-Sela SM, Glovinsky Y. A feasibility study of an Internet-based telemedicine system for consultation in an ophthalmic emergency room. *J Telemed Telecare.* 2007;13(3):119–124.

23. Bowman RJ, Kennedy C, Kirwan JF, Sze P, Murdoch IE. Reliability of telemedicine for diagnosing and managing eye problems in accident and emergency departments. *Eye (Lond).* 2003;17(6):743–746.

24. Blomdahl S, Maren N, Lof R. Tele-ophthalmology for the treatment in primary care of disorders in the anterior part of the eye. *J Telemed Telecare.* 2001;7(suppl. 1):25–26.

25. Association BD. *Retinal Photographic Screening for Diabetic Eye Disease.* London; 1997.

26. Banner Health. *Real-Time Remote Imaging Advances Banner Health Emergency Room Eye Care;* 2017. http://bannerhealth.mediaroom.com/2017-04-06-Real-time-remote-imaging-advances-Banner-Health-emergency-room-eye-care. Accessed 30.01.21.

27. UPMC. *Ophthalmology Telemedicine Services;* 2021. https://www.upmc.com/healthcare-professionals/physicians/telemedicine/services/ophthalmology. Accessed 30.01.21.

28. Nitkin K. *The (Remote) Eye Doctor Will See You Now;* 2017. https://www.hopkinsmedicine.org/news/articles/the-remote-eye-doctor-will-see-you-now. Accessed 30.01.21.

29. https://www.eyemergencymd.com/. Accessed 30.01.21.

30. Li JO, Thomas AAP, Kilduff CLS, et al. Safety of video-based telemedicine compared to in-person triage in emergency ophthalmology during COVID-19. *EClinicalMedicine.* 2021;34:100818.

31. Parel J-MA, Nankivil D, Gonzalez A, et al. Remote controlled stereo slit-lamp for imaging inaccessible patients. *Invest Ophthalmol Vis Sci.* 2012;53:3633.

CHAPTER 18

The Role of Data Analytics and Artificial Intelligence (AI) in Ocular Telehealth

MATTHEW S. HUNT, BS • STEPHANIE J. WEISS, DO • AARON Y. LEE, MD, MSCI

MACHINE LEARNING

Introduction

Within the field of artificial intelligence (AI), machine learning (ML) is a subgroup of algorithms that are not explicitly programmed in their final form but instead improve their performance on some task by learning through interaction with data relevant to the task. ML algorithms achieve this through optimization of a model given observed data. In general, a ML model can be thought of as a quantified description of patterns or relationships within data. For example, the equation for electrostatic forces between two charged particles,

$$Fe = \frac{k * q_1 * q_2}{r^2} \qquad (18.1)$$

is an example of a mathematical model that describes observations, or data, in the physical world. In this model, the relationship of force is fully constrained and known if the charges and distance between those charges are known. In the context of ML, models are given some type of mathematical structure, but the exact relationships within the model are mutable. Variables within the model, known as parameters, are altered using the data to optimally characterize relationships in the data. Many different types of models are used in ML, including linear regression, decision trees, Naive Bayes classifiers, support vector machines (SVM), and deep neural networks. These different models have different degrees of flexibility in their pattern-representing capabilities, with certain models being well-suited for capturing the patterns in different data distributions, a concept that will be explored in further depth.

Machine Learning Categories

ML algorithms in different settings have different objectives. ML algorithms can be organized by the kind of information present in the data into four major categories: supervised learning, unsupervised learning, semisupervised learning, and reinforcement learning (Table 18.1). In supervised learning, each data observation is assigned a ground-truth label that marks the observation as belonging to a certain class or having a certain value of interest. Typically the supervised-learning model's objective is to predict the label using

Ocular Telehealth. https://doi.org/10.1016/B978-0-323-83204-5.00018-4

TABLE 18.1
Types of Machine Learning

Category	Goal	Data	Example
Supervised learning	Predict labels or values	Observations with ground truth labels for training	Diabetic retinopathy (DR) severity prediction based on fundus images. Trained on images with severity categorized by a human expert
Unsupervised learning	Organize data by characterizing relationships between data attributes	Observations do not have labels associated with them	Exploratory analysis of DR images in order to group them into unnamed categories, none of which are labeled, but which share common pathologic features
Semisupervised learning	Predict labels or values	A portion of the data has labels	DR severity-prediction task, trained on many images, only a few of which are categorized by a human expert. The rest have no category labels
Reinforcement learning	Interact with environment in optimal manner	Observations of environment and history of actions taken in environment	Potential future applications include autonomous surgical robots, or systems for human-machine interaction with diagnostic tools

information about an observation's other attributes. Linear regression is an example of a supervised learning algorithm in which the labels are continuous variables that are predicted using some other attributes of each observation. In unsupervised learning, data observations do not have labels, and the model instead learns to perform characterization of relationships between attributes of each observation in order to organize the data. Clustering algorithms are examples of unsupervised learning. Data are grouped according to values of their attributes, but those groups are not explicitly named with meaningful categories. Components of both supervised learning and unsupervised learning are used in semisupervised learning, in which some data have labels provided. Without a large number of labeled data points it is typically more challenging for models to characterize the relationships between observation attributes and labels. Because of this, semisupervised algorithms leverage relationships between data attributes to create better representations of the data for more easily predicting labels. Reinforcement learning also has similarities to both supervised and unsupervised learning. It deals with the training of agents to interact optimally with environments. The agent takes actions in the environment, which alter the state of the environment and eventually deliver rewards (or punishments). The rewards act as noisy labels, suggesting which actions are best to take at given states of the environment. Explicit labels are not provided, but the agent learns through repeated interaction. Reinforcement

learning algorithms are used to teach computers to play games and are an area of research for autonomous vehicles. The majority of this chapter will discuss supervised learning.

ARTIFICIAL NEURAL NETWORKS
Introduction Through Logistic Regression
Artificial neural networks are a type of machine learning model in which relationships in data are modeled using distinct steps or "layers" of computations which are fed into subsequent layers. Neural networks are loosely inspired by the way biological neurons receive input from multiple neurons and transmit outputs to other neurons in networks of computation[1,2]. Artificial neural networks are related to simpler models such as linear or logistic regression, but extend their representational capabilities to be able to model nonlinear functions. A large enough neural network with properly set parameters is capable of modeling any function[3,4].

One way to gain an intuition for how artificial neural networks function and why they are beneficial is to consider logistic regression, a modeling technique commonly used in medical research. In its simplest form a one-neuron, one-layer neural network classification model is equivalent to a logistic regression. Logistic regression is used in classification tasks to predict the probability of class membership of a data point using some measured attributes (features) of that data point. After fitting or "training" the regression, it can be used with new

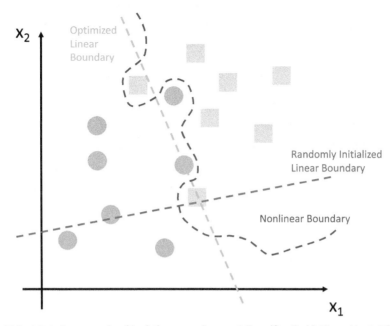

FIG. 18.1 An example of logistic regression modeling. (Credit: Matthew Hunt, BS)

data to predict the class, a process known as testing or "inference." Fig. 18.1 illustrates example data to be used in logistic regression. Each data point is represented by either a square or circle, and has two attributes, x_1 and x_2. The data are plotted in the "feature space" of x_1 and x_2. These observed data points are known as "training data" because their shapes are known (ground truth labels), and they will be used to fit the logistic regression using the x_1 and x_2 attributes. Test data have known x_1 and x_2 but unknown shape category, which will be predicted using the fitted regression. The label category (shapes in this example) is often represented as "y" in ML.

The logistic regression model for this example is represented by this equation:

$$\sigma(z) = \frac{1}{1+e^{-z}} \qquad (18.2)$$

$$z = x_1 * w_1 + x_2 * w_2 + b, \qquad (18.3)$$

where x_1 and x_2 are the input features to the model, and w_1, w_2, and b are the parameters of the model. Fig. 18.2 shows an illustration of the computations in the logistic regression model. The red unit in the "Current Layer" of Fig. 18.2A computes the sum of each input multiplied by its corresponding parameter, and that sum is subsequently put through "σ" the sigmoid nonlinearity, illustrated among other nonlinearities used in machine learning in Fig. 18.2B.

$\sigma(z)$ represents the probability of a data point belonging to class 1 ($P(y=1)$), and because the outcome is binary, $1-\sigma(z)$ represents the probability of that data point belonging to class 0. This model states that $P(y=1)$ is a linear combination of the input variables (Eq. 18.3) subsequently put through a nonlinear transformation to limit the output between zero and one. To make classifications, a probability threshold is set (often $\sigma(z)=0.5$), above which the data point will be categorized as class 1 (a square) and below which the data point will be categorized as class 0 (a circle). Setting a decision threshold for $\sigma(z)$ is equivalent to setting a (different) decision threshold based on "z." Given a constant threshold in "z," a linear decision boundary in feature space can be drawn which separates predictions of class 1 from class 0. Setting z = C, a constant, simple rearrangement of Eq. (18.3) gives the decision boundary:

$$C = x_1 * w_1 + x_2 * w_2 + b \rightarrow$$
$$x_2 = -w_1 / w_2 * x_1 + (C-b) / w_2 \qquad (18.4)$$

which has the form of a linear equation in x_1 and x_2.

Initially the mathematical form of the model is specified (Eq. 18.2) but the values of the model parameters are not. These parameters are typically initialized to some random values, which would yield a randomly oriented decision boundary in our data space (red dashed line in Fig. 18.1). The purpose of fitting, or "training," the model is to find the parameters which

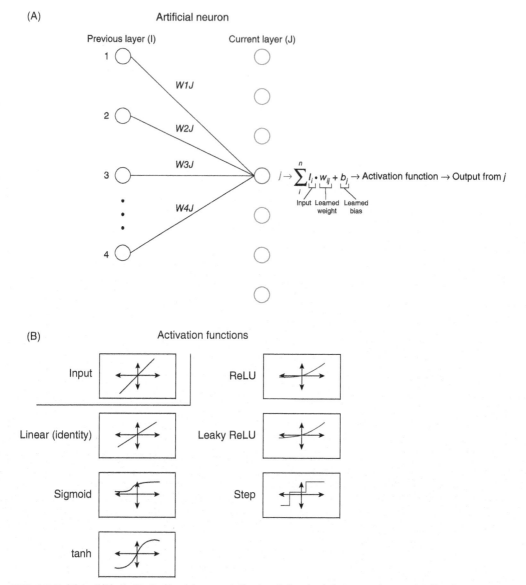

FIG. 18.2 (A) and (B): An illustration of computation levels in a logistic regression model.(Credit: Aaron Lee, MD and research team.)

give the best-fit decision boundary for the observed dataset. The goodness-of-fit of the parameters can be quantified using a cost function, also known as a "loss function." This loss function penalizes imperfect predictions in accordance with their difference from the correct prediction. The loss is a function of the model parameters given the observed training data.

In Fig. 18.3A a hypothetical shape of a loss function is shown, where the horizontal plane represents the w_1 and w_2 axes. The specific shape of this function depends on the specific training data observed, and each unique combination of parameter values gives a unique point on the loss surface. Finding the parameter values that minimize the loss corresponds to finding the best-fit parameters (and subsequently the optimal decision boundary). An ML method commonly used to find optimal parameters in more complex models is gradient descent, in which the parameter values are iteratively altered to approach better values. This function is designed to be differentiable such that a small

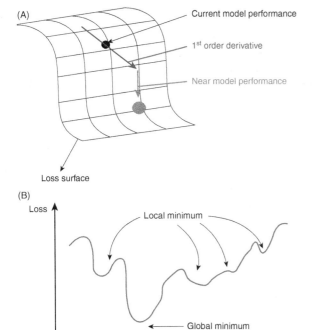

FIG. 18.3 (A) and (B): Hypothetical shapes of loss functions. (Credit: Aaron Lee, MD and research team.)

change in the parameters will yield a smooth change in the cost. A partial derivative of this function with respect to a parameter represents how much the loss changes as the parameter is increased by a tiny amount, while the other parameters are held constant. The gradient is the vector of partial derivatives with respect to each parameter, and the gradient at each location on the surface represents the direction of steepest increase in the BCE loss. The direction opposite the gradient thus gives the direction of steepest descent and most rapid decrease in cost. The process of gradient descent can be summarized by the repetition of two steps:

1. Calculate the gradient at the location of the current parameter values
2. Make a change in the parameters in the direction opposite of the gradient

The magnitude of change in the parameters is typically prespecified and is called the "learning rate" or "step size." The repetition of these two steps results in an approximate steepest descent along the loss surface to a minima (depicted in Fig. 18.3A). These two steps are repeated until a minima is reached and the value of the gradient is below some threshold. In this process, the full loss surface is not observed, as that would require calculating the BCE loss for every possible combination

of parameters. Thus, gradient descent may not find the best, or "global" minimum, but instead only a "local" minima or a suboptimal combination of parameters. Fig. 18.3B provides a one-dimensional illustration of a loss function with both global and local minima.

As the parameters are updated from their random initializations, the linear decision boundary shifts and rotates from its random initial position and orientation into the best-possible position, given our training data (green line in Fig. 18.1). If the underlying classes in the data are linearly separable, this would result in a perfect classification of all training data. However, in this example, the data are not linearly separable, and even the best-fit parameters at the global minimum of our loss surface cannot characterize the underlying phenomenon. This failure is known as "underfitting," one of the three major causes of ML model failure despite convergence of parameters to a minimal. Underfitting occurs when a model fails to capture relationships within the data due to insufficient model flexibility or capacity. In order to capture more complex patterns within data, nonlinear models are needed. Another major mode of failure in the setting of model convergence is overfitting, which is discussed later in the chapter.

Neural Networks and Modeling Nonlinear Relationships Within Data

Neural networks provide the representational capacity to model complicated, nonlinear relationships within data. A neural network model can be formed by computing successive layers of parallel multiple logistic regression models. In Fig. 18.4, each node in the hidden layer is the output of a logistic regression on the input features. Those hidden nodes then become the inputs to further logistic regressions. This composition of layers of logistic regression functions gives the network flexibility to draw complex decision boundaries, illustrated by the purple boundary in Fig. 18.1. The type of network illustrated in Fig. 18.4 is called a feedforward, fully connected network, otherwise known as a multilayer perceptron network. Each layer propagates its information only to the subsequent layer, and each unit in a layer is connected by a weight to each unit in the subsequent layer. Fully connected networks have high representational capacity, as each input feature and each hidden node can independently affect the next layer.

Neural networks can be trained using gradient descent, where the gradients are calculated efficiently using the backpropagation algorithm.

Framing neural networks as successive logistic regressions is accurate only for a small subset of neural

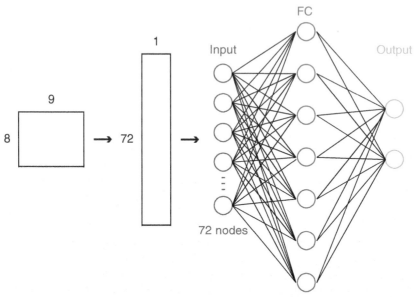

FIG. 18.4 An example of a neural network composed of multilayer, multiple linear regression models. (Credit: Aaron Lee, MD and research team.)

networks. More generally, neural network models are composed of successive linear transformations of an input vector, with nonlinear transformations interspersed between some (and often all) of the linear transformations. Each hidden layer is calculated as a linear transform of the previous layer typically followed by a nonlinearity. The rectified linear unit (ReLU) nonlinearity is typically used as the nonlinearity instead of the sigmoid function because it typically results in more stable gradient values throughout the network, which makes the network easier to optimize.

Deep Learning and Convolutional Neural Networks

Computer vision is a broad field that involves the processing of information in image-based data. Image processing tasks include classification (labeling an image as a single category), localization (defining a bounding box around a region or object of interest), semantic segmentation (categorizing each pixel in an image), regression (predicting continuous values), and image-to-image generation (creating a new or altered image using an image input). Traditionally the algorithms designed for these tasks used handcrafted features or heuristics. Advances in deep learning have resulted in dramatic improvements over these traditional methods and have

renewed interest in computationally analyzing the rich information in medical imaging studies.

Traditionally, images were represented as high-dimensional data, where each pixel in an image is treated as an independent feature. Fully connected networks suffer with such high-dimensional inputs because the model size increases dramatically as the image size increases. For example, for an 8×9 pixel image, there are 72 input dimensions (features), and each of these inputs is connected to every unit in the first hidden layer. This architecture discards the structural information inherent in the spatial arrangement of the pixels, and learning acceptable parameters via gradient descent may take a long time with many parameters. Having too many parameters in the network can also lead to model failure by enabling overfitting. Contrary to underfitting, in which the model does not have enough flexibility to find a function to represent a pattern in data, in overfitting, a model typically has too much flexibility. In this situation the model can find numerous functions that represent the relationships within the training data. The model might be able to perfectly classify all training observations using one of several functions. However, these different functions may have highly varying performance on the unseen test data. A comparison of overfitting and underfitting is illustrated in Fig. 18.5 using the same example data as previously.

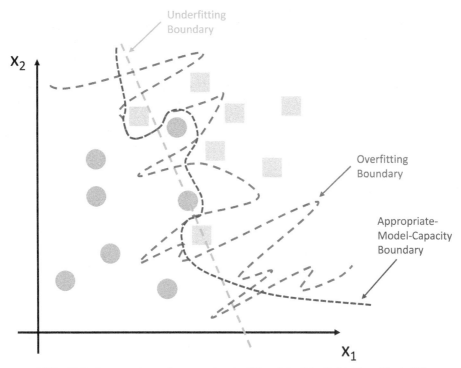

FIG. 18.5 A comparison of over and underfitting data. (Credit: Matthew Hunt, BS)

The green decision boundary represents an underfitting model (here a linear model) that cannot find a function that fits the entire training data without misclassification. The overfitting model represented by the red boundary can employ such a wide array of functions that it can perfectly fit the training data with many of them and may select a function that performs very poorly in regions of the feature space where there is not enough data density. A model with the purple boundary more appropriately matches representational capacity with the complexity of the underlying data being modeled and can result in easier training that avoids underfitting and overfitting.

For applications to imaging, one popular method to both reduce long training time and prevent overfitting is to replace the FC layers with convolution. The FC layers connect each unit in the input layer to each unit in the output layer with an independently learned weight, allowing the network to learn how each input should influence each output. Convolution is illustrated in Fig. 18.6, and can be thought of as sliding a small grid, or "kernel," of weights pixel-by-pixel across the input image, and generating the corresponding output by performing multiplication followed by summation at each position.

These convolutional neural networks, or CNNs, gain several desirable properties by substituting convolution for general matrix multiplication. Because the convolution kernel may be orders of magnitude smaller than the dimensions of the input image, the number of operations needed to compute the next layer can be drastically reduced compared to general matrix multiplication. Additionally, CNNs typically utilize weight-sharing, such that the kernel weights are the same at each pixel position, which drastically reduces model memory size. By applying the same weights to different image locations, the CNN effectively looks for features within the image that are picked up by the kernels. The kernels used to compute the first hidden layer can be thought of as local feature detectors, and the activations of the first hidden layer can thus be understood as representing the spatial locations of the sought-after features.

Interestingly, this method actually has parallels to the early stages of the human visual processing system. Retinal ganglion cells have classically been characterized as having on-surround- or off-surround receptive fields. An on-surround receptive field for a retinal ganglion cell means that the cell activates maximally when it is exposed to light and the surrounding region

Convolutional filter

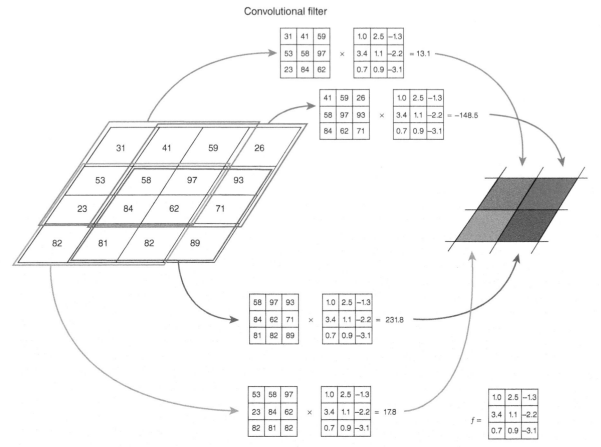

FIG. 18.6 An example of convolution.(Credit: Aaron Lee, MD and research team.)

of retina is exposed to darkness. This receptive field is the feature that is detected by an on-surround retinal ganglion cell. These receptive fields are local in that the activation of the retinal ganglion cells takes into account the strength of the light stimulus on nearby retina. Similarly, kernels in the early layers of CNNs are also conceptualized as detecting certain local features. CNNs typically have multiple kernels per layer, each of which produces a distinct output representing the location of the characteristic feature matching each kernel.

These constraints of convolution and weight sharing restrict the types of functions the network can use to model data. Convolution ensures the transformation function between subsequent layers only utilizes spatially local features. Weight sharing reduces model flexibility and ensures the same feature will be detected regardless of its location in the image. Importantly, these constraints tend to result in networks that are wellsuited for analyzing images. Local features in im-

ages are often informed by nearby pixels, and convolutions capture these interactions while ignoring more distant pixels, which tend to have less influence on the interpretation of image features, in the early layers of the network. Matching model structure to inherent structure within data is an effective technique in deep learning and is used in other data domains aside from imaging. Combined with recent improvements in hardware, such as increasing availability of graphics processing units, these efficient CNN architectural improvements enabled CNNs to achieve state-of-the-art performance on image classification tasks, beginning in 2012[5].

Despite the advantages to processing images with CNNs, there are still a number of technological limitations. CNNs still require large training datasets to generalize well to unseen testing data. These networks are still highly flexible, and thus may perform poorly in regions of the dataspace with few training examples.

Unfortunately medical imaging data can be costly to acquire, and for rare conditions sufficient training data may not exist. Data-focused techniques used to encourage model generalization include data augmentation and transfer learning. Training data augmentation refers to altering the training data in a reasonable manner such that more training examples can be observed by the model and the data space can be more evenly covered. In the domain of imaging, these augmentations commonly consist of affine transformations, such as rotations, vertical or horizontal shifting, and shearing. In transfer learning, a network is not trained from scratch on the training data, but instead a network that has already been trained on a different dataset is fine-tuned on the training data of interest. For instance, a CNN pretrained on the ImageNet dataset,[6] which consists of real-world images from the internet, may be further trained on medical image data. Natural images contain features in common with medical images, such as edges and curves. Pretraining a network on natural images gives the weights a headstart prior to exposing the network to medical images, and may allow the network to learn important basic concepts from a broad dataset.

DEEP LEARNING IN OPHTHALMOLOGY
Deep Learning in Retinal Imaging
Fundus photography
Many of the early applications of deep learning to retinal imaging applied existing computer vision neural network architectures to diagnose conditions using fundus photos, demonstrating their utility in medical imaging. Beginning in 2016, several groups have published work on the development of deep learning models for diagnosis of disease from fundus photos in various conditions, including diabetic retinopathy (DR)[7–12], age-related macular degeneration (AMD)[13–18], and retinopathy of prematurity[19–22]. With much of the groundwork laid by computer vision research and the emergence of CNNs like AlexNet as powerful image classifiers as early as 2012, progress in deep learning in retina was accelerated by the development of two factors: Large, standardized datasets of color fundus images with disease labels and clinical expert consensus on a DR severity grading system. Using 128,174 images from the EyePACS-1 dataset for training, a CNN developed by a research team associated with Google demonstrated a sensitivity of 90.3% and specificity of 98.1% in the classification of referable DR (defined as moderate NPDR or worse) on the 1748 images in the publicly available Messidor-2 dataset[8,23]. Public availability of a

dataset from EyePACS following a Kaggle competition on DR screening spurred the development of multiple models advancing state-of-the-art performance[9,24,25]. AI systems using deep learning have compared favorably to older AI systems, as illustrated by Abramoff et al.'s improvement in specificity by between 24% and 31.3% over the Iowa Detection Program's computer vision algorithm by including deep learning models in their automated algorithm[7]. Dataset availability has underpinned the surge of progress in this field.

More recent studies have utilized even larger datasets and have expanded the scope of the models to address multiple conditions. A 2017 study by Ting et al. used over 500,000 fundus images to train models to classify referable DR, glaucoma, and AMD and they attained (sensitivity, specificity) pairs of (90.5%, 91.6%), (96.4%, 87.2%), and (93.2%, 88.7%), respectively. This study also evaluated the performance of their model(s) on external testing data, with AUROC ranging from 0.889 to 0.983, which is an essential step toward investigating durability of these models in the real world.

The demonstration of disease classification performance by these models exhibited technological potential for AI employment in clinical care, but proof of safe and beneficial real-world application was needed prior to US Food and Drug Administration (FDA) approval of any AI algorithm for clinical care. That demonstration came in Abramoff et al.'s prospective study of 900 patients without a history of DR who had human grades from Wisconsin Fundus Photograph Reading Center compared with AI-predicted DR grades, without permitting any retraining of the AI model[26]. The AI system attained sensitivity and specificity of 87.2% and 90.7%, respectively, and has been approved by the FDA to detect diabetic macular edema and more than mild DR[26].

FDA approval is necessary prior to the incorporation of any AI algorithm into patient care. Even with FDA approval for certain clinical use cases, continuing to investigate the real-world performance of AI models in a range of use cases is a critical task to ensure long-term benefits to patients and to avoid unintended consequences. There are currently two FDA approved algorithms for the automated detection of DR[26,27], and several others are seeking FDA approval. These systems have potential to benefit patients with limited access to care and to aid physicians with the volume of DR screening. However, real-world data may have different image quality or characteristics from data used in research or even prospective studies, and such differences in data characteristics can influence model performance.

Lee et al. recently investigated the performance of several of these AI algorithms on their real-world performance using large retrospective analysis of fundus images taken at two VA hospitals[28]. Patient demographics, disease burden, and imaging parameters differed between the two hospitals, and the models exhibited differences in performance at two sites. Importantly, a real-world referral threshold different from the specific FDA indications for use was evaluated, and at this threshold, many commercial models differed substantially in performance. Adoption of these technologies into the clinic may first involve a hybrid screening strategy, in which providers and deep learning algorithms collaborate in grading. This could provide a check against unforeseen performance shortcomings in the models and might allow for a safer transition to giving the autonomous models more responsibility as their durability is confirmed. Additionally, a collaborative workflow may improve overall grading performance, though potentially at the cost of increased grading time, as suggested by a 2019 study by Sayres et al.[29].

The networks discussed so far have been used to diagnose disease, and they thus perform image classification, but image segmentation has also found numerous applications in fundus imaging. Image segmentation involves labeling each pixel in an image as belonging to one of multiple classes. Similar to the trend in classification tasks, a driver in the progress of retinal image segmentation was the development and availability of datasets of fundus images with corresponding expert labels. The initial datasets included DRIVE[30], STARE[31], HRF[32], and chase_db1[33], and were largely focused on retinal vessels.

Deep learning methods have come to play a major role in segmentation tasks as well as classification tasks. The ideal semantic segmentation model would perfectly label each pixel in an entire fundus image into several categories of normal or pathological retinal structures, and research has been progressing toward this end. This would give the precise locations and spatial relationships between pathologies, along with the pixel area of each pathology. Such a labeling system could be used for a downstream classification or decision output, further interpreted by a clinical expert to influence treatment, or used as quantitative endpoints for clinical trials. Using the aforementioned Kaggle DR dataset with additional annotations added, Lam et al. was able to perform pixel-level segmentation on smaller image patches[34].

Even when exact pixel predictions are not obtained, models can sometimes still be used to extract spatially localized information about categories in an image.

After training binary classification models to detect the presence or absence of 12 distinct retinal features (retinal hemorrhages, hard exudates, cotton wool spots, drusen, epiretinal membrane, macular hole, chorioretinal atrophy, vascular abnormality, retinal nerve fiber layer defect, glaucomatous disc changes, and nonglaucomatous disc changes), Son et al. applied model visualization methods to try to localize each feature[35]. Various visualization methods exist, but some attempt to demonstrate the degree of influence of each input pixel in the image has upon each output class, and thus may give an imprecise localization of that class within the image. Classification of DR disease severity from fundus photos requires attention to specific lesions. Wei et al. designed a multitask network to segment lesions, classify for the presence of eight different lesions types, and predict the DR disease severity grade for fundus images[36]. In their multitask architecture the prediction maps for each type of lesion were allowed to influence the overall image DR grading by interacting in an attention mechanism with the main grading backbone of the network.

OCT imaging

Classification and segmentation models have also been designed to perform clinical tasks using OCT scans. While OCT scans represent a rich source of clinical information, several aspects make deep-learning approaches to analyzing OCT scans more challenging than for fundus photo analysis. First, OCT scans are volumetric data composed of stacked planar B-scans. This could allow models to more accurately identify pathology, but analyzing structures in three dimensions requires nuanced approaches in neural network design. To capture structural relationships between all dimensions of the scan 3D CNNs can be used, in which the kernel is not a "patch," but rather a "cube" of weights. This typically increases computation cost. Second, there tends to be more variation between the images generated by different OCT scanners than between fundus photos taken using different cameras. Models may not generalize well between scanners of different types. Third, there has not been the same availability of large-scale, labeled data for training as there has been for fundus photos.

Even in the face of these challenges, deep learning approaches have shown success in the classification of diseases from OCT scans. In the first-ever application of deep learning to OCT scans, Lee et al. classified AMD with a sensitivity of 92.6% and a specificity of 93.7% (AUROC of 0.97)[37]. This study used approximately 100,000 OCT B-scan images. Additional achievement in classification was demonstrated by Kermany et al. using transfer learning to categorize OCT scans into normal, drusen, CNV, and DME[38]. Deep learning has also been used in segmentation tasks for OCT. Segmentation applications have included detecting boundaries of retinal layers[39-45], geographic atrophy[46], and hyperreflective foci[47], along with pixel segmentation of OCT features such as fluid[48-53] and pigment epithelial detachment[54]. The majority of these approaches used a "U-net" neural network architecture suited to capture both high-resolution details and general semantic information within images[55].

Segmentation and classification approaches have also been combined to analyze OCT volumes. In a 2018 study, De Fauw et al. developed an AI system that used two neural networks in series to both identify the presence of 10 different disease categories in OCT scans and to categorize referral urgency into urgent, semiurgent, routine, and observation[56]. The first network in the series took in a raw OCT as input and output a segmentation map in which each pixel was categorized as belonging to 1 of 15 different categories. That segmentation map was subsequently input into the classification network which predicted disease categories and referral urgency. The model matched or exceeded expert-level accuracy in referral urgency classification. This approach improves training-data efficiency and model interpretability. Different OCT devices produce images with different characteristics, which may cause AI models to perform poorly if they have not been exposed to these types of images during training. The two-stage approach allowed the authors to use a different OCT device by retraining only the segmentation network using a smaller amount of data and reusing the original classification network. This could help with diseases for which adequate training data is challenging to acquire. Additionally, the segmentation map provides more insight into how the AI system makes classifications compared to a single end-to-end neural network, as a clinician can visualize the model's understanding of the retinal tissues.

Deep learning for superhuman tasks

The classification and segmentation models discussed above were designed to perform routine clinical tasks. Deep learning models have also demonstrated performance on surprising tasks that were not thought to be clinically possible. One such example was the prediction of cardiovascular risk factors and biological sex and from color fundus photos alone[57]. This result suggests deep learning models can use image features of which clinicians are currently unaware. While some of these tasks may not have obvious clinical utility,

continued progress in model comprehensibility research may enable biological insight to be gleaned from parsing these models' mechanisms of classification.

Another task, typically considered beyond clinical ability, that deep learning models have shown promise is prediction of disease progression. Prediction of disease progression has been attempted both using fundus photos and OCT images. Using only color fundus photos, a deep learning model developed by Arcadu et al. demonstrated an AUROC of 0.79 for detecting a two-step progression in DR severity after 1 year[58]. Building upon the aforementioned 2018 work combining segmentation and classification architectures for the categorization of disease and referral urgency, a modified version of the same two-stage AI system was used to predict progression from dry to wet AMD in the ensuing 6 months in patients diagnosed with wet AMD in their fellow eye, using OCT scans alone[59]. The model outperformed five of six experts, both when experts had access to the single OCT scans alone and when they had access to serial OCT scans, fundus photos, and clinical information.

Cross-modality applications of deep learning have also demonstrated performance at tasks not performed clinically. Deep learning approaches benefit from large amounts of accurately-labeled data, and cross-modality approaches can be used to obtain a large amount of objective, ground-truth data. In these approaches, a model is used to generate a prediction of a structural output or objective functional measurement. Structural outputs could consist of generating synthetic structures or measurements from another type of scan. Lee et al. successfully generated OCTA B-scans from structural OCT B-scans[60]. Using OCTA B-scans as training targets eliminated the need for laborious expert annotation and provided a large volume of high-quality, objective data. In a different study, OCT central subfield thickness was predicted from color fundus photos with deep learning models using both a regression approach and a thresholded-classification approach[61]. Functional outcomes have also been predicted using cross-modality approaches. Kihara et al. was able to predict retinal sensitivity in the form of an en-face pseudo-perimetry map using single B-scan slices as input to a neural network by training on microperimetry values registered to the OCT B-scans[62].

Application of AI in Other Ophthalmic Subspecialties

While the utilization of various deep learning models into ocular telehealth has largely focused on retinal imaging, a variety of early models have been proposed to integrate deep learning into the fields of glaucoma, cataract, cornea, neuro-ophthalmology, oculoplastics, and pediatric ophthalmology. These models remain experimental but many have shown enhanced accuracy and sensitivity when compared to human models and existing nomograms.

Glaucoma

The vast majority of AI models developed within the field of glaucoma remain experimental. However, the emerging glaucoma-related DL models have shown significant promise in improving screening and predictive capabilities. Most of the DL algorithms developed to detect, stage, and predict glaucoma are based on either fundus photos or OCT images focusing on the optic disc and retinal nerve fiber layer (RNFL). Some groups have also been able to detect or predict glaucomatous visual field defects. There has also been some success in the development of AI models aimed at evaluating for angle closure or other angle abnormalities with anterior segment OCT or ultrasound biomicroscopy (UBM).

Several groups have been successful in showing that fundus photos can be used to detect glaucomatous optic neuropathy (GON). Experimental CNN models to detect GON in color fundus photos have been proposed as a sensitive, efficient and cost-effective screening method[63–66]. Many of these models utilize a CNN based on the Inception v3 architecture[63,66], while more recent models have employed a CNN algorithm based on a ResNet platform[64,65]. These models have been found to be as good as, or better than human graders in detecting referable GON. However, these models can be limited by confounding optic nerve abnormalities including peripapillary atrophy, tilted or myopic appearing discs and retinal pathology such as macular degeneration that can alter the appearance of the optic disc and distort the algorithm's ability to perform image processing[64,65]. Despite these limitations, these models are still capable of achieving high sensitivity and specificity in the detection of GON. Further modifications to these CNN-based algorithms have been suggested in an effort to further improve upon these capabilities. Gheisari et al. developed a combined CNN and recurrent neural network (RNN) to mine spatial features in a fundus image and combine those findings with temporal features in sequential fundus images or a fundus video[67]. This technique showed an improved ability to detect glaucomatous changes when compared to models that looked at spatial features alone. Ahn et al. developed a CNN based on Inception v3 and a custom CNN architecture using TensorFlow that were capable of distinguishing both early- and advanced-stage glaucoma from controls[68].

Some successful DL models have been developed based on a platform utilizing both OCT and fundus photos as part of the algorithm. For example, Thompson et al. developed a CNN that utilized SD-OCT and optic disc photos to evaluate the minimum rim width relative to Bruch's membrane opening (BMO-MRW). They found this measurement was capable of quantifying the amount of glaucomatous neuroretinal damage which in turn was highly accurate in detecting glaucoma. Another algorithm taking advantage of both OCT and fundus images was described by Medeiros et al. and consists of a CNN based on ResNet 34 architecture and trained on SD-OCT images to analyze fundus photographs and quantify structural optic nerve damage[69]. This model eliminates the need for human labeling of a reference training set and can be used to diagnose and stage glaucoma. The same group also developed a CNN based on ResNet 50 architecture trained to predict RNFL thickness on SD-OCT based on fundus photograph assessment that could be used to monitor for progressive glaucomatous changes[70].

While several models have been developed to utilize a combination of SD-OCT and fundus images, many models have focused on the analysis of OCT images alone. An early example of such a concept, proposed by Muhammad et al. is a hybrid deep learning model based on AlexNet and utilizing a random forest classifier designed to classify an image as healthy or glaucomatous based on a single widefield OCT[71]. This model was found to outperform traditional OCT metrics in detecting early glaucoma and was proposed as a screening model. As AI capabilities have become more sophisticated, several more recent models have been proposed that utilize segmentation-free deep learning algorithms based on OCT images[72–74]. These models have the distinct advantage of an improved ability to evaluate the RNFL on images with artifact or segmentation errors that are common with more conventional parameters. This adjustment therefore makes these models more accurate in detecting and staging glaucomatous damage.

Recently, DL models designed to manage glaucoma have turned to visual field defects. Several CNN algorithms utilize SD-OCT to predict and quantify glaucomatous visual field deficits[75–77]. For instance, Xu et al. was able to develop a CNN applying tensor regression to predict 10-2 visual field results based on RNFL thickness on OCT[78]. These models can reduce the need for visual fields in patients who have difficulty physically performing or accessing this type of study and can also help to further understand the correlation between SD-OCT and VF defects. While most algorithms designed to target glaucomatous visual field defects rely on OCT, alternative models employing other imaging modalities have also shown promise. Instead of OCT, Jammal et al. describe a machine-to-machine deep learning algorithm that relies on fundus photos to quantify RNFL damage and detect eyes with repeatable glaucomatous visual field damage[79]. This model was also found to be comparable to or better than a human model and was found to be good for screening programs. Conversely, Masumoto et al. developed a highly reliable DL model that utilizes an ultra-widefield scanning laser ophthalmoscope to detect glaucomatous damage and visual field defects[80]. While some DL models have successfully been shown to predict progressive VF damage, they often require multiple previous VF exams. Wen et al. was able to develop a unique DL algorithm capable of predicting future progressive HVF deficits from a single HVF as input[81]. This has the potential to quickly anticipate future glaucomatous progression.

In addition to glaucomatous optic nerve and visual field findings, AI models have also shown early success in evaluating intraocular pressure (IOP). Developed to analyze slit lamp video recordings, Spaide et al. described a DL model trained to localize and segment mires in order to automatically measure IOP using fixed force Goldmann applanation tonometry[82]. This concept shows promise as it could allow for more frequent, reliable and readily available IOP measurements without relying on highly trained personnel. Especially when considering the well-established importance of understanding individual IOP fluctuation as it relates to disease progression, the possibility of integrating AI-based IOP measurements into glaucoma management holds great potential.

Angle status is another important consideration in glaucoma management that has been targeted by recent AI development. Li et al. developed a ResNet-18-based CNN to distinguish between open and closed angles using UBM[83]. Anterior segment OCT has also been used to evaluate for angle closure with two models utilizing a CNN with transfer learning for improved convergence[84,85]. A ResNet-based CNN utilizing data augmentation and style transfer with paired images of anterior segment OCT and UBM has also been proposed to accurately detect plateau iris based on angle structure[86].

While glaucoma DL models are not yet used in mainstream ocular telehealth, the potential utility of these algorithms in programs to screen for glaucoma and monitor for progressive glaucomatous damage has increased as models have continued to become more sophisticated.

Cataract

The diagnosis and grading of cataract can be accomplished in telemedicine via several imaging modalities including slit lamp photographs, fundus photographs and anterior segment optical coherence tomography (OCT). Evaluation of cataract using artificial intelligence remains experimental, but several promising models have been proposed.

Several groups have suggested applying machine learning analysis of slit lamp photographs to diagnose and grade cataracts. Gao et al. proposed a convolutional neural network (CNN) with a recursive neural network to determine higher order features that replaces the typically utilized predefined set of image features with automatically learned features to enhance accuracy[87]. Xu et al. also proposed a model utilizing slit lamp photographs to grade nuclear sclerotic cataracts, though this was based on a group sparsity-based constraint for a linear regression model[88]. In addition to slit lamp photographs, fundus photographs have also been successfully used to evaluate cataracts. One efficacious model described by Zhang et al. is designed to detect and grade cataracts based on fundus photos. It extracts content features using a ResNet18 CNN and represents texture features using a gray level cooccurrence matrix. These features are input into two separate support vector machines (SVM), and final classification into severity categories is performed with a multilayer perceptron using SVM outputs[89]. Similarly, Yang et al.[90] also proposed a fundus-photo-based model employing an ensemble learning approach to improve accuracy with a combination of three independent feature sets (wavelet, sketch, and texture) and two base learning modules (SVM and back propagation neural network). These fundus photograph-based methods demonstrate the potential for expansion of traditional ocular telehealth programs to include cataract evaluation without additional photography requirements.

The utilization of machine learning models has also been suggested to assist with pre- and postcataract surgery concerns. Brant et al.[91] suggested a model designed to optimize the intraocular lens (IOL) inventory prior to a global cataract surgery campaign based on review of prior records. IOL design has also been targeted by AI models. A region-based fully convolutional network model developed by Xin et al.[92] using anterior segment OCT and capable of evaluating IOL position, lens tilt relative to scleral spur, and lens eccentricity has been proposed. Finally, a ResNet-CNN-based algorithm has been proposed to define not only cataractous lens changes but also to detect posterior capsular opacification within the visual axis[93].

While all of the aforementioned models have been shown to be comparable to or superior to existing technology currently employed, the utilization of AI-based models to assist with cataract management has yet to reach its full potential.

Cornea

The proposed value of AI in the field of cornea and refractive surgery is varied and shows promise in clinical practice as well as expansion of cornea care within the realm of ocular telehealth. Several CNN algorithms have been proposed to utilize confocal microscopy to evaluate corneal nerve fibers[94-96]. ACCMetrics is a widely used experimental algorithm designed to detect and quantify corneal nerve fibers as well as morphological descriptors of the individual nerves[95]. These models are particularly useful in the diagnosis of diabetic neuropathy and have been suggested as a screening tool for more peripheral neuropathy.

Corneal ectasia and keratoconus have also been significant areas of development that have shown promise with respect to integration of AI into the world of ocular telehealth. For example, a potential deep learning model using color-coded maps of swept source anterior segment OCT to diagnose and classify keratoconus and a three-step algorithm, utilizing principal component analysis, followed by manifest learning, and then density-based clustering to successfully stage keratoconus patients in an automated fashion have both been described as potential models to improve keratoconus management.[97,98] Additionally, a CNN algorithm known as KeratoDetect has been put forth as a program to rapidly screen for and diagnose keratoconus.[99] These proposed models can help to risk stratify patients and determine need for in person evaluation, thus demonstrating promise for future integration within ocular telehealth programs. While less applicable to the world of ocular telehealth as it currently stands, Fariselli et al.[100] proposed a successful artificial neural network capable of improved predictability of intracorneal ring segment implantation and improved visual outcomes when compared to the existing nomogram.

An additional target of AI research within the field of cornea has been the corneal endothelium. Several U-Net based CNN models have been suggested to evaluate the density of corneal endothelial cells[101-103]. The potential automation of a task which was previously inaccurate and tedious to perform manually has the potential to significantly improve accuracy and efficiency and enable remote management of corneal pathology.

While corneal surgery considerations are not immediately ready for implementation within ocular telehealth programs, this subject has been a point of interest for AI development. Yousefi et al.[104] proposed a machine learning mechanism to assess corneal shape, thickness, and elevation and predict the risk for future keratoplasty. Additionally, models designed to determine the need for rebubbling following Descemet Membrane Endothelial Keratoplasty (DMEK) and to automatically detect graft detachment following DMEK have also been put forth[105,106].

Additionally, a variety of other corneal and ocular surface pathology have been the subject of development with AI-based models. These include a deep learning model designed to detect meibomian gland dysfunction in dry eye syndrome patients[107], a SVM and artificial neural network-based model designed to screen for pterygia in rural patient populations[108] and an AlexNet CNN based model designed to diagnose fungal keratitis via confocal microscopy[109].

The success of these models and the broad range of pathology represented is a testament to the promise of future implementation of AI within corneal ocular telehealth.

Neuroophthalmology

While the implantation of AI in the field of neuroophthalmology remains largely unexplored, future possibilities have largely focused on evaluating the optic nerve for signs of papilledema or optic neuropathy. Several models have been shown to successfully evaluate the optic nerve, suggesting promise in remote automated diagnosis of optic disc pathology.

Examples of these models include a deep learning model utilizing fundus photos to diagnose papilledema[110] and a deep learning system using a U-Net CNN segmentation model to detect the location of the optic disc along with a DenseNet model to classify the optic disc as normal, papilledema or other abnormality using fundus photographs[111]. Finally, Ahn et al.[112] demonstrated at least 95% accuracy in delineating optic neuropathy from pseudopapilledema and normal optic discs via four models including a unique algorithm as well as three commercially available CNNs (GoogleNet Inception v3, VGG19 and ResNet).

While the success of these experimental models shows significant promise for future implementation, further research will be necessary before AI can be utilized in mainstream telemedicine and neuroophthalmology.

Oculoplastics

As with many other subspecialties, the utility of AI in the field of ocular telehealth and oculoplastics has yet to be well established. Few experimental models have been proposed to assist in the remote automated management of lid and orbital disease.

One successful model proposed by Thomas et al.[51,113] suggested the use of OpenFace, an open-source AI-driven facial analysis system capable of landmarking and analyzing lid position as a system to evaluate vertical palpebral aperture in pre- and post-ptosis repair patients from full facial photographs. The success of this model shows promise for this still undeveloped field.

Pediatric ophthalmology

Development of AI integration in the field of pediatric tele-ophthalmology has largely focused on retinopathy of prematurity (ROP).

One example of a promising AI model, described by Coyner et al.[21], is an algorithm employing a CNN to distinguish acceptable screening fundus photos from poor-quality photos that cannot be used in an effort to improve the image acquisition quality in remote ROP screening programs. Several models have been proposed that demonstrate the ability to stage ROP and detect the presence of plus disease with accuracy comparable to or better than human graders in a more efficient manner. These models include a model that performed well in the detection of type 2 or worse ROP based on ETROP treatment guidelines[114], as well as a dual-model based on a ResNet CNN to stratify urgency of ROP disease management and a faster region-based CNN (Faster-RCNN) to determine ROP stage and detect the presence of plus disease[115]. Brown et al. and the i-ROP group[19] developed a U-Net CNN-based model to successfully diagnose plus and pre-plus disease. Additionally, Tan et al.[116] utilized the TensorFlow Inception v3 CNN to develop an algorithm known as ROP.AI that is capable of successfully diagnosing plus disease with high sensitivity.

As with most other AI-related models designed for the field of ocular telehealth, the implementation of AI algorithms in the field of pediatric ophthalmology remains experimental at this time.

Applications of AI and Big Data in Ocular Telehealth

The successes thus far in these various applications of AI to ophthalmic subspecialties indicate potential for eventual utilization in clinical settings, following FDA approval. Ocular telehealth is a domain where these AI technologies have potential to decrease cost and increase efficiency of care. As an example, eye telehealth for diabetic retinopathy (DR) screening stands to benefit from AI. The use of a telemedicine paradigm for DR screening, in which a central fundus-photo grading center has human image graders evaluating remotely-acquired images, has been indicated to be both cost effective and provide more effective screening for DR[117]. A meta-analysis analyzing the sensitivity and specificity of teleretinal screening for macular edema and DR found high sensitivity and specificity for the absence of DR (87% and 91%, respectively). An economic analysis by Xie et al., evaluated two ways of integrating deep learning models into a workflow where only patients with suspected DR beyond mild disease are referred to specialists, both of which were projected to cut costs[118]. A hybrid approach with fundus-image grading performed by both AI and human graders at the grading center was projected to deliver the greatest cost savings (19.5% savings). A fully automated grading approach, with no human grader involvement at the grading-center stage, was also projected to cut costs, but to a lesser degree (14.3% savings). The reason for the superiority of the hybrid approach over the fully automated approach was the higher rate of false positives by the AI-only system resulting in a greater number of unnecessary referrals. As suggested by the previously mentioned study by Lee et al.[28], the performance of AI models involved in DR telehealth screening should be evaluated in their real-world context prior to deployment, as different referral thresholds or image characteristics (such as dilation) may alter model performance.

Other potential applications of AI to eye-telehealth have been suggested[119]. Applications designed to improve efficiency include use of AI for front-office tasks, including invoice generation and patient scheduling. Integration of AI with robotics could enable ophthalmic devices to interact autonomously with patients, which could reduce provider burden in busy clinics and enable patient data acquisition in remote or underserved settings where an experienced telehealth facilitator may not be available. As medical remote smart-devices are further developed, steady streams of temporal data could be acquired while patients are at home. Continual analysis of this data will require AI integration with devices, either on-board the device, or in a central server which receives data from the devices. In this setting, the AI system could alert the patient's physician if more urgent intervention is necessary and could provide recommendations taking into account the patient's longitudinal data.

Along with the potential for massive amounts of data to be collected by these smart-devices, the use of electronic medical records (EMR) will continue to increase the amount of medical data available for patients. The scale of this data ("big data") will make full analysis beyond the capabilities of a clinician. AI methods have already shown promise in the analysis of EMR data in glaucoma, cataract, AMD, and DR to provide insight into individual patients[120]. EMR data alone was used to predict progression to surgical intervention in patients with primary open-angle glaucoma. Natural language processing in conjunction with supervised learning was used to predict postoperative and intraoperative complications from cataract surgery. Regression has been used to predict the response of visual acuity to anti-VEGF treatment in AMD patients. A decision support system achieved an AUC of 98% in predicting the risk of type I diabetic patients developing diabetic retinopathy. AI techniques show potential for augmenting the capabilities of physicians to deliver precise and personalized care based on a patient's longitudinal health data.

CONCLUSION

The development of AI in the field of eye care is still in its infancy but is progressing in several areas, especially retinal imaging. These technologies hold potential to improve healthcare by increasing access to care while decreasing costs, objectively and accurately quantifying disease, reducing repetitive tasks for providers, and achieving clinical insights not previously possible with big data analytics. One specific way AI will increase access to care is by augmenting ocular telehealth—enabling continuous analysis of remotely-acquired patient data, increasing efficiency of disease screening, and improving patient interaction with imaging devices. FDA approval is a necessary step before realizing any of these benefits, and continued study of the performance characteristics will be necessary to ensure long-term positive impact for all patients.

REFERENCES

1. Bain A. *Mind and Body: The Theories of Their Relation.* Henry S. King; 1873.
2. James W. *The Principles of Psychology.* vol. I; 1890. https://doi.org/10.1037/10538-000. Published Online.
3. Csáji BC. *Approximation With Artificial Neural Networks.* vol. 24. Hungary: Faculty of Sciences, EtvsLornd University; 2001:48. 7.
4. Cybenko G. *Approximations by Superpositions of a Sigmoidal Function.* University of Illinois at Urbana-Champaign, Center for Supercomputing Research and Development; 1989.
5. Krizhevsky A, Sutskever I, Hinton GE. ImageNet classification with deep convolutional neural networks. In: Pereira F, Burges CJC, Bottou L, Weinberger KQ, eds. *Advances in Neural Information Processing Systems 25.* Curran Associates, Inc.; 2012:1097–1105.
6. Russakovsky O, Deng J, Su H, et al. ImageNet large scale visual recognition challenge. *Int J Comput Vis.* 2015;115(3):211–252. https://doi.org/10.1007/s11263-015-0816-y.
7. Abràmoff MD, Lou Y, Erginay A, et al. Improved automated detection of diabetic retinopathy on a publicly available dataset through integration of deep learning. *Invest Ophthalmol Vis Sci.* 2016;57(13):5200–5206.
8. Gulshan V, Peng L, Coram M, et al. Development and validation of a deep learning algorithm for detection of diabetic retinopathy in retinal fundus photographs. *JAMA.* 2016;316(22):2402–2410.
9. Gargeya R, Leng T. Automated identification of diabetic retinopathy using deep learning. *Ophthalmology.* 2017;124(7):962–969.
10. Ting DSW, Cheung CY-L, Lim G, et al. Development and validation of a deep learning system for diabetic retinopathy and related eye diseases using retinal images from multiethnic populations with diabetes. *JAMA.* 2017;318(22):2211–2223.
11. Abbas Q, Fondon I, Sarmiento A, Jiménez S, Alemany P. Automatic recognition of severity level for diagnosis of diabetic retinopathy using deep visual features. *Med Biol Eng Comput.* 2017;55(11):1959–1974.
12. Takahashi H, Tampo H, Arai Y, Inoue Y, Kawashima H. Applying artificial intelligence to disease staging: deep learning for improved staging of diabetic retinopathy. *PLoS One.* 2017;12(6), e0179790.
13. Burlina PM, Joshi N, Pekala M, Pacheco KD, Freund DE, Bressler NM. Automated grading of age-related macular degeneration from color fundus images using deep convolutional neural networks. *JAMA Ophthalmol.* 2017;135(11):1170–1176.
14. Keenan TD, Dharssi S, Peng Y, et al. A deep learning approach for automated detection of geographic atrophy from color fundus photographs. *Ophthalmology.* 2019;126(11):1533–1540.
15. Chen Q, Peng Y, Keenan T, et al. A multi-task deep learning model for the classification of age-related macular degeneration. *AMIA Jt Summits Transl Sci Proc.* 2019;2019:505–514.
16. Peng Y, Dharssi S, Chen Q, et al. DeepSeeNet: a deep learning model for automated classification of patient-based age-related macular degeneration severity from color fundus photographs. *Ophthalmology.* 2019;126(4):565–575.
17. Burlina PM, Joshi N, Pacheco KD, Freund DE, Kong J, Bressler NM. Use of deep learning for detailed severity characterization and estimation of 5-year risk among patients with age-related macular degeneration. *JAMA Ophthalmol.* 2018;136(12):1359–1366.
18. Grassmann F, Mengelkamp J, Brandl C, et al. A deep learning algorithm for prediction of age-related eye disease study severity scale for age-related macular degeneration from color fundus photography. *Ophthalmology.* 2018;125(9):1410–1420.

19. Brown JM, Campbell JP, Beers A, et al. Automated diagnosis of plus disease in retinopathy of prematurity using deep convolutional neural networks. *JAMA Ophthalmol.* 2018;136(7):803–810.

20. Redd TK, Campbell JP, Brown JM, et al. Evaluation of a deep learning image assessment system for detecting severe retinopathy of prematurity. *Br J Ophthalmol.* 2018. https://doi.org/10.1136/bjophthalmol-2018-313156. Published Online.

21. Coyner AS, Swan R, Brown JM, et al. Deep learning for image quality assessment of fundus images in retinopathy of prematurity. *AMIA Annu Symp Proc.* 2018;2018:1224–1232.

22. Taylor S, Brown JM, Gupta K, et al. Monitoring disease progression with a quantitative severity scale for retinopathy of prematurity using deep learning. *JAMA Ophthalmol.* 2019;137:1022–1028. https://doi.org/10.1001/jamaophthalmol.2019.2433. Published Online.

23. Decencière E, Zhang X, Cazuguel G, et al. Feedback on a publicly distributed image database: the Messidor database. *Image Anal Stereol.* 2014;33(3):231.

24. Raju M, Pagidimarri V, Barreto R, Kadam A, Kasivajjala V, Aswath A. Development of a deep learning algorithm for automatic diagnosis of diabetic retinopathy. *Stud Health Technol Inform.* 2017;245:559–563.

25. Quellec G, Charrière K, Boudi Y, Cochener B, Lamard M. Deep image mining for diabetic retinopathy screening. *Med Image Anal.* 2017;39:178–193.

26. Abràmoff MD, Lavin PT, Birch M, Shah N, Folk JC. Pivotal trial of an autonomous AI-based diagnostic system for detection of diabetic retinopathy in primary care offices. *NPJ Digit Med.* 2018;1:39.

27. Eyenuk Announces FDA. *Clearance for EyeArt Autonomous AI System for Diabetic Retinopathy Screening.* Eyenuk; 2021. Accessed 16.04.21 https://www.eyenuk.com/us-en/articles/diabetic-retinopathy/eyenuk-announces-eyeart-fda-clearance/.

28. Lee AY, Yanagihara RT, Lee CS, et al. Multicenter, head-to-head, real-world validation study of seven automated artificial intelligence diabetic retinopathy screening systems. *Diabetes Care.* 2021. https://doi.org/10.2337/dc20-1877. Published Online.

29. Sayres R, Taly A, Rahimy E, et al. Using a deep learning algorithm and integrated gradients explanation to assist grading for diabetic retinopathy. *Ophthalmology.* 2019;126(4):552–564.

30. Niemeijer M, Staal JJ, Ginneken B, Loog M, Abramoff MD. DRIVE: digital retinal images for vessel extraction. In: *Methods for Evaluating Segmentation and Indexing Techniques Dedicated to Retinal Ophthalmology;* 2004. Published Online.

31. Goldbaum MH, Katz NP, Nelson MR, Haff LR. The discrimination of similarly colored objects in computer images of the ocular fundus. *Invest Ophthalmol Vis Sci.* 1990;31(4):617–623.

32. Köhler T, Budai A, Kraus MF, Odstrčilik J, Michelson G, Hornegger J. Automatic no-reference quality assessment for retinal fundus images using vessel segmentation. In: *Proceedings of the 26th IEEE International Symposium on Computer-Based Medical Systems;* 2013:95–100.

33. Fraz MM. *CHASE_DB1.* Kingston Univ Res; 2011. Tech Rep. Published Online.

34. Lam C, Yu C, Huang L, Rubin D. Retinal lesion detection with deep learning using image patches. *Invest Ophthalmol Vis Sci.* 2018;59(1):590–596.

35. Son J, Shin JY, Kim HD, Jung K-H, Park KH, Park SJ. Development and validation of deep learning models for screening multiple abnormal findings in retinal fundus images. *Ophthalmology.* 2020;127(1):85–94.

36. Wei Q, Li X, Yu W, et al. *Learn to Segment Retinal Lesions and Beyond.* arXiv [csCV]; 2019. Published Online http://arxiv.org/abs/1912.11619.

37. Lee CS, Baughman DM, Lee AY. Deep learning is effective for the classification of OCT images of normal versus age-related macular degeneration. *Ophthalmol Retina.* 2017;1(4):322–327.

38. Kermany DS, Goldbaum M, Cai W, et al. Identifying medical diagnoses and treatable diseases by image-based deep learning. *Cell.* 2018;172(5):1122–1131.e9.

39. Fang L, Cunefare D, Wang C, Guymer RH, Li S, Farsiu S. Automatic segmentation of nine retinal layer boundaries in OCT images of non-exudative AMD patients using deep learning and graph search. *Biomed Opt Express.* 2017;8(5):2732–2744.

40. He Y, Carass A, Yun Y, et al. Towards topological correct segmentation of macular OCT from cascaded FCNs. *Fetal Infant Ophthalmic Med Image Anal (2017).* 2017;10554:202–209.

41. Pekala M, Joshi N, Liu TYA, Bressler NM, DeBuc DC, Burlina P. Deep learning based retinal OCT segmentation. *Comput Biol Med.* 2019;114:103445.

42. Kugelman J, Alonso-Caneiro D, Read SA, et al. Automatic choroidal segmentation in OCT images using supervised deep learning methods. *Sci Rep.* 2019;9(1):13298.

43. Maloca PM, Lee AY, de Carvalho ER, et al. Validation of automated artificial intelligence segmentation of optical coherence tomography images. *PLoS One.* 2019;14(8), e0220063.

44. Shah A, Zhou L, Abràmoff MD, Wu X. Multiple surface segmentation using convolution neural nets: application to retinal layer segmentation in OCT images. *Biomed Opt Express.* 2018;9(9):4509–4526.

45. Hamwood J, Alonso-Caneiro D, Read SA, Vincent SJ, Collins MJ. Effect of patch size and network architecture on a convolutional neural network approach for automatic segmentation of OCT retinal layers. *Biomed Opt Express.* 2018;9(7):3049–3066.

46. Xu R, Niu S, Chen Q, Ji Z, Rubin D, Chen Y. Automated geographic atrophy segmentation for SD-OCT images based on two-stage learning model. *Comput Biol Med.* 2019;105:102–111.

47. Saha S, Nassisi M, Wang M, et al. Automated detection and classification of early AMD biomarkers using deep learning. *Sci Rep.* 2019;9(1):10990.

48. Lee CS, Tyring AJ, Deruyter NP, Wu Y, Rokem A, Lee AY. Deep-learning based, automated segmentation of macular

edema in optical coherence tomography. *Biomed Opt Express.* 2017;8(7):3440–3448.

49. Bogunovic H, Venhuizen F, Klimscha S, et al. RETOUCH: the retinal OCT fluid detection and segmentation benchmark and challenge. *IEEE Trans Med Imaging.* 2019;38(8):1858–1874.

50. Gao K, Niu S, Ji Z, et al. Double-branched and area-constraint fully convolutional networks for automated serous retinal detachment segmentation in SD-OCT images. *Comput Methods Prog Biomed.* 2019;176:69–80.

51. Lu D, Heisler M, Lee S, et al. Deep-learning based multi-class retinal fluid segmentation and detection in optical coherence tomography images using a fully convolutional neural network. *Med Image Anal.* 2019;54:100–110.

52. Roy AG, Conjeti S, Karri SPK, et al. ReLayNet: retinal layer and fluid segmentation of macular optical coherence tomography using fully convolutional networks. *Biomed Opt Express.* 2017;8(8):3627–3642.

53. Schlegl T, Waldstein SM, Bogunovic H, et al. Fully automated detection and quantification of macular fluid in OCT using deep learning. *Ophthalmology.* 2018;125(4):549–558.

54. Xu Y, Yan K, Kim J, et al. Dual-stage deep learning framework for pigment epithelium detachment segmentation in polypoidal choroidal vasculopathy. *Biomed Opt Express.* 2017;8(9):4061–4076.

55. Ronneberger O, Fischer P, Brox T. U-Net: convolutional networks for biomedical image segmentation. In: *Medical Image Computing and Computer-Assisted Intervention—MICCAI 2015.* Springer International Publishing; 2015:234–241.

56. De Fauw J, Ledsam JR, Romera-Paredes B, et al. Clinically applicable deep learning for diagnosis and referral in retinal disease. *Nat Med.* 2018;24(9):1342–1350.

57. Poplin R, Varadarajan AV, Blumer K, et al. Prediction of cardiovascular risk factors from retinal fundus photographs via deep learning. *Nat Biomed Eng.* 2018;2(3):158–164.

58. Arcadu F, Benmansour F, Maunz A, Willis J, Haskova Z, Prunotto M. Deep learning algorithm predicts diabetic retinopathy progression in individual patients. *NPJ Digit Med.* 2019;2:92.

59. Yim J, Chopra R, Spitz T, et al. Predicting conversion to wet age-related macular degeneration using deep learning. *Nat Med.* 2020;26(6):892–899.

60. Lee CS, Tyring AJ, Wu Y, et al. Generating retinal flow maps from structural optical coherence tomography with artificial intelligence. *Sci Rep.* 2019;9(1):5694.

61. Arcadu F, Benmansour F, Maunz A, et al. Deep learning predicts OCT measures of diabetic macular thickening from color fundus photographs. *Invest Ophthalmol Vis Sci.* 2019;60(4):852–857.

62. Kihara Y, Heeren TFC, Lee CS, et al. Estimating retinal sensitivity using optical coherence tomography with deep-learning algorithms in macular telangiectasia type 2. *JAMA Netw Open.* 2019;2(2), e188029.

63. Phene S, Dunn RC, Hammel N, et al. Deep learning and glaucoma specialists: the relative importance of optic disc features to predict glaucoma referral in fundus photographs. *Ophthalmology.* 2019;126(12):1627–1639.

64. Liu H, Li L, Wormstone IM, et al. Development and validation of a deep learning system to detect glaucomatous optic neuropathy using fundus photographs. *JAMA Ophthalmol.* 2019. https://doi.org/10.1001/jamaophthalmol.2019.3501. Published Online.

65. Yang HK, Kim YJ, Sung JY, Kim DH, Kim KG, Hwang J-M. Efficacy for differentiating nonglaucomatous versus glaucomatous optic neuropathy using deep learning systems. *Am J Ophthalmol.* 2020;216:140–146.

66. Li Z, He Y, Keel S, Meng W, Chang RT, He M. Efficacy of a deep learning system for detecting glaucomatous optic neuropathy based on color fundus photographs. *Ophthalmology.* 2018;125(8):1199–1206. https://doi.org/10.1016/j.ophtha.2018.01.023.

67. Gheisari S, Shariflou S, Phu J, et al. A combined convolutional and recurrent neural network for enhanced glaucoma detection. *Sci Rep.* 2021;11(1). https://doi.org/10.1038/s41598-021-81554-4.

68. Ahn JM, Kim S, Ahn K-S, Cho S-H, Lee KB, Kim US. A deep learning model for the detection of both advanced and early glaucoma using fundus photography. *PLoS One.* 2018;13(11), e0207982.

69. Medeiros FA, Jammal AA, Thompson AC. From machine to machine: an OCT-trained deep learning algorithm for objective quantification of glaucomatous damage in fundus photographs. *Ophthalmology.* 2019;126(4):513–521.

70. Medeiros FA, Jammal AA, Mariottoni EB. Detection of progressive glaucomatous optic nerve damage on fundus photographs with deep learning. *Ophthalmology.* 2020. https://doi.org/10.1016/j.ophtha.2020.07.045. Published Online.

71. Muhammad H, Fuchs TJ, De Cuir N, et al. Hybrid deep learning on single wide-field optical coherence tomography scans accurately classifies glaucoma suspects. *J Glaucoma.* 2017;26(12):1086–1094.

72. Mariottoni EB, Jammal AA, Urata CN, et al. Quantification of retinal nerve fibre layer thickness on optical coherence tomography with a deep learning segmentation-free approach. *Sci Rep.* 2020;10(1):402.

73. Thompson AC, Jammal AA, Berchuck SI, Mariottoni EB, Medeiros FA. Assessment of a segmentation-free deep learning algorithm for diagnosing glaucoma from optical coherence tomography scans. *JAMA Ophthalmol.* 2020;138(4):333–339.

74. Petersen CA, Mehta P, Lee AY. Data-driven, feature-agnostic deep learning vs retinal nerve fiber layer thickness for the diagnosis of glaucoma. *JAMA Ophthalmol.* 2020;138(4):339–340.

75. Mariottoni EB, Datta S, Dov D, et al. Artificial intelligence mapping of structure to function in glaucoma. *Transl Vis Sci Technol.* 2020;9(2):19.

76. Christopher M, Bowd C, Belghith A, et al. Deep learning approaches predict glaucomatous visual field damage from OCT optic nerve head en face images and retinal nerve fiber layer thickness maps. *Ophthalmology.* 2020;127(3):346–356.

77. Park K, Kim J, Lee J. A deep learning approach to predict visual field using optical coherence tomography. *PLoS One.* 2020;15(7), e0234902.

78. Xu L, Asaoka R, Kiwaki T, et al. Predicting the glaucomatous central 10-degree visual field from optical coherence tomography using deep learning and tensor regression. *Am J Ophthalmol.* 2020;218:304–313.

79. Jammal AA, Thompson AC, Mariottoni EB, et al. Human versus machine: comparing a deep learning algorithm to human gradings for detecting glaucoma on fundus photographs. *Am J Ophthalmol.* 2020;211:123–131.

80. Masumoto H, Tabuchi H, Nakakura S, Ishitobi N, Miki M, Enno H. Deep-learning classifier with an ultrawide-field scanning laser ophthalmoscope detects glaucoma visual field severity. *J Glaucoma.* 2018;27(7):647–652.

81. Wen JC, Lee CS, Keane PA, et al. Forecasting future humphrey visual fields using deep learning. *PLoS One.* 2019;14(4), e0214875.

82. Spaide T, Wu Y, Yanagihara RT, et al. Using deep learning to automate Goldmann applanation tonometry readings. *Ophthalmology.* 2020;127(11):1498–1506.

83. Li W, Chen Q, Jiang Z, et al. Automatic anterior chamber angle measurement for ultrasound biomicroscopy using deep learning. *J Glaucoma.* 2020;29(2):81–85.

84. Xu BY, Chiang M, Chaudhary S, Kulkarni S, Pardeshi AA, Varma R. Deep learning classifiers for automated detection of gonioscopic angle closure based on anterior segment OCT images. *Am J Ophthalmol.* 2019;208:273–280.

85. Fu H, Baskaran M, Xu Y, et al. A deep learning system for automated angle-closure detection in anterior segment optical coherence tomography images. *Am J Ophthalmol.* 2019;203:37–45.

86. Wanichwecharungruang B, Kaothanthong N, Pattanapongpaiboon W, et al. Deep learning for anterior segment optical coherence tomography to predict the presence of plateau iris. *Transl Vis Sci Technol.* 2021;10(1):7.

87. Gao X, Lin S, Wong TY. Automatic feature learning to grade nuclear cataracts based on deep learning. *IEEE Trans Biomed Eng.* 2015;62(11):2693–2701.

88. Xu Y, Gao X, Lin S, et al. Automatic grading of nuclear cataracts from slit-lamp lens images using group sparsity regression. *Med Image Comput Comput Assist Interv.* 2013;16(pt. 2):468–475.

89. Zhang H, Niu K, Xiong Y, Yang W, He Z, Song H. Automatic cataract grading methods based on deep learning. *Comput Methods Prog Biomed.* 2019;182:104978.

90. Yang J-J, Li J, Shen R, et al. Exploiting ensemble learning for automatic cataract detection and grading. *Comput Methods Prog Biomed.* 2016;124:45–57.

91. Brant AR, Hinkle J, Shi S, et al. Artificial intelligence in global ophthalmology: using machine learning to improve cataract surgery outcomes at Ethiopian outreaches. *J Cataract Refract Surg.* 2020. https://doi.org/10.1097/j.jcrs.0000000000000407. Published Online.

92. Xin C, Bian G-B, Zhang H, Liu W, Dong Z. Optical coherence tomography-based deep learning algorithm for quantification of the location of the intraocular lens. *Ann Transl Med.* 2020;8(14):872.

93. Wu X, Huang Y, Liu Z, et al. Universal artificial intelligence platform for collaborative management of cataracts. *Br J Ophthalmol.* 2019;103(11):1553–1560.

94. Williams BM, Borroni D, Liu R, et al. An artificial intelligence-based deep learning algorithm for the diagnosis of diabetic neuropathy using corneal confocal microscopy: a development and validation study. *Diabetologia.* 2020;63(2):419–430. https://doi.org/10.1007/s00125-019-05023-4.

95. Chen X, Graham J, Dabbah MA, Petropoulos IN, Tavakoli M, Malik RA. An automatic tool for quantification of nerve fibers in corneal confocal microscopy images. *IEEE Trans Biomed Eng.* 2017;64(4):786–794.

96. Scarpa F, Colonna A, Ruggeri A. Multiple-image deep learning analysis for neuropathy detection in corneal nerve images. *Cornea.* 2020;39(3):342–347.

97. Kamiya K, Ayatsuka Y, Kato Y, et al. Keratoconus detection using deep learning of colour-coded maps with anterior segment optical coherence tomography: a diagnostic accuracy study. *BMJ Open.* 2019;9(9), e031313.

98. Yousefi S, Yousefi E, Takahashi H, et al. Keratoconus severity identification using unsupervised machine learning. *PLoS One.* 2018;13(11), e0205998.

99. Lavric A, Valentin P. KeratoDetect: keratoconus detection algorithm using convolutional neural networks. *Comput Intell Neurosci.* 2019;2019:8162567.

100. Fariselli C, Vega-Estrada A, Arnalich-Montiel F, Alio JL. Artificial neural network to guide intracorneal ring segments implantation for keratoconus treatment: a pilot study. *Eye Vis (Lond).* 2020;7:20.

101. Daniel MC, Atzrodt L, Bucher F, et al. Automated segmentation of the corneal endothelium in a large set of "real-world" specular microscopy images using the U-Net architecture. *Sci Rep.* 2019;9(1). https://doi.org/10.1038/s41598-019-41034-2.

102. Vigueras-Guillén JP, van Rooij J, Engel A, Lemij HG, van Vliet LJ, Vermeer KA. Deep learning for assessing the corneal endothelium from specular microscopy images up to 1 year after ultrathin-DSAEK surgery. *Transl Vis Sci Technol.* 2020;9(2):49.

103. Fabijańska A. Segmentation of corneal endothelium images using a U-Net-based convolutional neural network. *Artif Intell Med.* 2018;88:1–13.

104. Yousefi S, Takahashi H, Hayashi T, et al. Predicting the likelihood of need for future keratoplasty intervention using artificial intelligence. *Ocul Surf.* 2020;18(2):320–325.

105. Hayashi T, Tabuchi H, Masumoto H, et al. A deep learning approach in rebubbling after descemet's membrane endothelial keratoplasty. *Eye Contact Lens.* 2020;46(2):121–126.

106. Treder M, Lauermann JL, Alnawaiseh M, Eter N. Using deep learning in automated detection of graft detachment in descemet membrane endothelial keratoplasty: a pilot study. *Cornea.* 2019;38(2):157–161.

107. Zhou YW, Yu Y, Zhou YB, et al. An advanced imaging method for measuring and assessing meibomian glands based on deep learning. *Zhonghua Yan Ke Za Zhi.* 2020;56(10):774–779.

108. Wan Zaki WMD, Mat Daud M, Abdani SR, Hussain A, Mutalib HA. Automated pterygium detection method of anterior segment photographed images. *Comput Methods Prog Biomed.* 2018;154:71–78.

109. Liu Z, Cao Y, Li Y, et al. Automatic diagnosis of fungal keratitis using data augmentation and image fusion with deep convolutional neural network. *Comput Methods Prog Biomed.* 2020;187:105019.

110. Biousse V, Newman NJ, Najjar RP, et al. Optic disc classification by deep learning versus expert neuro-ophthalmologists. *Ann Neurol.* 2020;88(4):785–795.

111. Milea D, Najjar RP, Zhubo J, et al. Artificial intelligence to detect papilledema from ocular fundus photographs. *N Engl J Med.* 2020;382(18):1687–1695.

112. Ahn JM, Kim S, Ahn K-S, Cho S-H, Kim US. Accuracy of machine learning for differentiation between optic neuropathies and pseudopapilledema. *BMC Ophthalmol.* 2019;19(1):178.

113. Thomas PBM, Gunasekera CD, Kang S, Baltrusaitis T. An artificial intelligence approach to the assessment of abnormal lid position. *Plast Reconstr Surg Glob Open.* 2020;8(10), e3089.

114. Greenwald MF, Danford ID, Shahrawat M, et al. Evaluation of artificial intelligence-based telemedicine screening for retinopathy of prematurity. *J AAPOS.* 2020;24(3):160–162.

115. Tong Y, Lu W, Deng Q-Q, Chen C, Shen Y. Automated identification of retinopathy of prematurity by image-based deep learning. *Eye Vis (Lond).* 2020;7:40.

116. Tan Z, Simkin S, Lai C, Dai S. Deep learning algorithm for automated diagnosis of retinopathy of prematurity plus disease. *Transl Vis Sci Technol.* 2019;8(6):23.

117. Whited JD, Datta SK, Aiello LM, et al. A modeled economic analysis of a digital teleophthalmology system as used by three federal healthcare agencies for detecting proliferative diabetic retinopathy. *Telemed J E Health.* 2005;11(6):641–651.

118. Xie Y, Nguyen QD, Hamzah H, et al. Artificial intelligence for teleophthalmology-based diabetic retinopathy screening in a national programme: an economic analysis modelling study. *Lancet Digit Health.* 2020;2(5):e240–e249.

119. Klyce S, Barnebey H, Brown T, Habash R, Lyons C. *Introduction to Tele-Ophthalmology a Guide for Ophthalmologists*; 2019. Published Online https://ascrs.org/-/media/ascrs-website/government-relations/pdfs/introduction-to-teleophthalmology-2019.pdf.

120. Lin W-C, Chen JS, Chiang MF, Hribar MR. Applications of artificial intelligence to electronic health record data in ophthalmology. *Transl Vis Sci Technol.* 2020;9(2):13.

CHAPTER 19

Education of Future Providers on Ocular Telehealth and Integration of Telehealth Into Future Practice

XIAOQIN ALEXA LU, MD

INTRODUCTION

The advent of ocular telehealth has presented both new challenges and opportunities for medical education. This was especially true in the Spring of 2020 when the COVID-19 pandemic closed clinics and cancelled elective surgeries across the world. Student clinical rotations were cancelled. Residents were limited in their patient exposure. In light of the sudden change in the hands-on, in-person, educational landscape, educators scrambled to develop new courses utilizing telehealth and provide meaningful learning opportunities remotely. This chapter will focus on opportunities for ocular telehealth education and how ocular telehealth programs can be used to increase ophthalmic knowledge and supplement traditional in-person teaching.

Ocular telehealth courses are best developed by following the four general principles of virtual learning: clearly defined goals or objectives, the use of innovative tools and technology, engagement of the trainees' attention and building interest in the subject, and prompt feedback. Optometry and ophthalmology are both visual specialties where diagnoses are made by recognizing specific features/patterns, or where specific findings generate a short differential diagnosis. Exposure to ocular telehealth programs, therefore, since many are based on images, offers learners the opportunity to view and be exposed to a variety of ocular disease through photographs, which enhances pattern recognition learning. This type of learning may be particularly beneficial early on in a student's learning pathway because the student can focus on interpreting the findings and learning the medical decision-making process (discussed in detail later on) without the initial struggle of learning to use the equipment. Both aspects of training—telehealth and traditional clinic rotations—are important, however, to educate students and ocular telehealth rotations can

Ocular Telehealth. https://doi.org/10.1016/B978-0-323-83204-5.00019-6

help lay a solid foundation for clinical pattern recognition and subsequent patient management.

In addition, ophthalmology has an established practice of using videos to teach surgery, so incorporating videos and images into a remote telehealth rotation is not a foreign concept to attending teachers or student learners. Furthermore, established ocular telehealth courses are often more conveniently accessible for both learners and teachers. They may be more interactive than a traditional classroom or clinic setting and may be better able to keep the learner's attention, especially when the student and the teacher are located remotely and interacting one on one. Finally, given the rising utilization of ocular telehealth programs, it is important that future providers in the field understand how to incorporate telemedicine techniques into their practice. This chapter will address different groups of trainees and their specific goals. Where applicable, the Veteran Affairs (VA) Technology-based Eye Care Services (TECS), ocular telehealth student rotation, (see Chapter 2) is used as an index case example.

SECTION I: TEACHING MEDICAL STUDENTS, OPTOMETRY STUDENTS, OR ALLIED HEALTH STUDENTS

Due to the pandemic, medical student ophthalmology clinical hours were reduced, a troubling problem that only compounded the general national trend of declining ophthalmology exposure. Overall, the number of medical schools requiring ophthalmic education for graduation in the United States is declining.[1] By utilizing ocular telehealth, however, more exposure and learning prospects were created. For medical students, optometry students, and allied health students, ophthalmic education utilizing telehealth techniques should be combined with didactic lectures. This provides the students a solid foundation about the eye using a variety of learning platforms, flexibility of recorded lectures and self-directed learning, and exposure to the field of eye care. Below, the author outlines some best practices to consider when planning to teach about ocular telehealth. Students are divided into two groups as the goals of each group are different. The first group has no previous exposure to eyes and mainly need a basic understanding of the eye and how to triage clinical complaints; and the second group of students are hoping to pursue ophthalmology or optometry as a future career.

Group A: Initial Exposure to Eye Care

Examples given in this subsection focus on medical students, however, the same principles apply for allied health students or any novice ophthalmic student provider. When organizing a course for the novice student, it is best to start with clear objectives. These represent the goals to achieve and the framework on which to build the curriculum. As an example, for a 3rd-year medical student pursuing a career outside of ophthalmology, the course objectives might be the pre-existing guidelines endorsed by the Association of University Professors of Ophthalmology (AUPO) and the American Academy of Ophthalmology (AAO). They list the ophthalmic knowledge that every graduating medical student should possess, whether they go into the field of ophthalmology or not.[2] These objectives can be modified to address the need of each student (see Table 19.1).

Using the latest technology, the familiar didactic courses remain a good way to acquire basic knowledge that can be taught through meeting platforms, various video websites (YouTube, Eyetube), and online content developed and available on various education websites. For example, there are three downloadable chapters addressing vision loss, red eye, and eye trauma on the AAO website.[3,4] AAO also has a website of interactive ophthalmic figures to familiarize learners with eye anatomy.[5] The learner clicks on various parts of the

---

TABLE 19.1
Ophthalmology Objectives for Graduating Medical Student

The 12 main objectives the medical students should know on graduation from medical school are:

(1) Describe the anatomy of the eye and the visual system
(2) Perform a basic eye examination
(3) Evaluate a patient with acute painless vision loss
(4) Evaluate a patient with chronic vision loss
(5) Evaluate a patient with a red or painful eye
(6) Evaluate a patient with eye trauma
(7) Evaluate a patient with an eye movement abnormality or diplopia
(8) Describe the important causes of vision loss in children
(9) Describe the ocular manifestations of systemic disease
(10) List the most important ocular side effects of systemic drugs
(11) List the common ocular medications that can have systemic side effects
(12) Describe when it is necessary to refer a patient urgently to ophthalmology

Adapted from Graubart EB, Waxman EL, Forster SH, et al. Ophthalmology objectives for medical students: revisiting what every graduating medical student should know. *Ophthalmology*. 2018;125(12):1842–1843, with permission.

eye anatomy and can perform self-quizzes. The same website also contains two YouTube video links for the learners to watch examinations of both adult and pediatric patients.[6]

To make the curriculum more hands-on and interactive, students can take advantage of skill transfer labs without an actual patient encounter. Especially during COVID-19, social distancing requirements meant students could not practice direct ophthalmoscopy on patients due to the proximity of the examiner and the patient. There is a simulator for direct ophthalmoscopy, Eyesi Direct, which offers the trainees a lifelike visualization of optic nerve and retina (see Fig. 19.1).

The training module has different difficulty levels with performance feedback. The curriculum is designed for medical students of all specialties and contains a collection of the most common pathologies. The downside of the simulator is the high cost, which might be less daunting if shared between clinical departments.

To engage the learner, interactive cases are highly encouraged, such as the eight interactive student cases present on the AAO website. They address topics like red eye, trauma, and systemic diseases that affect the eyes. The cases were written together by both ophthalmologists and medical students. Each case starts with a short but pertinent review of the

eye conditions, a pre-test, and chart-like tabs listing the patient's complaints and medical history. There are "clickable" interactive exam rooms to obtain the findings as a primary care physician and as an ophthalmologist. Along with interactive quizzes on diagnosis and additional testing, there is also a post-test to check knowledge retention.[7]

For students who lost the opportunity to observe surgery due to the reduced operating schedules, there are numerous websites with surgery videos. YouTube and Eyetube websites contain many videos of routine cataract surgeries, laser procedures, eyelid procedures, and glaucoma procedures with narration. While observing live surgery is irreplaceable, eye surgery is sometimes more educational and interesting for the students when they can clearly visualize the surgery, with the added benefit of having the different steps and rational for action clearly explained.

To foster collegiality and team work, especially during a socially isolating time, programs should consider small group virtual meetings. Through different meeting platforms, education programs could consider student peer-to-peer presentation of interesting cases, weekly faculty discussion time on a specific topic, and weekly grand rounds to exchange information virtually and allow questions and concerns to be addressed.

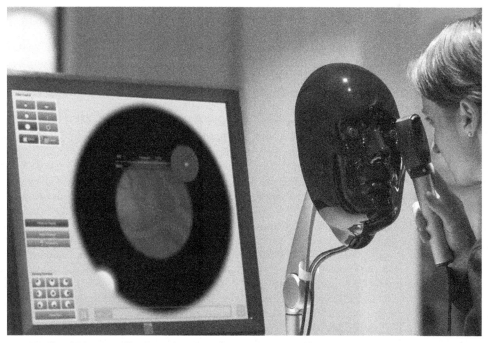

FIG. 19.1 Eyesi Direct—a Simulator for Direct Ophthalmoscopy. (Credit: Used with permission from VRmagic, Mannheim, Germany)

The VA ocular telehealth program, TECS, was used in virtual education for both medical and allied health students. Rotators were educated real-time, using photographs of actual patients that were going through the program that day. Several interesting cases were reviewed, such as: diabetic retinopathy, cataracts, macular degeneration, and papilledema. These photographs added to the student's base knowledge of ophthalmology by providing visual pictures of these serious disease findings. The students provided feedback that the session was engaging and they felt more comfortable asking clarifying questions and could study eye anatomy without causing discomfort to real patients.

Group B. Students Who are Interested in Pursuing a Career in Ophthalmology or Optometry

For medical students who wish to pursue a career in eye care, their main objectives are both to acquire more ophthalmic knowledge and to get to know the profession. Ideally, they would have basic knowledge of ophthalmology already, using the aforementioned methods. While the case example below highlights an ophthalmology rotation, a similar set up and similar principles can be utilzed for students in optometry school. Optometric students can perform virtual exams with their attendings, either through a synchronous or asynchronous visit, thereby learning how to use ocular telehealth as part of their future practice.

Case Example: TECS 4th year medical student rotation

TECS offered a more in-depth and interactive study of common comprehensive ophthalmology cases using an ocular telehealth platform. In the TECS program patients receive a standard eye work up including vision and refraction, and then have external photos and fundus photos taken. The patient may also obtain a visual field or ocular coherence tomography (OCT) photo, depending on the reason for the visit. The medical students have a multi-week rotation where they visit a TECS patient site (pre-pandemic), interpret TECS studies, and then perform a "read out" with the attending readers. The students gain critical clinical knowledge through detailed assessment and clinical data integration of pertinent history, eye exam elements (e.g., vision, eye pressure), through the technician's record. They then begin to develop pattern recognition skills, viewing, and examining ocular structures with external and fundus photographs. They make their own

assessment and plan, learn abbreviations, and then present the case to an attending, similar to an in-person clinic. There are additional opportunities to learn how to interpret ancillary testing, such as visual fields and OCT, especially through the TECS specialty arms, tele-glaucoma, and tele-macula clinics.

Through the reading rotation, students not only learn to distinguish normal and abnormal, they can do so without struggling to "get" the exam. The telehealth rotation can be an excellent first rotation for those interested in ophthalmology because it allows the student to first focus on information processing—developing good clinical thought processes and focused differentials based on ocular findings. This is a good foundation before an in-person clinical rotation, where much of the time may be spent learning to use the slit lamp, the indirect, etc. The rotation is very interactive and individually focused, as one student is paired with one attending. Moreover, during the TECS clinical rotation, the student is expected to work on a scholarly project with an ophthalmologist mentor, either doing research or reporting an interesting case they may have seen through telehealth. TECS attendings also offer supplemental lectures on topics related to ocular telehealth such as implementation science, quality assurance/improvement, and big data/artificial intelligence. If circumstances permit, the student might also work with an attending in-person during clinic to see follow ups from the TECS exam and apply the skills he/she has learned remotely. The virtual aspect of this ophthalmology rotation makes it conducive as an "away" rotation as it can be done from anywhere in the country and might also be offered to students without home ophthalmology departments.

SECTION II: OPHTHALMOLOGY RESIDENTS

During the COVID-19 pandemic, ophthalmology residency training was disrupted by clinical closures and elective surgery cancellation. The ingenuity and flexibility of residents' capacity for learning are commendable. They continued to care for patients in the emergency room and on the hospital floors while risking exposure to the viral infection. They embraced opportunities to practice ocular telehealth through telemedicine appointments, and learned new telemedicine codes. Their main goals were to continue learning advanced clinical skills, improving surgical proficiencies, and searching for research opportunities.

The residents practiced in wet labs to learn and maintain their surgery skills when surgical cases disappeared. The traditional surgical wet lab utilized animal eyes, which are relatively easy and cheap to obtain. Human cadaveric eyes are scarcer and more expensive. However, animal eyes are not entirely similar to human eyes and cannot fully simulate human tissue. Another option for wet lab is using synthetic model eyes, such as the series from Phillips Studio, which are nonperishable. The current models offer specific eyes designed for practicing cataract surgery, cornea surgery, strabismus surgery, glaucoma surgery, and retina procedures. These eyes do have the downside of being more expensive than animal eyes. They are also made of plastic structures which do not behave like human tissue. The third option for surgery simulation is to use the latest technology, such as: the Eyesi Surgical System from VRmagic (see Fig. 19.2). The system has both cataract and vitreoretinal surgery simulations. There are ports for instrument insertion and realistic virtual interaction with intraocular tissue. Each simulated surgery is graded and the trainees can attempt to improve their scores with subsequent practices.

New research opportunities also emerged from new ways of practicing medicine. In the TECS program, the residents who are interested in ocular telehealth participate in study design, program implementation, and publish research projects with data generated by the telemedicine program. There is a great deal of interest in how patient care was affected by the pandemic and integration of telemedicine with traditional practice.

Aside from creative ways to improve surgery skills and participation in more research projects, one of the best education modalities emerging from the pandemic is the webinar. Webinars are recorded lectures, such as Grand Rounds, from different eye institutions and virtual annual eye conferences. Most of them are free of charge and can be accessed from anywhere, as long as the learner has an internet connection. This means more affordability and efficiency for the residents to attend meetings. Residents can also learn from experts across the world, thus promoting increased inclusivity in the field. The recorded sessions are also available for repeated viewing and studying of information.

SECTION III: RESIDENTS FROM OTHER MEDICAL SPECIALTIES
Case Example: TECS Session for Primary Care Providers

As a part of the VA Tele-Primary Care Rotation, residents from Family Medicine and Preventive Medicine rotate through TECS for an ocular telehealth experience. Prior to the pandemic, this rotation was done in-person. During the pandemic, the attending meets the resident remotely through a virtual platform. Prior to the session, the resident receives the course objectives based on the American Association of Family Medicine recommendations of eye knowledge for graduating residents. They also receive a handout on the systematic interpretation of photographs with pictures of common ocular disease findings. The ocular telehealth teaching sessions are designed to be an interactive, engaging, informative 90-min session. During the session, the attending gives a brief introduction of the TECS program and ocular telehealth. A normal patient is first presented with the history and the photographic eye exam. The photographs are interpreted with the resident. The attending interprets the right eye systematically while the resident follows along with the handout. The resident is then asked to read the second eye prompted by the attending. After the normal patient, the attending has two additional patient cases with severe diabetic retinopathy and other

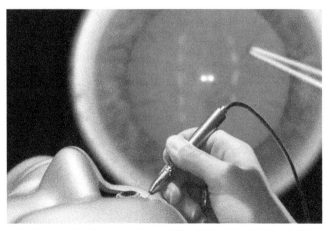

FIG. 19.2 Eyesi Surgical System for Cataract Surgery Simulation. (Credit: Used with permission from VRmagic, Mannheim, Germany)

interesting eye findings to share with the resident. Along the way, the resident is free to ask clarifying questions. The last 30 min in the session is a slide presentation of red eye and its differential diagnoses. Red eye was chosen as an additional topic as it is the most common ocular complaint presenting to a primary care clinic. The attending also tries to tailor the session to the future career goals of the residents. Residents have expressed that the session was both interesting and informative in post-course evaluations.

SECTION IV: ATTENDING OPHTHALMOLOGISTS OR OPTOMETRISTS

Most attending eye care specialists would like to include ocular telehealth as a part of their practice. In 2015, Woodward et al. surveyed a group of eye care providers: ophthalmology residents, optometrists, and ophthalmologists, at Kellogg Eye Center in Michigan. They found that while a majority would be interested in providing care through telehealth (82%) and felt ocular telehealth would be a positive addition (60%), over half of the providers (59%) had low confidence in making medical decisions through ocular telehealth. One of the reasons for this hesitation at Kellogg specifically, was theorized to be a lack of an excellent and creditable ocular telehealth program at their institution at the time of publication of the paper, so eye providers did not have experience making medical diagnoses through images and clinical information.[8] While eye providers are familiar with diagnosing ocular disease in-person, there are nuances to skilled image interpretation. Training new eye telehealth readers about image display tools, artifacts versus true findings, and reading 'best practices' increases both reader accuracy and consistency. Furthermore, providing a new reader a solid foundation on how to give care through telehealth methods, speeds up the learning curve while improving buy-in and confidence in the ocular telehealth program. The TECS program, developed and started in 2015, has a validated program protocol[9-12] and includes a strict quality assessment and quality control component. One of these quality controls is a standardized training and certification process for reading ophthalmologists and optometrists. The training protocol at TECS will be detailed below and could be used as a blueprint for other ocular telehealth reader training programs.

Case Example: TECS Reader Certification Course

Potential readers are board-certified ophthalmologists and optometrists with extensive in-person clinical experience. The readers already have all the necessary knowledge to make clinical decisions through telehealth; the goal of the training is therefore geared towards teaching skills that will help readers be more successful and feel more confident about their clinical decision-making utilizing photographs instead of the typical in-person exam. The entire process is summarized in a flow sheet (see Fig. 19.3).

First, the readers-in-training are required to review and become familiar with the program protocols from the National TECS Handbook, and the tele-glaucoma and tele-macula supplemental protocols, if applicable to their site. The handbooks contain instructions on grading ocular findings, guidelines on determining disease severity, and general recommendations for follow ups for different diagnoses. The participants also receive a PowerPoint course on the image viewing platform, in this case, Vista Imaging Display. The course highlights several image manipulation tools, available in Vista Imaging, that aid with photograph interpretation, e.g., red, green filters, changing contrast, side-by-side image display. Correct electronic medical record documentation and correct coding are other items emphasized in the initial didactic information. All of the above information is then illustrated in four practice patients that the readers-in-training can review and try to apply their knowledge.

Each trainee is then scheduled with an experienced reader for a one-on-one session while they work through a regular day of TECS patient care and photo interpretation ("buddy reads"). This can be done remotely through a meeting platform with shared screens. It is useful for the new TECS doctor to experience the TECS read process in a real-life clinic and in real time to learn how remote supervision and guidance of the ophthalmic technicians is done. The experienced reader can then address questions that the training doctor might have regarding patient care, triage, follow up, documentation, and charting.

Once the training doctor is ready, the final step in the certification process is an "exam" with 10 model patients. These patients with different diseases are presented with history, exam, and photographs similar to the TECS format. A successful reader is required to have a passing score of 100% by identifying all of the major diagnoses and correct follow up for the patients. If the score is not 100%, the training doctor is requested to review the patients again and re-submit the answers. If the second attempt is not fully correct, the education director would discuss the case with the training doctor and relay the discrepancy to the site director. The site

TECS Reader Training Process

Readers-in-training are encouraged to reach out with questions during the entire process.

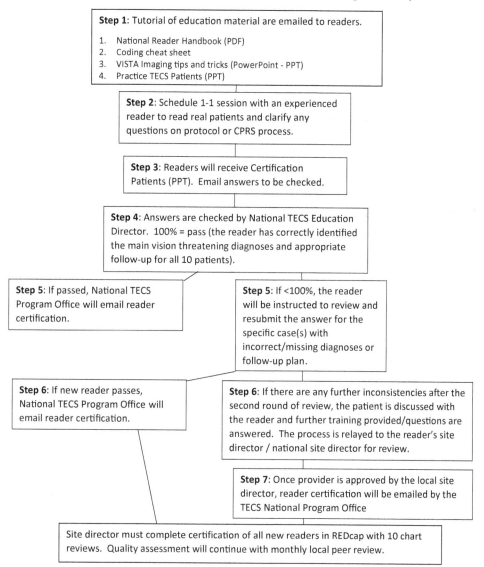

Step 1: Tutorial of education material are emailed to readers.

1. National Reader Handbook (PDF)
2. Coding cheat sheet
3. VISTA Imaging tips and tricks (PowerPoint - PPT)
4. Practice TECS Patients (PPT)

Step 2: Schedule 1-1 session with an experienced reader to read real patients and clarify any questions on protocol or CPRS process.

Step 3: Readers will receive Certification Patients (PPT). Email answers to be checked.

Step 4: Answers are checked by National TECS Education Director. 100% = pass (the reader has correctly identified the main vision threatening diagnoses and appropriate follow-up for all 10 patients).

Step 5: If passed, National TECS Program Office will email reader certification.

Step 5: If <100%, the reader will be instructed to review and resubmit the answer for the specific case(s) with incorrect/missing diagnoses or follow-up plan.

Step 6: If new reader passes, National TECS Program Office will email reader certification.

Step 6: If there are any further inconsistencies after the second round of review, the patient is discussed with the reader and further training provided/questions are answered. The process is relayed to the reader's site director / national site director for review.

Step 7: Once provider is approved by the local site director, reader certification will be emailed by the TECS National Program Office

Site director must complete certification of all new readers in REDcap with 10 chart reviews. Quality assessment will continue with monthly local peer review.

FIG. 19.3 TECS Reader Training Flowsheet. (Credit: Xiaoqin Alexa Lu, MD.)

director can then approve the trainee's certification at his/her discretion.

Quality control efforts continue once a reader is certified. The site director reviews 10 patient interpretations at random of the new reader. In addition, TECS also has a peer review process for on-going quality control—for more details about quality assurance and monitoring, please refer to Chapter 16.

QUALITY ASSESSMENT AND IMPROVEMENT IN OCULAR TELEHEALTH EDUCATION

As mentioned before, one of the principles of developing a new course is prompt feedback from the trainees. As many of the education methods and materials involving ocular telehealth are relatively novel, improvement specifically in virtual education

TABLE 19.2
Postcourse Survey Questions

A. Survey questions for participants of Tele-
   ophthalmology Teaching Session:
   1. How helpful was the hand out?
   2. How educational was the session?
   3. How interesting was the session?
   4. Was the duration of the session too short, too
      long, or just right?
   5. What are some suggestions you have to make
      the session better?
B. Survey questions for participants of the TECS
   Certification Course
   1. Did the certification process meet your
      expectations?
   2. How would you rate the quality of your
      certification process?
   3. Was the initial tutorial suitable?
   4. How would you rate the quality of the 1-1
      session with the experience reader?
   5. How would you rate the quality of the
      Certification Patients PowerPoint?
   6. Did you learn any new?
   7. What other training materials should be included
      in the certification process?
   8. Please give us any suggestions on improving the
      certification process.

Credit: Xiaoqin Alexa Lu, MD.

is a constant pursuit. Some of the most valuable and useful enhancements to the ocular telehealth rotation and educational experience of the TECS rotation were based on survey feedback from the participants. A survey was sent to every participant of the remote teaching sessions and the reader training and certification program, through a third-party survey website, Survey Monkey. To encourage participation, these anonymous surveys were designed to be short and simple to answer. (see Table 19.2) The anonymity makes the participants more comfortable in giving honest feedback. The results have helped to refine both the TECS remote teaching rotation and the reader certification process.

The survey results also provided some indication on the quality of the TECS tele-education programs. With regard to the education session for residents and healthcare students, 7 out of 14 participants, who completed the course from March of 2020 to January of 2021, responded to the survey. The results showed that the eye handout was scored 96 out of 100 in helpfulness. The teaching session was valued at 96 out of 100 on being educational, and 95 out of 100 on being interesting. For the reader training and certification program, 10 out of 10 participants from June of 2020 to January 2021 returned their surveys. The results showed that 100% of the participants thought the initial tutorials were appropriate and the course met their expectations. The quality of the overall course was rated 4.8 out of 5. The quality of individual session with an experienced reader was evaluated at 4.9 out of 5; and the Certification Patients PowerPoint was valued at 4.8 out of 5.

INCREASING ADOPTION AND BUY-IN FOR OCULAR TELEHEALTH THROUGH EDUCATION

A high quality, reliable ocular telehealth program that has active participation and buy-in from providers will add another motivator for eye doctors to include ocular telehealth as part of their careers. Providers participating in ocular telehealth appear to have an increase in optimism regarding job satisfaction and career longevity. A poster was presented at Women in Ophthalmology Annual Conference in August of 2020. The results were based on anonymous survey responses from 22 TECS reading ophthalmologists and optometrists. Data showed that a career that included ocular telehealth improved the overall job satisfaction in 46% of the participants; 15% of the participants expressed that they hope to retire later than previously planned; 38% of the participants reported improved work–life balance. The top reasons cited for these changes were flexibility, feelings of accomplishment, teamwork, improved commute, and better work environment. None reported decreased job satisfaction, earlier retirement, or decreased work–life balance.[13] Ocular telehealth has multiple demonstrated benefits for patients. While these findings are preliminary, telemedicine may also provide benefits for providers in terms of greater career longevity and satisfaction. In an era where provider wellness and burnout are of high concern, telehealth may be one tool to help mitigate the stresses of the "daily grind," helping eye providers achieve a good balance which ultimately benefits society as a whole.

CONCLUSION

In conclusion, ocular telehealth programs offer great opportunities for medical education of healthcare students, residents, and attendings. Due to social distancing restrictions, caused by the COVID-19 pandemic, creative solutions have been developed to help acquire and distribute new information. With clearly defined objectives tailored to different groups of trainees, programs can develop effective, innovative, and engaging new courses. Webinars and patient simulators will continue to augment learning. Due to the flexibility, convenience, and inclusive nature of these changes, many of these virtual education solutions will likely remain after the end of the pandemic. As more ophthalmologists and optometrists explore adding ocular telehealth to their practices, the training and certification process such as the one deployed by TECS might serve as a model for other programs to ensure quality and safe patient care, along with increasing provider buy-in and confidence in the telehealth care delivery method. By exposing the next generation of non-eye and eye providers to ocular telehealth, the field encourages both future advancement and long-term sustainability/use of eye telemedicine programs. Ocular telehealth helps both the patient and the eye provider reach their visual goals.

REFERENCES

1. Chadha N, Gooding H. Twelve tips for teaching ophthalmology in the undergraduate curriculum. *Med Teach.* 2021;43(1):80–85.
2. Graubart EB, Waxman EL, Forster SH, et al. Ophthalmology objectives for medical students: revisiting what every graduating medical student should know. *Ophthalmology.* 2018;125(12):1842–1843.
3. American Academy of Ophthalmology. *Basic Ophthalmology Samples PDF*; 2021. [Online]. Available: https://www.aao.org/Assets/ebeb77be-b306-4651-bf6f-d7b8feab-c3fb/637255651055970000/basic-ophthalmology-sample-pdf?inline=1. Accessed 11.02.21.
4. Duong AT, Van Tassel SH, Fernandez AG, et al. Medical education and path to residency in ophthalmology in the COVID-19 era: perspective from medical student educators. *Ophthalmology.* 2020;127(11):e95–e98.
5. American Academy of Ophthalmology. *Interactive Figures for Medical Students*; 2021. [Online]. Available: https://www.aao.org/interactive-figures. Accessed 11.02.21.
6. American Academy of Ophthalmology. *Guide to the Bedside Ophthalmic Exam*; 2021 [Online]. Available: aao.org/medical-students. [Accessed 11.02.21].
7. American Academy of Ophthalmology. *Interactive Medical Student Cases*; 2021. [Online]. Available: https://www.aao.org/interactive-cases. Accessed 11.02.21].
8. Woodward MA, Ple-plakon P, Blachley T, et al. Eye care providers' attitudes towards tele-ophthalmology. *Telemed J E Health.* 2015;21(4):271–273.
9. Maa AY, Medert CM, Lu X, et al. Diagnostic accuracy of technology-based eye care services: the technology-based eye care services compare trial part I. *Ophthalmology.* 2020;127(1):38–44.
10. Maa AY, McCord S, Lu X, et al. The impact of OCT on diagnostic accuracy of the technology-based eye care services protocol: part II of the technology-based eye care services compare trial. *Ophthalmology.* 2020;127(4):544–549.
11. Maa AY, Wojciechowski B, Hunt KJ, et al. Early experience with technology-based eye care services (TECS): a novel ophthalmologic telemedicine initiative. *Ophthalmology.* 2017;124(4):539–546.
12. Maa AY, Wojciechowski B, Hunt K, Dismuke C, Janjua R, Lynch MG. Remote eye care screening for rural veterans with technology-based eye care services: a quality improvement project. *Rural Remote Health.* 2017;17(1):4045.
13. Lu X, Maa AY. Teleophthalmology improves job satisfaction, career longevity, and work–life balance. In: *Women in Ophthalmology Annual Conference, Virtual*; 2020.

Index

Note: Page numbers followed by *f* indicate figures and *t* indicate tables.